Davis's

PA Exam Review
Focused Review for the PANCE and PANRE

Second Edition

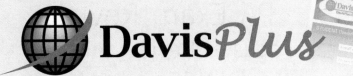

DavisPlus

Online Resource Center

DavisPlus is your online source for a wealth of learning resources and teaching tools, as well as electronic and mobile versions of our products.

Visit **DavisPlus.FADavis.com**

STUDENTS
FREE access.
Sign up today to see what's available for your title.

INSTRUCTORS
Upon Adoption.
Password-protected library of title-specific, online course content.

Easy, personalized access to your resources is just a click away.

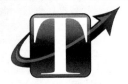

Taber's online resources are now available across many of the **DavisPlus** resource pages.

Look for this icon to find Taber's resources!

Explore more online resources from F.A. Davis

Taber's Online
www.Tabers.com

The power of Taber's® Cyclopedic Medical Dictionary on the web.
Find more than 60,000 terms, 1,000 images, and more.

powered by
unbound
MEDICINE

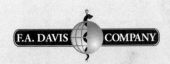

Davis's
PA Exam Review
Focused Review for the PANCE and PANRE

Second Edition

Morton A. Diamond, MD, FACP, FAHA, FACC(E)
2012 Distinguished Professor
College of Health Care Sciences
Medical Director
Physician Assistant Program
Nova Southeastern University
Fort Lauderdale, Florida

 F.A. Davis Company • Philadelphia

F. A. Davis Company
1915 Arch Street
Philadelphia, PA 19103
www.fadavis.com

Copyright © 2013 by F. A. Davis Company

Printed in the United States of America

Last digit indicates print number: 10 9 8 7 6 5 4 3

Acquisitions Editor: Andy McPhee
Manager of Content Development: George W. Lang
Developmental Editor: Angela Norton
Art and Design Manager: Carolyn O'Brien

As new scientific information becomes available through basic and clinical research, recommended treatments and drug therapies undergo changes. The author(s) and publisher have done everything possible to make this book accurate, up to date, and in accord with accepted standards at the time of publication. The author(s), editors, and publisher are not responsible for errors or omissions or for consequences from application of the book, and make no warranty, expressed or implied, in regard to the contents of the book. Any practice described in this book should be applied by the reader in accordance with professional standards of care used in regard to the unique circumstances that may apply in each situation. The reader is advised always to check product information (package inserts) for changes and new information regarding dose and contraindications before administering any drug. Caution is especially urged when using new or infrequently ordered drugs.

Library of Congress Cataloging-in-Publication Data

Diamond, Morton A.
  Davis's PA exam review : focused review for the PANCE and PANRE / Morton A. Diamond. — 2nd ed.
      p. ; cm.
  PA exam review
  Includes index.
  ISBN 978-0-8036-2951-6
  I. Title. II. Title: PA exam review.
  [DNLM: 1. Physician Assistants—Examination Questions. 2. Certification—Examination Questions. W 18.2]

  610.73'72069076—dc23
                              2012039181

To my precious wife, Louise
Whose love is my most powerful medicine

And to my darling granddaughters
Yael Leah, Shira Bracha, and Aviva Michal
Who are the sunshine of my life

Foreword

Recently a new physician assistant (PA) graduate of my program replied to a question about her preparation for the Physician Assistant National Certifying Examination (PANCE) by saying that she bought "every review text I could find." Not a surprising answer, given the importance of the examination to her career as a PA, and not surprising that she was able to find a number of review texts on the market. So what makes this text different?

Morton Diamond, a PA educator since 1994 and previously a practicing cardiologist, has constructed a unique and highly effective system that reviews medical concepts while at the same time teaches critical thinking. Rather than taking a body system approach he splits his book into two sections, the second building off the first.

In the first section, *Essentials*, he poses specific clinical scenarios and questions using a multiple-correct answer methodology. This approach allows for specific, detailed feedback on the range and depth of one's knowledge. The likelihood of answering the questions accurately just by guessing is significantly reduced using this method because the test-taker must select the correct *combination* of answers. Further, this method avoids the "one right answer," lower-order mentality so antithetical to the real world of medicine.

Answers in the text are provided alongside specific teaching points central to understanding the material. This approach ensures the integration of key concepts into the review of each subject. He also provides body system classification labels so that students can focus on the content they most need to review.

The second section, *Performance*, takes a more traditional approach to questions, with single correct answers for each, just as one would encounter on the PANCE and PANRE. However, even in this section, the correct answer is keyed back to its earlier discussion in *Essentials*, an approach that provides excellent testing as well as critical review.

Included with every book is a CD-ROM with even more questions, none of which are repeated in the book. The testing software on the CD-ROM allows users to take practice tests using a large pool of questions from a variety of topic areas or a smaller pool of questions from specific topic areas. Highly flexible and customizable, the testing software adds one more tool to the test-taker's arsenal of exam preparation weapons.

Dr. Diamond seems to understand exactly what a new graduate PA needs to know, as well as what practicing PAs need to know to recertify and remain in practice. New graduates and recertifying PAs will find this book-and-software package an invaluable tool in preparing for their next, critical examination.

DANA SAYRE-STANHOPE, EDD, PA-C
Associate Professor and Director
Physician Assistant Program Emory University School of Medicine
Atlanta, Georgia
Former Chair of the Accreditation Review Commission on Education
for the Physician Assistant

Reviewers

Jane Arenas, MS, PA-C
Clinical Coordinator
Physician Assistant Program
DeSales University
Center Valley, Pennsylvania

Cynthia Bunde, MPAS, PA-C
Physician Assistant
Pocatello Women's Health Clinic
Pocatello, Idaho

Anna M. Choo, MD, JD
Resident Physician
Department of Physical Medicine
    and Rehabilitation
Emory University Hospital
Atlanta, Georgia

Tom Colletti, MPAS, PA-C
Assistant Consulting Professor
Physician Assistant Program
Duke University School of Medicine
Durham, North Carolina

Kathleen L. Ehrhardt, MMS, PA-C
Assistant Professor, Academic Coordinator
Physician Assistant Program
DeSales University
Center Valley, Pennsylvania

Katherine M. Erdman, MPAS, PA-C
Assistant Director and Assistant Professor
Physician Assistant Program
School of Allied Health
Baylor College of Medicine
Houston, Texas

Alison C. Essary, MHPE, PA-C
Program Director
Physician Assistant Program
College of Health Sciences
Midwestern University
Glendale, Arizona

Kaesa Footracer, PA-C
Physician Assistant
Complete Care
Tarzana, California

Richard Gicking, MD, FACP
Department of Medicine
Emanuel Hospital
Portland, Oregon

Karen Graham, MPAS, PA-C
Clinical Associate Professor
Physician Assistant Program
University of Wisconsin–La Crosse
La Crosse, Wisconsin

Kenneth Harbert, PhD, MCHES, PA-C,
DFAAP
Dean and Program Director
School of Physician Assistant Studies
South College
Knoxville, Tennessee

Bernadette Howlett, PhD
Research Director
Research Office
Bingham Memorial Hospital
Blackfoot, Idaho

Diana Kharbat, DO
Resident Physician
Department of Physical Medicine
    and Rehabilitation
Emory University Hospital
Atlanta, Georgia

Naghmeh Khodai, MD
Resident Physician
Obstetrics/Gynecology
Rush University Medical Center
Chicago, Illinois

Adam J. Kinninger, DO
Intern
Osteopathic Medicine
St. Vincent Mercy Hospital
Toledo, Ohio

Clara LaBoy, PA-C, MS
Assistant Professor
Physician Assistant Program
Pacific University
Forest Grove, Oregon

Mary Ann Laxen, PA-C, MAB
Director
Physician Assistant Program
University of North Dakota
Grand Forks, North Dakota

Allison A Morgan, MPA, PA-C
Instructor
Department of Physician Assistant Studies
Duquesne University
Pittsburgh, Pennsylvania

Charlene Morris, MPAS, PA-C, DFAAPA
Physician Assistant
Pamlico Medical Center
Bayboro, North Carolina

John Tobias Musser, MD
Resident Physician
Physical Medicine & Rehabilitation Residency
   Program
Department of Rehabilitation Medicine
Emory University School of Medicine
Atlanta, Georgia

Manali Indravadan Patel, MD, MPH
Resident Physician
Internal Medicine Residency Program
Stanford University School of Medicine
Stanford, California

Tammy Dowdell Ream, MPAS, PA-C
Coordinator of Clinical Education
Physician Assistant Program
Texas Tech University Health Sciences Center
Midland, Texas

Megan Rourke, PA-C
Physician Assistant
Dermatology Practice
Avon, Connecticut

John M. Schroeder, PA-C, JD
Associate Professor
Department of Physician Assistant Studies
Idaho State University
Pocatello, Idaho

Erica Young, PA-C
Physician Assistant
Correctional Managed Care
The University of Texas Medical Branch
Galveston, Texas

Kevan Zipin, MD
Resident
Emergency Medicine
Lincoln Medical and Mental Health Center
Bronx, New York

The Author

Morton A. Diamond, MD, FACP, FAHA, FACC(E), is a clinical cardiologist with four decades of experience in the education of physician assistant students and medical students. Since 1994 he has been the full-time Medical Director of the Nova Southeastern University Physician Assistant Program in Ft. Lauderdale, Florida.

For several years Dr. Diamond served on the national PANCE test-writing committee and was considered to be a skilled and prolific writer of test questions. He has published many articles in peer-reviewed medical journals and has authored chapters in medical textbooks. He has presented lectures at 71 state and national medical meetings.

Dr. Diamond is the author of the book entitled *Medical Insights: From Classroom to Patient* in addition to the 1st edition of *Davis's PA Exam Review: Focused Review for the PANCE and PANRE.*

Preface

While this, the 2nd edition of *Davis's PA Exam Review: Focused Review for the PANCE and PANRE,* is more expansive than the 1st edition, having many more questions and explanations, the successful guiding principles of the 1st edition are unchanged. First, the medical content of the book remains FOCUSED, emphasizing the information that you must know in order to pass the examination.

Secondly, this unique book is carefully constructed to promote your success on the national Physician Assistant (PA) certifying examinations PANCE and PANRE by employing a novel and highly efficient educational structure. *Davis's PA Exam Review* is distinctively different from other review books in both its goals and format. Its goals are the following:

- To challenge you to think critically,

- To encourage you to compare and contrast diseases with similar clinical presentation, and

- To enrich your medical knowledge base

In its format this book is divided into two sections, **Essentials** and **Performance. Essentials** will challenge you to think critically, for most questions have *more than one correct answer.* Thus, you must carefully consider each possible answer (distracter). For example, if the question asks which condition is a risk factor for acute dissection of the aorta, *correct answers include* Marfan syndrome, chronic hypertension, and cocaine use.

Each **Essentials** question is followed by the correct answers with a succinct exposition called *You Should Know.* These *You Should Know* sections explain why the answers are correct and are followed by key information critical to your understanding of the material.

You should consider Essentials as a bridge to **Performance,** the section of the book that gives you the sense of an actual certifying examination. In Performance there is *only one correct answer.* Performance questions are crafted with patient vignettes similar to PANCE and PANRE questions. The answer to each Performance question is linked (see **Performance Answer section**) to *You Should Know* sections in **Essentials.** Clearly, every question in the book enriches your knowledge and promotes your success on the certifying examination.

No Logical Order

Davis's PA Exam Review is intentionally not structured in a logical order. Specifically, test items are not colligated by organ system, such as cardiovascular and endocrine, nor are they compiled by task, such as health maintenance, formulating the most likely diagnosis, pharmaceutical therapeutics, and clinical intervention. The chaotic order of test items in the book mimics the certifying examination and forces you to maintain an agile, fast-moving mind so you can move quickly and effectively from a gastroenterology question to a reproductive question to a pharmacology item; or from making the correct diagnosis to proper preventive medicine counseling to selecting the most appropriate medication in therapy.

The book strives to present an equal distribution of items in the knowledge and skill areas being tested by the exams. These areas include history taking and physical examination, using laboratory and diagnostic studies, formulating most likely diagnoses, clinical interventions, clinical therapeutics, health maintenance, and applying scientific concepts.

Test Item Breakdown

Test items related to disorders by organ systems will be generally formulated as follows:

- 30% to 35% of the items relate to cardiovascular or pulmonary disorders
- 15% to 20% of the items relate to musculoskeletal or gastrointestinal disorders
- 20% to 25% of the items relate to EENT, reproductive, endocrine, or neurological disorders
- 20% to 25% of the items relate to psychiatric, genitourinary, dermatological, or hematological disorders, or infectious diseases

These percentage breakdowns roughly approximate the breakdown used for actual certifying examinations.

The NCCPA website states that 3% of PANCE exam content is Infectious Disease. However, you should expect many more questions that relate to infections. Why? you may ask. In the NCCPA Content Blueprint pyelonephritis is considered Genitourinary, not an Infectious Disease; meningitis is considered Neurologic, not an Infectious Disease; and pneumonia is considered Pulmonary, not an Infectious Disease.

Advantages

If you've examined other PANCE/PANRE review books, you no doubt know that their test items offer only one correct answer. For instance, a review book might have a test item on therapy of atrial fibrillation in which diltiazem is the correct response in order to slow the ventricular rate. In the patient with atrial fibrillation, slowing of the ventricular response is an essential element in treatment. Several medications may thus be used, including verapamil, diltiazem, propranolol, and digoxin. In no way does a test item that requires only one correct answer probe the test taker's ability to define the proper medication in a specific clinical setting, such as atrial fibrillation in a patient with heart failure.

This book, on the other hand, probes your knowledge in depth. It helps you to think critically and respond clinically, which the PANCE and PANRE both require.

You have undoubtedly found as well that other exam review books provide medical information *after* a test item has been answered. In contrast, this book enriches your information base in **Essentials,** well before you encounter test items in **Performance.** It is educationally more effective to inform first and, thereafter, to test, rather than to initially test and then, later, offer an explanation.

Please read the Appendix. Succinctly, it provides you with important information that is likely to be tested in your examinations. The Appendix includes the features that:

- Summarize several adult immunizations.
- List the most common infecting organism in patients who have certain diseases.
- Correlate autoimmune diseases with their antibodies.
- Provide counseling tips related to disease or medicine administration.
- Describe new, important diagnostic tests.
- Define important clinical concepts (e.g., negative and positive neurological symptoms).

Last and most important, you will find that the test items here mirror exactly the format and structure of test items in actual certifying examinations. The author is a veteran item-writer for PA certifying examinations and has carefully crafted the test items in this book and CD-ROM to fit the items you will actually encounter on your examination.

About the CD-ROM

The CD-ROM that accompanies the book contains an electronic question bank in the flexible interactive Quiz (iQ) software. With this self-paced testing and teaching software, you can choose from the available bank of test items by specifying areas to be tested. For instance, you can choose to be tested on just cardiovascular items, neurological and pulmonary items, or any combination of body system chapters.

The CD-ROM contains a test bank of more than 950 test items. After a test is graded, the score shows the test items broken down by chosen categories. In that way, you can identify weak areas and then focus on them in your studies.

Preparing for the Exam

If you are preparing for the Physician Assistant National Certifying Exam (PANCE), you already know that the test is a milestone in your Physician Assistant career. You have a sense of pride and accomplishment for having successfully completed rigorous academic training. The PANCE is the final hurdle before you fulfill your bright promise of service, commitment, and caring.

If you are preparing for the Physician Assistant National Recertifying Exam (PANRE), you are seeking recertification that will demonstrate your having the requisite knowledge to meet the standard of your profession. Success on the PANRE affords you the satisfaction of knowing you are a member of an elite medical profession that sets recertification standards.

Either way, you will want to read through this special section. It covers key test-taking tips for these examinations and also highlights exactly how test-item writers—the people who made the test you are about to take—craft questions, answers, and distracters. (See *What Experienced Test Writers Do*.) The more you know about how test items are built, the better prepared you will be to answer each item correctly.

Tips for Success

To pass either the PANCE or PANRE, you will need to prepare wisely, develop clear and efficient test-taking strategies, and know what to expect on test day.

Preparing Wisely

Before you do anything else, visit the National Commission on Certification of Physician Assistants (NCCPA) Web site at www.nccpa.net. It offers information on test eligibility requirements, registration information, examination content blueprint, sample questions, and other important guidelines concerning the PANCE and PANRE. In addition, you may take a practice exam (http://www.nccpa.net/SelfAssessment.aspx).

Read the NCCPA Content Blueprint, and learn as much as you can about the diseases and disorders that are listed. Use this book and accompanying CD-ROM for enriching your information base and practicing your test-taking skills.

For instance, you can practice your time-management skills by selecting a number of questions and then giving yourself an average of 1 minute per question to respond. By taking timed tests, you can become comfortable working under actual test-taking conditions.

Just Before Test Day

Make sure that you get to the test site on time. If you will be traveling to an unfamiliar location, obtain directions to the site. Then make a test drive before the day of the test. Remember to bring the directions with you on exam day.

If you live a considerable distance from the test site, arrive the day before the exam and stay overnight in the area. You will need a good night's rest to ensure your being as relaxed as possible.

Do not cram the night before taking the test. You need rest at this point, not more study. Bring a small snack with you for refreshment during break periods.

Test-taking Strategies

Here are a few strategies to employ when taking the test

- Read each question carefully. Be aware of words and phrases such as *indicated, contraindicated, preferred initial* (therapy), and *except. Except* questions are generally rare, but be alert for their appearance nonetheless.

- Read all responses (*A* through *E*) before making your decision. Try to systematically exclude responses you know are incorrect.

- Do not spend an excessive amount of time on a single question. If you find that you have spent 2 minutes on a question, it is probably best to flag that question and return to it later, in the block-time period.

Exam Day

You should arrive at least 30 minutes before your test is scheduled to begin. If you arrive late, you may have to forfeit your breaks or pay a late fee to reschedule the examination.

Upon arrival at the test center you will present your scheduling permit. You must be prepared to show two forms of identification, including a driver's license or passport. Both must be original and valid (not expired). No one is permitted to take the examination without the permit and personal identification. A digital fingerprint or palm scan and photo will be taken at the center. Refer to NCCPA website for more details related to identification.

You are not allowed to bring personal belongings into the testing room. Examples of prohibited personal property include book bags, handbags, brimmed hats, books, notes, study materials, watches, electronic devices, and food or beverages. A locker will be assigned for storage of these items.

Staff members at the testing center will provide instructions to assist in use of the computer equipment. You will have the opportunity to complete a brief tutorial before starting the formal testing session. The examination will be observed by testing center staff members who will use audiovisual monitors and recording equipment.

Examination Structure

PANCE and PANRE examinations are administered in blocks. The PANCE consists of five blocks, each having 60 multiple-choice test items (see "Parts of a Test Item"), for a total of 300 test items. You will have 60 minutes to complete each block, a time-frame that represents an average of 1 minute per question.

PANRE consists of four blocks, each having 60 multiple-choice test items, for a total of 240 test items. You will have 60 minutes to complete each block, a time frame that represents an average of 1 minute per question.

In both PANCE and PANRE, test items may be answered in any order within a block. You may review questions, and answers may be changed within a block during the time allotted for that block. You will have a total of 45 minutes for breaks between blocks. You are solely responsible for managing your break time, so manage it well.

NCCPA now offers a Certificate of Added Qualifications (CAQ) for those who seek recognition in certain specialty areas. Successful completion of a CAQ examination is one of NCCPA's core requirements for specialty credentialing. CAQ examinations are given in the following specialties: Cardiovascular and Thoracic Surgery; Emergency Medicine; Orthopaedic Surgery; and Psychiatry. The 2-hour examination has 120 questions in 2 blocks of 60 questions with 60 minutes to complete each block.

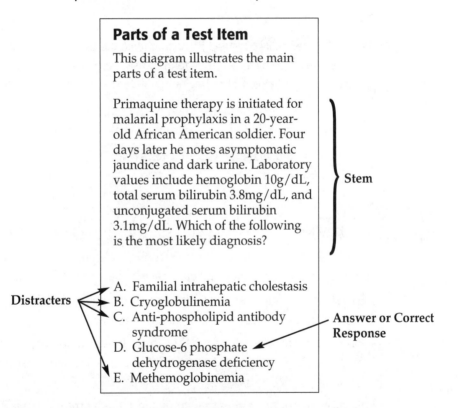

Parts of a Test Item

This diagram illustrates the main parts of a test item.

Primaquine therapy is initiated for malarial prophylaxis in a 20-year-old African American soldier. Four days later he notes asymptomatic jaundice and dark urine. Laboratory values include hemoglobin 10g/dL, total serum bilirubin 3.8mg/dL, and unconjugated serum bilirubin 3.1mg/dL. Which of the following is the most likely diagnosis?   **Stem**

A. Familial intrahepatic cholestasis
Distracters   B. Cryoglobulinemia
C. Anti-phospholipid antibody   **Answer or Correct**
  syndrome   **Response**
D. Glucose-6 phosphate
  dehydrogenase deficiency
E. Methemoglobinemia

What Experienced Test Writers Do

Experienced test-writers commonly use certain terms or phrases for consistency and clarity in presentation. Your familiarity with those terms or phrases will make you more comfortable during the exam. Here are four key tips for understanding what experienced test writers do and what you can learn from it.

Tip #1: Worry Not About the Small Stuff

Item writers, when constructing a clinical vignette, typically write that the patient has a symptom rather than complains of a symptom. For example, an item stem might read, "A 52-year-old man has a 1-hour history of chest pressure," or "A 42-year-old woman has a 3-week history of nausea and weight loss." You should understand that "has" is essentially equivalent to "complains of."

Here's another example. In clinical vignettes, item writers often use the phrase "Examination shows" when describing physical signs of a disease or disorder. For instance, you might see something like "Examination shows the apical impulse to be in the fifth intercostal space," or "Examination shows hyperpigmentation in the skin creases." Yes, there are other ways to say the same thing, but PANCE and PANRE item writers tend to use just this one.

Tip #2: Differentiation

Item writers generally construct items that force the test candidate to clinically distinguish between two diseases. They tend to use the phrase "Presence of which of the following differentiates" at the beginning of item stems. Here's a typical example:

Presence of which of the following differentiates heart failure in hyperthyroidism from heart failure in chronic mitral regurgitation?

   A. Elevated systemic vascular resistance
   B. Pulmonary crackles
   C. Peripheral edema
   D. Elevated cardiac output
   E. Atrial fibrillation

This item asks you to define which condition is present only in heart failure associated with hyperthyroidism. Your analysis, then, might flow something like this:

• Elevated systemic vascular resistance is not characteristic of heart failure in hyperthyroidism and, therefore, is incorrect.

• Pulmonary crackles may be heard in both conditions (hyperthyroidism and mitral regurgitation) and does not differentiate between them. This response is therefore incorrect.

• Peripheral edema and atrial fibrillation are common in both conditions. Therefore, both C and E are incorrect responses.

• An elevated cardiac output is found only in hyperthyroid heart failure and, thus, D is the correct response.

Tip #3: Management Distracters

Many test items deal with the initial management of a disease or disorder. These items may contain responses beginning with "Consultation with," followed by a physician-specialist, such as vascular surgeon, gastroenterologist, or dermatologist.

Be careful of these items; there are many conditions in which the initial management involves first a medication, and then a consultation. Here's an example:

A 65-year-old man has the sudden onset of a painful, cold left arm. Examination shows the left arm to be pale, cold, and numb. No brachial, radial, or ulnar pulses are felt in the affected arm. Electrocardiography shows atrial fibrillation. Which of the following is the preferred initial management?

    A. Administration of oral aspirin
    B. Administration of intravenous heparin
    C. Application of warm compresses to the left arm
    D. Consultation with a vascular surgeon
    E. Administration of phentolamine into the brachial artery

This patient has suffered an embolus to the brachial artery related to his atrial fibrillation. Consultation with a vascular surgeon is indicated, but consultation is not the initial step in management. Initial management involves administration of intravenous heparin prior to arrival of the surgeon.

Tip #4: Assume Nothing

Experienced item writers do not use trick questions. Their items are specifically designed to find out what you know. They don't "hide" critical information, so test takers shouldn't assume that they do. Many test takers, for instance, erroneously assume that a patient has a particular disorder when in fact the test item stem indicates no such disorder. Here's an example:

A 66-year-old man has angina pectoris associated with ventricular premature beats. Vital signs are normal. Heart and lung examination is normal. Which of the following is the preferred therapy?

This test item is trying to determine whether the test taker knows that beta-adrenergic blockers are preferred when a patient has myocardial ischemia associated with ventricular ectopy. If the test taker mistakenly assumes that the patient has Type 1 diabetes mellitus, he or she might answer that a calcium channel blocker is preferred.

The lesson: Do not make assumptions.

Contents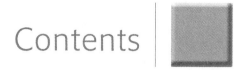

Part One

Essentials: Your Medical Information Base

ESSENTIALS is the resource that is carefully designed to enhance your clinical skills in the most important aspects of disease:

- Symptoms and signs
- Pathophysiology
- Pharmacology
- Anatomy
- Laboratory/imaging diagnostic studies
- Clinical therapeutics

ESSENTIALS is composed of didactic questions that will strengthen your medical information base. The questions are constructed to enable you to *compare and contrast* medical data. Therefore, many questions in **ESSENTIALS** have **more than one correct answer.** Your skill in critical thinking will be improved. Each **ESSENTIALS** question will be followed by the correct answer(s) and **You Should Know.**

 ESSENTIALS is the medical information bridge to **PERFORMANCE**.

Section One

Essentials Review

Organ Classification System

Although the questions are presented in random order to simulate the actual structure of the PANCE and PANRE examinations, each question has a tag identifying the organ system or systems to which that question relates. For example, a question on endocarditis will be tagged for both Infectious Disease (ID) and Cardiovascular (CV); a question on melasma will be tagged Reproductive (REPRO) and Dermatology (DERM). In this way, you may self-assess your knowledge in each of the following categories.

Cardiovascular	CV
Pulmonary	PUL
Endocrine	ENDO
Eye, Ear, Nose, and Throat	EENT
Gastrointestinal/Nutritional	GI/N
Genitourinary	GU
Musculoskeletal	MS
Reproductive	REPRO
Neurologic	NEURO
Psychiatric/Legal and Ethics	PSY/LE
Dermatologic	DERM
Hematologic/Oncology	HEME/ONC
Infectious Disease	ID

CV

E 001   Diastolic heart failure is associated with which of the following?
- A. Increased afterload
- B. Left ventricular hypertrophy
- C. Decreased left ventricular ejection fraction
- D. Systemic hypotension
- E. Mitral valve regurgitation

Essentials is designed to promote critical thinking and enrich your knowledge base. Therefore, many questions will have more than one correct answer.

Answer: A and B

A and B are correct because increased afterload causes left ventricular hypertrophy (LVH). The left ventricular hypertrophy causes the ventricle to be stiff resulting in diastolic heart failure with its associated dyspnea.

▨ You should know:

1. Diastolic heart failure is due to increased stiffness (decreased compliance) of the left ventricle. In order to effectively fill the LV during diastole, left atrial pressure must increase. This increased pressure is transmitted backward to the lung. Therefore, the cardinal symptom of diastolic heart failure is *dyspnea* that is treated with diuretics.

2. Diastolic heart failure is most often associated with left ventricular hypertrophy. LVH is the compensatory response to increased afterload caused by systemic hypertension or aortic valve stenosis. The physical sign of LVH is an apical lift or heave, often accompanied by an S4 gallop if the patient is in sinus rhythm.

3. The left ventricular hypertrophy may be secondary to *acquired* disease (e.g., hypertension or aortic valve stenosis) or due to *congenital* disease (e.g., hypertrophic cardiomyopathy or coarctation of the aorta).

4. Other causes of increased left ventricular stiffness *not associated with left ventricular hypertrophy* include infiltrative myocardial disease (e.g., amyloidosis and myocardial ischemia). Myocardial ischemia causes a *transient* increase in ventricular stiffness, thus explaining the brief dyspnea that often accompanies angina pectoris.

5. "Anginal equivalent" is dyspnea *without anginal discomfort* of brief duration that is caused by myocardial ischemia. In a patient who has only dyspnea, the clinician must consider myocardial ischemia as the underlying cause. Provocative cardiac stress testing may be indicated.

6. In addition to diuretics, diastolic heart failure is treated with beta-adrenergic blockers, which improve ventricular filling by slowing the heart rate, and with nondihydropyridine calcium channel blockers (verapamil and diltiazem), which improve ventricular compliance.

NEURO, PSY/LE, GI/N

E 002   Which of the following is a cause of dementia?

    A. Alzheimer's disease
    B. Folic acid deficiency
    C. Chronic alcohol abuse
    D. Parkinson's disease
    E. Huntington's chorea

Answer: A, C, D, and E

A, C, D, and E are correct because dementia occurs in Alzheimer's disease, chronic alcohol abuse, Huntington's chorea, and Parkinson's disease.

▨ You should know:

1. Dementia is a syndrome characterized by deterioration of cognitive abilities manifest by memory loss and impairment in calculation, judgment, and

problem solving. It is often associated with social deficits including depression, agitation, hallucinations, and insomnia.

2. Dementia due to chronic alcohol abuse is related to malnutrition, especially of the B vitamins, and particularly thiamine. Dementia is six times more common in patients with Parkinson's disease than in the general population.

3. Normally, there is a balance between the neurotransmitters acetylcholine and dopamine in the basal ganglia. In Parkinson's disease, there is a depletion of dopamine resulting in exaggerated acetylcholine effect. This is the basis of *anticholinergic* therapy in this disease. Anticholinergic medications are used primarily when tremor is the most troubling manifestation. However, they may worsen the cognitive deficits in the patient.

4. Huntington's disease, also associated with dementia, is inherited in an autosomal dominant manner. It is associated with chorea, characterized by involuntary rapid, jerky motions.

5. A *cholinesterase inhibitor* (donepezil, rivastigmine, galantamine) is the preferred initial treatment of dementia associated with Alzheimer's disease, vascular dementia, dementia with Lewy bodies, and dementia associated with Parkinson's disease. The pharmacologic mechanism of action is an increase in cerebral production of acetylcholine.

6. Cholinesterase inhibitors do not improve the psychiatric symptoms, including depression, aggression, and delusions, that are commonly observed in the patient with dementia.

7. Common adverse effects of cholinesterase inhibitor medications include nausea, vomiting, and diarrhea.

PSY/LE, ENDO, HEME, NEURO

E 003 Which of the following is a cause of *reversible* dementia?
A. Hypothyroidism
B. Depression
C. Pernicious anemia
D. Bismuth poisoning
E. Normal pressure hydrocephalus

Answer: A, B, C, D, and E
A, B, C, D, and E are correct because dementia may be the result of endocrine (hypothyroidism), hematologic (pernicious anemia), psychiatric (depression), and neurologic (normal pressure hydrocephalus) disease. If diagnosed early and treated, the dementia is reversible. Further, bismuth poisoning is potentially reversible.

■ **You should know:**

1. The clinician must always search for treatable (reversible) causes of dementia.

2. Depression may masquerade as dementia with apparent memory loss and impaired judgment ("pseudodementia"). Treatment of the depression results in improved cognitive function.

3. Vitamin B_{12} deficiency may cause dementia while the blood elements are *completely normal* (i.e., normal hemoglobin, red blood cell indices, and

number of segments in the neutrophils). The patient's dementia may make examination of the posterior spinal columns (proprioception and vibratory sensation) impossible. A serum vitamin B_{12} level should be obtained. Be aware, however, that even a normal serum vitamin B_{12} level does not completely rule out this diagnosis. An increased serum level of methylmalonic acid appears to be more sensitive for the diagnosis of vitamin B_{12} deficiency.

4. Patients who take metformin in treatment of diabetes mellitus have impaired absorption of vitamin B_{12} and lowered serum levels. This can be reversed with oral calcium intake.

5. Patients having normal pressure hydrocephalus will have dementia plus an abnormal gait and urinary incontinence or urinary urgency. Ventricular shunting surgery will improve the mental faculty in half of the operated patients. Assessment of gait is essential in evaluation of every patient who has dementia.

6. Considerable intake of oral bismuth, as in treatment of *Helicobacter pylori* infection, may cause dementia, particularly in the patient who has underlying renal insufficiency.

7. Hypothyroid patients often have memory loss and depression, in addition to cold intolerance, weight gain, and weakness. Serum thyroid-stimulating hormone (TSH) is elevated in primary hypothyroidism and normal or low in secondary hypothyroidism.

8. Patients who have *autoimmune* primary hypothyroidism have increased serum titers of antibodies to thyroid peroxidase and thyroglobulin.

9. Hypothyroidism *not on an autoimmune basis* may occur in patients who are taking lithium in treatment of bipolar disorder or amiodarone in treatment of supraventricular or ventricular arrhythmias. There is a significant incidence of *hypothyroidism* in those patients who have received radioactive iodine (RAI) months or years earlier in treatment of hyperthyroidism. Patients who have received RAI should have monitoring of serum TSH levels for the rest of their lives.

10. Other important adverse effects of amiodarone therapy include interstitial pneumonitis, corneal deposits, optic nerve atrophy, hepatitis, and rash ("blue man" face).

GI/N, HEME

E 004   Which of the following conditions may cause jaundice?

A. Hemolysis
B. Pancreatic carcinoma
C. Acute viral hepatitis
D. Gilbert's disease
E. Pulmonary infarction

Answer: A, B, C, and D
A, B, C, and D are correct because jaundice may be due to hematologic disease (hemolysis) or hepatobiliary disease (intrahepatic or extrahepatic obstruction to bilirubin excretion).

▓ **You should know:**

1. Jaundice may be due to *either* increased unconjugated ("indirect") or increased conjugated ("direct") serum bilirubin levels.

2. Carcinoma of the pancreas causes jaundice when it obstructs the biliary tree.

3. Viral hepatitis produces jaundice in the obstructive phase of the illness.

4. Gilbert's disease, an inherited disorder of bilirubin conjugation in the liver, causes jaundice due to accumulation of indirect (unconjugated) bilirubin in the serum.

GI/N, HEME

E 005   Which of the following conditions is associated with an increase in serum unconjugated ("indirect") bilirubin?

A. Hemolysis
B. Physiologic jaundice in the newborn
C. Gilbert's disease
D. Dubin-Johnson syndrome
E. Metastatic tumor in the liver

Answer: A, B, and C
A is correct because both extravascular hemolysis and intravascular hemolysis result in increased levels of serum unconjugated bilirubin. B is correct because physiologic jaundice in the newborn is unconjugated hyperbilirubinemia due to increased bilirubin production and decreased bilirubin clearance. C is correct because Gilbert's disease is an inherited disorder in which there is a defect in conjugation of bilirubin.

▓ **You should know:**

1. Both *extravascular* hemolysis (destruction of red blood cells in the spleen, bone marrow, and liver) and *intravascular* hemolysis result in increased levels of serum unconjugated bilirubin.

2. Gilbert's disease is more common in males. Other routine laboratory tests in the patient are usually normal. Prognosis appears to be the same as the general population.

HEME, GI/N

E 006   Which of the following conditions is associated with an increase in serum conjugated ("direct") bilirubin?

A. Dubin-Johnson syndrome
B. Biliary tract obstruction
C. Intrahepatic cholestasis
D. Glucose-6-phosphate dehydrogenase deficiency
E. Metastatic tumor in the liver

Answer: A, B, C, and E
A is correct because Dubin-Johnson syndrome is a hereditary disorder in which there is an elevation in serum conjugated bilirubin. B, C, and E are correct because in intrahepatic cholestasis, biliary tract obstruction, and metastatic tumor in the liver the hepatocytes are able to conjugate the bilirubin but not to normally remove it in

Essentials is designed to promote critical thinking and enrich your knowledge base.
Therefore, many questions will have more than one correct answer.

the biliary system. Therefore, conjugated bilirubin spills from the hepatocytes into the serum causing jaundice from conjugated hyperbilirubinemia.

▨ **You should know:**

1. Glucose-6-phosphate dehydrogenase (G-6-PD) deficiency of red blood cells is an X-linked disorder in which patients may have acute hemolysis related to infection, medications, or stress. In these patients, hemolysis would cause an increase in unconjugated serum bilirubin.

2. Dubin-Johnson syndrome is an inherited disorder in which the patient has mild icterus but is usually otherwise asymptomatic. Although the serum direct bilirubin level is elevated, the remainder of liver function tests—namely, prothrombin time, aminotransferases, and alkaline phosphatase—are normal.

3. Cholangitis is a serious disease manifest by the triad of *abdominal pain, jaundice* associated with an increased serum conjugated bilirubin level due to obstruction in the common bile duct (CBD), and *fever* with chills. Most commonly, the biliary obstruction is caused by a stone. Bacteria ascend from the gut into the biliary tree from which they enter the bloodstream causing gram-negative bacteremia.

4. Emergency treatment of cholangitis includes endoscopic retrograde cholangiopancreatography (ERCP) with sphincterotomy and stone removal plus intravenous antibiotic therapy. Antibiotics, used alone or in combination, include ciprofloxacin, metronidazole, ampicillin, gentamicin, sulbactam, ceftriaxone, and piperacillin.

CV

E 007   Which of the following may cause a patient to have myocardial ischemia?

     A. Atherosclerosis
     B. Coronary artery spasm
     C. Left ventricular hypertrophy
     D. Anomalous coronary artery
     E. Infiltrative myocardial disease

Answer: A, B, C, and D
A is correct because atherosclerotic narrowing of a coronary artery causes myocardial ischemia when myocardial oxygen demand exceeds oxygen delivery through the stenotic artery (e.g., with physical effort or emotional distress). B is correct because coronary artery spasm can provoke ischemia without increased oxygen demand on the heart. C is correct because left ventricular hypertrophy can cause myocardial ischemia in the absence of coexistent atherosclerosis or coronary spasm. D is correct because infants born with an anomalous coronary artery (e.g., the right coronary artery arising from a pulmonary artery) have myocardial ischemia starting at birth.

▨ **You should know:**

1. Coronary artery spasm is the mechanism causing variant angina (Prinzmetal's angina), a condition more common in women and causing anginal discomfort during the very early morning hours. The acute myocardial ischemia is treated with calcium channel blockers and nitrates. The

same medications are prescribed in an effort to prevent future attacks of coronary artery spasm.

2. Left ventricular hypertrophy may be secondary to acquired disease (e.g., aortic valve stenosis) or due to congenital disease (e.g., hypertrophic cardiomyopathy).

3. Children with an anomalous coronary artery may begin to experience angina pectoris during childhood or young adult years. Remember: Children may have angina pectoris!

4. In variant angina, electrocardiography performed *during the anginal discomfort* shows ST segment *elevation*. In contrast, the classic electrocardiographic expression of myocardial ischemia caused by atherosclerotic coronary artery stenosis is horizontal ST segment *depression*.

DERM, GI/N, NEURO

E 008   Which of the following is a side effect of niacin therapy?

A. Flushing
B. Pruritus
C. Nausea
D. Paresthesias
E. Peripheral edema

Answer: A, B, C, and D
A, B, C, and D are correct because flushing is the most common side effect, affecting approximately 75% of patients; pruritus, paresthesias, and nausea affect approximately 20%.

■ **You should know:**

1. Niacin reduces serum cholesterol, low-density lipoprotein (LDL) cholesterol, very low-density lipoprotein (VLDL), and triglycerides. It increases serum high-density lipoprotein (HDL) cholesterol levels.

2. The onset of hepatotoxicity is not predictable; therefore, serial monitoring of liver function tests is essential.

3. Short-acting niacin preparations appear to have less hepatotoxicity than long-acting preparations.

4. Additional side effects of niacin include hyperglycemia and elevation of serum uric acid. Niacin should not be given to a patient who has a history of gout.

5. In a brief summary, hepatotoxicity may occur during therapy with the following medications:
   • Methotrexate
     (1) Given in treatment of malignancy, including leukemias and solid tumors
     (2) Given in treatment of nonmalignant disorders, including psoriasis and rheumatoid arthritis
     (3) Folate (leucovorin), given prophylactically, reduces the incidence of methotrexate-related hepatotoxicity
   • Amiodarone
     (1) Given in treatment of supraventricular and ventricular arrhythmias

Essentials is designed to promote critical thinking and enrich your knowledge base.
Therefore, many questions will have more than one correct answer.

- Isoniazid (INH)
  (1) Given in treatment of tuberculosis or latent tuberculous infection
- HMG CoA reductase inhibitors ("statins")

Patients receiving these medicines should have serial monitoring of liver function tests.

CV

E 009   Which of the following is a cardiovascular complication of cocaine use?

A. Acute myocardial infarction
B. Dissection of the aorta
C. Ventricular tachycardia
D. 1st degree atrioventricular block
E. Myocarditis

Answer: A, B, C, and E
A, B, C, and E are correct because cocaine causes stimulation of both alpha- and beta-adrenergic receptors. Cocaine usage results in hypertension and tachycardia and may provoke angina pectoris and myocardial infarction due to coronary artery spasm, myocarditis, supraventricular and ventricular arrhythmias, and dissection of the aorta.

■ **You should know:**

1. Administration of a pure beta-adrenergic blocker (e.g., propranolol) may worsen cocaine-induced hypertension. Beta blocker administration would result in unopposed alpha-adrenergic stimulation by the cocaine resulting in higher systemic arterial pressure.

2. Treatment of myocardial ischemia/infarction secondary to cocaine use includes a benzodiazepine anxiolytic agent, aspirin, nitrates, calcium blocker, and alpha-adrenergic blocker. Alternatively, a combined alpha-adrenergic and beta-adrenergic blocker (e.g., labetalol) may be administered.

3. Myocardial infarction is usually due to profound cocaine-induced coronary artery spasm. Myocardial infarction most often occurs in patients with normal coronary arteries. In some cases, infarction is related to thrombus formation. Coronary angiography is often performed on an emergent basis in these patients.

4. Cardiovascular effects of ephedrine-containing substances (e.g., "herbal ecstasy") cause similar adrenergic hyperactivity.

GI/N, MS

E 010   Which of the following is an extraintestinal manifestation of Crohn's disease?

A. Arthritis
B. Cholelithiasis
C. Cerebral berry aneurysm
D. Clubbing
E. Pulmonary fibrosis

Answer: A, B, and D
A is correct because Crohn's disease (and ulcerative colitis) has arthritic manifestations including large joint arthritis and spondylitis. B is correct because cholelithiasis

(cholesterol stones) is common in Crohn's disease due to malabsorption of bile salts from the terminal ileum. D is correct because clubbing occurs in inflammatory bowel disease.

■ **You should know:**

1. Clubbing of the fingers and toes may be noted in patients with lung abscess, idiopathic pulmonary fibrosis, bronchiectasis, primary and metastatic lung malignancy, cyanotic congenital heart disease, and endocarditis.

2. The intraocular inflammatory disease uveitis is often associated with systemic disease. Crohn's disease, ulcerative colitis, reactive arthritis, ankylosing spondylitis, psoriasis, and sarcoidosis are associated with uveitis.

3. Chronic hemolytic anemias, particularly sickle cell disease (SCD), are associated with development of *bilirubin* gallstones. Gallstones occur in SCD patients as early as age 3 years.

HEME

E 011   Which of the following laboratory values would be expected in a patient who has hemolysis?

A. Decreased serum haptoglobin
B. Increased serum lactate dehydrogenase
C. Increased reticulocyte percentage
D. Decreased serum gamma-glutamyl transpeptidase
E. Decreased serum ferritin

Answer: A, B, and C
A is correct because haptoglobin binds to the free hemoglobin that is released during hemolysis. This binding leads to a decrease in the level of circulating haptoglobin. B is correct because lactate dehydrogenase enzyme is found in erythrocytes. Therefore, hemolysis would cause release of this enzyme into the serum. C is correct because reticulocytes are relatively immature erythrocytes that are released into the circulation in response to hemolysis or blood loss.

■ **You should know:**

1. Ferritin is the major iron *storage protein.* A serum level less than 35 ng/mL is indicative of iron deficiency.

2. The reticulocyte count is expressed as an "index"; a value greater than 2 suggests hemolysis or blood loss.

GI/N, NEURO

E 012   Which of the following is a complication of cirrhosis of the liver?

A. Esophageal varices
B. Spontaneous bacterial peritonitis
C. Encephalopathy
D. Hepatocellular carcinoma
E. Spontaneous arterial thrombosis

Answer: A, B, C, and D
A is correct because the portal hypertension associated with cirrhosis causes development of esophageal varices. B is correct because chronic liver disease increases the

Essentials is designed to promote critical thinking and enrich your knowledge base.
Therefore, many questions will have more than one correct answer.

risk of the patient developing spontaneous bacterial peritonitis, an infection of ascites without an apparent intra-abdominal source of infection. C is correct because the cirrhotic patient has impaired ability to detoxify products of intestinal origin. The pathogenesis of hepatic encephalopathy is complex. Increased blood levels of ammonia can only partly explain the mental disturbances in the patient who has advanced liver disease. D is correct because cirrhotic patients have a markedly increased risk of developing hepatocellular carcinoma (HCC).

▨ **You should know:**

1. Ascites is the most common complication of portal hypertension that occurs in the cirrhotic patient.

2. Spontaneous bacterial peritonitis (SBP) should be suspected in the patient with cirrhosis and ascites who has fever, abdominal pain or tenderness, and altered mental status; however, some patients are asymptomatic. Most cases develop from gram-negative infection, most commonly *E. coli,* without an apparent source of infection. SBP may be caused by a gram-positive organism, particularly in those patients who have an indwelling vascular line that is complicated by bacteremia.

3. When SBP is suspected paracentesis should be performed. An absolute neutrophil count of greater than 250/microL is an indication to start antibiotic therapy before results of ascitic fluid culture are known. Without early treatment, mortality is high. Nearly 70% of those who have had SBP will have a recurrence; therefore, prophylactic antibiotics are indicated.

4. The clinician must carefully search for a primary source of abdominal infection before the diagnosis of SBP is established. Infection of ascitic fluid may be caused by perforated ulcer, diverticulitis, or appendicitis.

5. Hemorrhage from esophageal or gastric varices is a major complication of portal hypertension. Intravenous octreotide is the preferred medicinal therapy of active bleeding. Endoscopic measures are employed in addition to octreotide administration. When hemorrhage has ceased, beta-adrenergic blocker therapy is given in an effort to prevent recurrent variceal hemorrhage.

6. Although not specific, increasing levels of serum alpha-fetoprotein (AFP) in the patient with cirrhosis should raise concern that hepatocellular carcinoma (HCC) has developed.

7. Additionally, an increased serum AFP level may be noted in males who have gonadal tumors. In the pregnant woman an abnormally high level suggests a congenital neural tube abnormality in the fetus. Maternal screening starts at 15 to 20 weeks of gestation.

CV

E 013   Which of the following medications slows atrioventricular conduction?

A. Digoxin
B. Metoprolol
C. Nifedipine
D. Captopril
E. Diltiazem

Answer: A, B, and E

A is correct because digoxin slows atrioventricular (AV) conduction via its parasympathetic effect on the atrioventricular (AV) node. B and E are correct because beta-adrenergic blockers and the nondihydropyridine calcium channel blockers verapamil and diltiazem slow conduction velocity in the atrioventricular node. Thus, these agents are used to slow the ventricular response in patients who have atrial fibrillation (AF) or atrial flutter.

■ **You should know:**

1. Digoxin is preferred for rate slowing in those atrial fibrillation patients who are hypotensive or who are in systolic heart failure. When clinically appropriate, therapy with a beta-adrenergic blocker is added, both to further slow the ventricular rate and to improve left ventricular function. (Systolic heart failure is treated with the basic triad of a beta-adrenergic blocker, loop diuretic, and angiotensin-converting enzyme inhibitor [ACEI].)

2. Nifedipine, a dihydropyridine calcium blocker, does not slow atrioventricular conduction, nor does an ACEI.

3. In the atrial fibrillation patient who has chronic obstructive lung disease or claudication secondary to peripheral arterial disease, verapamil and diltiazem are preferred treatment because beta-adrenergic blockers may worsen both the pulmonary function and the claudication symptoms.

4. Patients with atrial fibrillation or atrial flutter who have poor control of the ventricular response, specifically, with ventricular rates chronically greater than 100/min, may develop a dilated cardiomyopathy with its associated reduced cardiac output and systolic heart failure. This is called *tachycardia cardiomyopathy*. Ambulatory monitoring should be performed in patients who are in chronic atrial fibrillation in order to assess control of the ventricular rate.

5. In the patient who is in *diastolic heart failure*, the onset of atrial fibrillation often provokes acute pulmonary edema. Immediate restoration of normal sinus rhythm is preferred. If this cannot be accomplished, a beta-adrenergic blocker or verapamil is administered to control the ventricular response.

6. In the patient who is in normal sinus rhythm, toxic doses of digoxin, beta-adrenergic blockers, verapamil, or diltiazem may cause 2nd-degree or 3rd-degree atrioventricular block.

CV, GU

E 014   Which of the following conditions is associated with increased jugular venous pressure?

A. Superior vena cava syndrome
B. Right heart failure
C. Constrictive pericarditis
D. Nephrotic syndrome
E. Cirrhosis

Answer: A, B, and C

A is correct because superior vena cava (SVC) syndrome caused by obstruction in superior vena cava flow into the right atrium results in elevation of the jugular venous pressure (JVP). B and C are correct because the hemodynamic sequelae of right heart failure and constrictive pericarditis increase jugular venous pressure.

▓ You should know:

1. Superior vena cava syndrome is manifest by facial and upper arm swelling and cyanosis. *It does not cause edema of the lower extremities.* The etiology of SVC syndrome most commonly is small cell carcinoma of the lung or non-Hodgkin's lymphoma. An additional important cause is thrombosis around an indwelling central venous catheter.

2. Both right heart failure and constrictive pericarditis (CP) are manifest by bilateral peripheral edema, ascites, and hepatomegaly. The most common cause of right heart failure (RHF) is *chronic systolic left heart failure.* Another important etiology of RHF is pulmonary hypertension caused by pulmonary vascular obstruction (pulmonary embolism) or pulmonary parenchymal disease (pulmonary fibrosis or chronic bronchitis).

3. The most common cause of constrictive pericarditis in the United States is prior chest radiation for malignant disease. CP may also be related to cardiac surgery, connective tissue disease, and bacterial pericarditis including tuberculosis. Only rarely does acute viral pericarditis lead to CP.

4. Nephrotic syndrome and advanced cirrhosis of the liver both cause hypoalbuminemia, which is clinically manifest as ascites and bilateral peripheral edema. The edema commonly involves the periorbital area, the presacral area, and both lower legs. Anasarca is severe edema involving the entire body. However, it is important to note that in these patients the jugular venous pressure is normal. With loss of intravascular volume related to the low oncotic pressure, the blood pressure in patients with nephrotic syndrome or advanced cirrhosis is normal or low.

CV

E 015   Which of the following is the preferred initial test to confirm the diagnosis of an acute thoracic dissection of the aorta?

A. Chest radiography
B. Magnetic resonance imaging (MRI) of the thorax
C. Transesophageal echocardiography
D. Computed tomography (CT) of the thorax
E. Contrast aortography

Answer: **B, C, and D**
B, C, and D are correct because transesophageal echocardiography (TEE), computed tomography scan, and magnetic resonance imaging of the thorax are all considered to be valuable in diagnosis of dissection and are considered by different medical authorities to be the preferred initial diagnostic test.

▓ You should know:

1. *Transthoracic* echocardiography and chest radiography have a lower sensitivity.

2. Aortography is not considered to be the initial diagnostic test.

3. Complications of acute dissection of the ascending aorta include pericardial tamponade, left hemothorax, acute aortic valve regurgitation, stroke, and acute myocardial ischemia or infarction.

4. Acute dissection of the thoracic aorta is typically associated with tearing or ripping chest pain. Risk factors include the following:
   • Collagen diseases including Marfan syndrome and Ehler-Danlos syndrome
   • Chronic systemic hypertension
   • Inflammatory diseases of the aorta (vasculitis) including giant cell arteritis and Takayasu arteritis
   • Use of crack cocaine
   • Bicuspid aortic valve

DERM, HEME, GI/N

E 016   Which of the following may cause pruritus?
   A. Polycythemia rubra vera
   B. Primary biliary cirrhosis
   C. Nonsteroidal anti-inflammatory medications
   D. Legionnaires' disease
   E. Renal cell carcinoma

Answer: A, B, and C
A is correct because polycythemia rubra vera often causes the patient to experience itching after a warm shower or bath. B is correct because primary biliary cirrhosis, occurring in middle-aged women, often has itching as the initial symptom. C is correct because nonsteroidal anti-inflammatory medications (NSAIDs) may cause itching without a rash.

■ **You should know:**

1. Polycythemia rubra vera (PRV) is a myeloproliferative disease in which there is overproduction of all blood elements. Hematologic abnormalities include increased hemoglobin and hematocrit, increased white blood cell count, and variably increased platelet count. The treatment of choice is phlebotomy.

2. In PRV, the arterial oxygen saturation is normal and the serum erythropoietin level is *low*. In contrast, disorders in which systemic arterial oxygen saturation is low (hypoxemia) have a *secondary* erythrocytosis related to increased production of erythropoietin.

3. To differentiate PRV from secondary erythrocytosis: in PRV, serum erythropoietin is low; in secondary erythrocytosis caused by hypoxemia, the erythropoietin level is high.

4. In primary biliary cirrhosis, the serum alkaline phosphatase is elevated. Antimitochondrial antibodies are present in the serum in 95% of patients.

5. Antinuclear antibodies in the serum are found in primary biliary cirrhosis, systemic lupus erythematosus (SLE), rheumatoid arthritis, Sjögren's syndrome, scleroderma, and polymyositis.

6. Anti-double-stranded DNA antibodies (anti-dsDNA) are much more specific for SLE but are less sensitive.

7. Other common adverse effects of NSAIDs include elevation of blood pressure, peptic ulcer, and peripheral edema. A less frequent effect is psychosis (or other mental change), especially in the elderly patient. Remember,

NSAIDs have antiplatelet activity and therefore should be discontinued before elective surgery.

8. NSAIDs, in addition to sulfonamides, tetracycline, and hydrochlorothiazide, may cause the patient to develop a lichen planus–like rash. Lichen planus is an inflammatory pruritic disease of the skin and mucous membranes characterized by violaceous papules and lacy white streaks.

CV, GU, ENDO

E 017   In which of the following diseases is angiotensin-converting enzyme inhibitor therapy indicated?

A. Diabetic nephropathy
B. Systolic heart failure
C. Acute interstitial nephritis
D. Primary hyperaldosteronism
E. Pheochromocytoma

Answer: A and B
A is correct because angiotensin-converting enzyme inhibitors (ACEIs) and angiotensin-receptor blockers (ARBs) both reduce intraglomerular pressure and slow progression of diabetic nephropathy to end-stage renal disease. B is correct because ACEIs and ARBs reduce blood pressure (afterload) and therefore are used in treatment of systolic heart failure in an effort to improve left ventricular ejection fraction.

▪ **You should know:**

1. Primary hyperaldosteronism and pheochromocytoma are preferably treated with surgical removal of the tumors.

2. Primary hyperaldosteronism is characterized by hypertension and hypokalemia. Although the hyperaldosteronism causes marked renal conservation of sodium and water by the kidney, the patient does not become edematous.

3. Pheochromocytoma may cause intermittent paroxysmal hypertension or chronic sustained hypertension.

4. Acute interstitial nephritis (AIN) is most commonly caused by medicines, including penicillins and cephalosporins, NSAIDs, sulfonamides, and allopurinol. Infrequently, infection may cause AIN. Fever, rash, eosinophilia, and arthralgia are clinical features. Urinalysis may show microscopic hematuria, white blood cell casts, eosinophils, and slight proteinuria.

CV, GU

E 018   Which of the following conditions is associated with acute pericarditis?

A. Isoniazid therapy
B. Systemic lupus erythematosus
C. Uremia
D. Angiotensin-converting enzyme inhibitor therapy
E. Levodopa therapy

Answer: A, B, and C
A is correct because isoniazid is one of several medicines that may cause acute pericarditis. B is correct because acute pericarditis is common in systemic lupus

erythematosus (SLE) and may be the presenting manifestation of the disease. C is correct because uremia is a common cause of acute pericarditis.

■ **You should know:**

1. Isoniazid, procainamide, phenytoin, hydralazine, and the penicillins may cause acute pericarditis.

2. Anemia, leukopenia, and thrombocytopenia are common hematologic abnormalities in the patient who has SLE.

3. SLE must be suspected in a *female of any age* who has acute pericarditis.

4. Pericardial tamponade is a fairly common complication of uremia-induced pericarditis. Tamponade is characterized by hypotension, tachycardia, elevated jugular venous pressure, and paradoxical pulse. Emergency needle cardiac pericardiocentesis may be performed, followed by surgical pericardiectomy.

5. Dialysis is an effective modality in therapy of uremia-associated acute pericarditis.

CV, ENDO

E 019   Which of the following is a cause of orthostatic hypotension?
   A. Chronic adrenal insufficiency
   B. Diabetic autonomic insufficiency
   C. Hypovolemia due to blood loss
   D. Pheochromocytoma
   E. Subclavian steal syndrome

Answer: A, B, C, and D
A is correct because orthostatic hypotension (OH) in chronic adrenal insufficiency is caused by hypotension related to a deficiency in the mineralocorticoid effect of aldosterone and cortisol. The diminished mineralocorticoid effect results in decreased renal reabsorption of sodium, hypovolemia, and hyperkalemia. (Although cortisol is primarily a glucocorticoid, it does have a significant mineralocorticoid effect.) B is correct because patients with diabetes mellitus often have an autonomic neuropathy that results in orthostatic hypotension. C is correct because hypovolemia from blood loss may be associated with orthostatic hypotension. D is correct because pheochromocytoma causes hypertension, but in contrast to other hypertensive disorders, it is often associated with orthostatic hypotension.

■ **You should know:**

1. Hypovolemia of any etiology, including chronic adrenal insufficiency (Addison's disease), blood loss, or excessive diuresis, may cause orthostatic hypotension. In these patients, the decrease in blood pressure with assumption of the standing position is associated with a *compensatory increase* in heart rate.

2. Addison's disease patients commonly have hyperpigmentation of the skin. Hyponatremia is noted in 90% and hyperkalemia in 65% of cases. The cosyntropin stimulation test is performed for diagnosis. Cosyntropin is synthetic adrenocorticotropic hormone (ACTH). The response of the serum cortisol level to cosyntropin is the basis of the diagnostic test.

Essentials is designed to promote critical thinking and enrich your knowledge base. Therefore, many questions will have more than one correct answer.

3. Diabetic autonomic insufficiency is a common cause of orthostatic hypotension. In contrast to hypovolemia, the orthostatic decrease in blood pressure is *not associated with a compensatory increase* in heart rate.

4. Always check sitting blood pressure *and* heart rate followed by standing blood pressure *and* heart rate in a patient who has orthostatic hypotension. The heart rate response differentiates hypovolemia from autonomic (sympathetic) insufficiency.

5. Hypovolemia causes immediate orthostatic hypotension upon assumption of the standing position. In contrast, the orthostatic hypotension associated with autonomic neuropathy may be manifest only after 3 to 4 minutes of standing.

GI/N, MS

E 020   Which of the following medications causes painful swallowing due to esophagitis?

A. Doxazosin
B. Amoxicillin
C. Sumatriptan
D. Digoxin
E. Alendronate

Answer: E
E is correct because the bisphosphonate alendronate used in the treatment of osteoporosis is a fairly common cause of retrosternal pain and painful swallowing due to medication-induced esophagitis.

▓ **You should know:**

1. Patients starting alendronate should be advised to take the pill with at least 8 ounces of water and to stand or sit upright at least 30 minutes after ingestion.

2. The mechanism of action of bisphosphonates is inhibition of osteoclastic bone resorption.

3. Bisphosphonates are also used in therapy in Paget's disease of bone, multiple myeloma, and metastatic bone disease.

NEURO

E 021   Which of the following is associated with an intention tremor?

A. Myasthenia gravis
B. Parkinson's disease
C. Amyotrophic lateral sclerosis
D. Cerebellar infarction
E. Multiple sclerosis

Answer: D and E
D is correct because cerebellar disease causes an intention tremor, usually in conjunction with other neurologic defects including nystagmus, ataxia, and dysmetria. E is correct because multiple sclerosis commonly involves cerebellar pathways. Impaired cerebellar function may be caused by stroke, midbrain tumor, mercury poisoning, Wilson's disease, and hereditary cerebellar degeneration.

■ **You should know:**

1. Familial (essential) tremor, often with an autosomal dominant inheritance character, is an intention and postural tremor—the latter signifying tremor when an extremity is outstretched (e.g., holding a glass with an extended arm). Neurologic examination is otherwise normal. If therapy is indicated, propranolol is usually the preferred initial medication.

2. Multiple sclerosis often involves cerebellar pathways. As a result, gait ataxia, intention tremor, slurred speech, and nystagmus are neurologic manifestations.

3. Parkinson's disease causes a resting tremor. The tremor disappears during active motion, only to reappear when the extremity is again in a position of rest.

4. Myasthenia gravis, an autoimmune disorder characterized by the presence of anti–acetylcholine receptor antibodies, causes variable weakness of skeletal muscles. Diagnosis is established by response to a short-acting anticholinesterase (e.g., edrophonium or neostigmine).

CV

E 022 An increased serum level of C-reactive protein is associated with increased risk of which of the following?

A. Acute myocardial infarction
B. Rupture of cerebral aneurysm
C. Antiphospholipid antibody syndrome
D. Carcinoma of the colon
E. Glaucoma

Answer: A
A is correct because C-reactive protein is a potent predictor of future coronary events (e.g., unstable angina pectoris and acute myocardial infarction) and ischemic stroke.

■ **You should know:**

1. C-reactive protein (CRP) is an acute phase reactant that accompanies inflammation. Serum CRP measurement is used in rheumatoid arthritis, giant cell arteritis, and polymyalgia rheumatica to monitor disease activity.

2. In addition to being a predictor of increased risk, C-reactive protein itself is prothrombotic, thus promoting occlusive thrombosis in an artery.

3. Increased serum C-reactive protein levels in apparently healthy individuals are used to determine which patients are in need of more intensive therapy (e.g., use of statins to lower LDL cholesterol).

4. Increased serum CRP is a risk indicator for recurrent ischemic events after coronary artery bypass grafting (CABG) and percutaneous coronary artery intervention (PCI) with stenting.

5. Antiphospholipid antibody (APA) syndrome may be primary or may be associated with systemic lupus erythematosus. Patients with APA syndrome have increased risk of arterial and venous thrombosis. Spontaneous abortion after the first trimester is common. Lifelong anticoagulation is indicated in those patients who have recurrent thrombosis.

Essentials is designed to promote critical thinking and enrich your knowledge base. Therefore, many questions will have more than one correct answer.

E 023   Which of the following is characteristic of a vasovagal faint?

A. Palpitations
B. Cold sweat
C. Headache
D. Wheezing
E. Diarrhea

Answer: B
B is correct because the increased parasympathetic tone associated with a vasovagal reaction is characterized by cold sweat, nausea and, commonly, fainting.

■ **You should know:**

1. A vasovagal reaction is commonly precipitated by stress, either emotional or somatic (e.g., pain). Hypotension and bradycardia are typical hemodynamic features. The initial therapy is to have the person lie flat, preferably with elevation of the legs.

2. The common denominator in patients who faint is *generalized* cerebral ischemia and may be due to vasovagal reflex, orthostatic hypotension, arrhythmia, structural heart disease (e.g., aortic valve stenosis, hypertrophic obstructive cardiomyopathy, or atrial myxoma), pulmonary embolism or pulmonary hypertension, and acute myocardial infarction.

3. *Focal* cerebral ischemia causes a transient ischemic attack, not syncope.

4. Syncope due to cardiac arrhythmia, either bradycardia or tachyarrhythmia, often occurs *without the premonitory symptoms* of lightheadedness or blurred or darkened vision.

E 024   Which of the following may cause syncope in an 80-year-old man?

A. Acute myocardial infarction
B. Sick sinus syndrome
C. Orthostatic hypotension
D. Acute mesenteric ischemia
E. Subarachnoid hemorrhage

Answer: A, B, and C
A is correct because sudden fainting without chest pain may be a presentation of acute myocardial infarction. It is in the elderly patient that syncope is most likely to be associated with infarction. B is correct because sick sinus syndrome (brady-tachy syndrome), characterized by intermittent paroxysms of supraventricular tachycardia interspersed with periods of bradycardia (e.g., marked sinus bradycardia or sinus arrest), commonly causes syncope. C is correct because orthostatic hypotension of any etiology can provoke syncope upon assumption of the upright position. (Please refer to question E 019).

■ **You should know:**

1. In the patient with sick sinus syndrome, the cerebral ischemia responsible for the faint may be due to either the supraventricular arrhythmia with a fast ventricular rate or, obversely, the period of bradycardia.

2. Any elderly patient who faints, even without associated chest pain, must be evaluated for acute myocardial infarction.

3. Syncope due to arrhythmia is often not associated with premonitory symptoms.

4. Subarachnoid hemorrhage may cause coma or impaired consciousness; this is not syncope. Similarly, loss of consciousness caused by profound hypoglycemia may be transient, but this is not syncope.

5. Hypoglycemia may be clinically manifest in several ways. These include the following:
   - Autonomic (hyperadrenergic), with tremulousness, sweating, palpitations, hunger, and paresthesias
   - Neuroglycopenic, with confusion, fatigue, generalized seizure, or coma. Rarely, hypoglycemia may be manifest by a *focal neurologic deficit* (e.g., hemiparesis).

PUL, CV

E 025 Which of the following is a typical clinical finding in the patient who has chronic bronchitis complicated by right heart failure?

A. Systemic arterial hypoxemia
B. Pulmonary hypertension
C. Anemia
D. Leukocytosis
E. Peripheral edema

Answer: A, B, and E
A, B, and E are correct because the chronic bronchitis patient with heart failure (the "blue bloater") has hypoxemia and elevated pulmonary artery pressure. The pulmonary hypertension is caused by obliteration of the pulmonary vascular bed and hypoxia-induced pulmonary arteriolar constriction and leads to development of right heart failure and peripheral edema.

■ **You should know:**

1. In contrast to patients with emphysema, patients with chronic bronchitis have greater systemic arterial *desaturation* (lower PaO_2) and often exhibit central cyanosis. Additionally, they have pulmonary hypertension that may lead to right heart failure (cor pulmonale) manifest by peripheral edema, congestive hepatomegaly, and elevated jugular venous pressure.

PSY/LE, NEURO, ENDO

E 026 Which of the following is a side effect of lithium therapy?

A. Tremor
B. Hypothyroidism
C. Cogwheel rigidity
D. Diarrhea
E. Hyperchloremic acidosis

Answer: A, B, and C
A is correct because lithium may cause tremor. B is correct because lithium inhibits thyroid hormone synthesis and release resulting in hypothyroidism. C is correct because cogwheel rigidity may occur with long-term lithium therapy.

Essentials is designed to promote critical thinking and enrich your knowledge base.
Therefore, many questions will have more than one correct answer.

■ **You should know:**

1. The tremor associated with lithium therapy, if persistent, may be treated with propranolol.

2. Hypothyroidism is common. Thyroid function studies should be performed approximately every 3 months during therapy.

3. Thiazide diuretics, but not loop diuretics, increase serum lithium levels. Therefore, lithium dosage should be reduced in the patient taking a thiazide.

4. There is increased risk of fetal abnormalities in women taking lithium during early pregnancy. A pregnant woman should not take lithium. Women of childbearing age must be informed of this risk before lithium therapy is initiated.

5. Lithium should be taken with meals in order to lessen nausea.

6. Other medicines that can cause hypothyroidism include amiodarone, interferon alfa, and interleukin-2. Serum thyroid-stimulating hormone (TSH) levels should be serially monitored in patients who take these medicines.

7. Amiodarone is used to prevent recurrent, paroxysmal atrial fibrillation and to suppress ventricular ectopy. Other toxic effects include pulmonary interstitial pneumonitis, chemical hepatitis, corneal deposits, and optic neuropathy.

NEURO

E 027   Which of the following is a clinical symptom associated with atherosclerotic stenosis of a carotid artery?

A. Vertigo
B. Urinary incontinence
C. Transient visual loss in one eye
D. Fatigue
E. Transient difficulty in speaking

Answer: C
C is correct because carotid atherosclerotic disease commonly causes amaurosis fugax, a transient, monocular, ipsilateral (on the same side as the carotid narrowing) visual disturbance due to retinal emboli.

■ **You should know:**

1. Amaurosis fugax generally does not last more than 1 to 2 minutes. A patient who has amaurosis fugax should undergo duplex ultrasonography of the carotid artery.

2. Vertebrobasilar artery insufficiency frequently is manifest by impaired speech, double vision (or blurred vision in both eyes), vertigo, ataxia, and weakness.

3. Fatigue and dysarthria (impaired speech) are not characteristic symptoms of carotid artery disease.

4. Cerebral ischemia resulting from very low cardiac output due to bradycardia (e.g., 3rd-degree atrioventricular block or sinus arrest) typically causes syncope rather than localized neurologic symptoms.

5. Neurologic symptoms may be *positive* or *negative*. Positive symptoms indicate that a nerve is *irritated*. Irritation of a sensory nerve may cause burning, tingling, or visual hallucinations. Irritation of a motor nerve may cause muscle jerking or repetitive rhythmic movements. Irritation of an autonomic nerve may cause excessive sweating known as hyperhydrosis.

6. *Negative* neurologic symptoms indicate that a nerve is *not functioning*. Negative symptoms may involve sensory, motor, or autonomic nerves. Weakness, loss of somatic sensation, and visual loss are all negative symptoms. Negative symptoms should be associated with loss of that sense upon neurologic examination. Negative autonomic symptoms include impotence, anhydrosis, and lightheadedness caused by orthostatic hypotension.

7. Migraine typically starts with *positive* neurologic symptoms. As a result, the patient with migraine has light flashes, sparks, and stars in both visual fields lasting longer than 1 to 2 minutes. Following positive neurologic symptoms, the patient with migraine may have *negative* neurologic symptoms. The patient then has *loss* of a sensation, noting visual loss or numbness in extremities.

8. In contrast to migraine, a transient ischemic attack (TIA) always has *negative* neurologic symptoms.

PSY/LE

E 028   Which of the following is a characteristic of attention-deficit hyperactivity disorder?
   A. Impulsivity
   B. Inattention
   C. Urinary incontinence
   D. Association with congenital heart anomalies
   E. Association with other psychiatric conditions

Answer: A, B, and E
A and B are correct because the central manifestations of attention-deficit hyperactivity disorder (ADHD) are impulsivity, inattention, and hyperactivity. E is correct because attention-deficit hyperactivity disorder (ADHD) in the child commonly occurs in conjunction with other psychiatric disorders, including mood disorders (20%), conduct disorders (20%), oppositionally defiant disorder (40%), and Tourette's syndrome (25%).

■ **You should know:**

1. In children stimulants such as methylphenidate (Ritalin) are the first-line treatment of ADHD.

2. Children with ADHD have impaired academic performance in school and as adolescents are more likely to be involved in motor vehicle accidents.

3. Up to 50% of children with ADHD continue to have symptoms as adults, particularly antisocial personality disorder.

4. Tourette's syndrome is characterized by tics, barking of obscenities, and often echolalia (repetition of words or sentences said by others). Haloperidol is generally regarded as the medication of choice. However, in view of potential long-term extrapyramidal adverse effects of haloperidol, therapy may be initiated with clonazepam, clonidine, or the dopamine blocker pimozide.

Essentials is designed to promote critical thinking and enrich your knowledge base. Therefore, many questions will have more than one correct answer.

DERM, PUL

E 029   Which of the following is a common food allergen in a 3-year-old child?

A. Wheat
B. Eggs
C. Milk
D. Oats
E. Beef

Answer: A, B, and C
A, B, and C are correct because eggs, milk, peanuts, soy, and wheat are common food allergens in young children.

▩ **You should know:**

1. In older children and adolescents, fish, shellfish, and nuts are common allergens.

2. Oats and beef are not allergens.

3. Children whose allergic response includes respiratory distress or anaphylaxis should carry injectable epinephrine.

4. The differential diagnosis of food allergy includes cystic fibrosis, celiac disease, lactase deficiency, congenital intestinal malformations, and chronic bowel infection.

GI/N

E 030   Which of the following is the pathophysiologic abnormality in infants who have Hirschsprung's disease?

A. Deficiency of bile salts in the ileum
B. Absence of ganglion cells in the colon
C. Presence of an abnormal transmitter at neuromuscular junctions
D. Presence of autoimmune receptor blockers in colonic mucosa
E. Hypersecretion of Brunner's glands in the duodenum

Answer: B
B is correct because Hirschsprung's disease, due to absence of ganglion cells in the colonic mucosa, results in the affected segment being unable to relax. Therefore, functional bowel obstruction results.

▩ **You should know:**

1. Hirschsprung's disease is characterized by failure of the newborn to pass meconium, followed by abdominal distention and vomiting.

2. Suction biopsy and rectal manometry are preferable to contrast radiography (barium enema) in making the diagnosis.

3. The definitive treatment is surgical.

4. Meconium ileus is the presenting clinical problem in approximately 15% of newborns who have cystic fibrosis (CF). Newborn screening for CF is via assay for immunoreactive trypsin (IRT). An elevated blood IRT level is positive for CF and is followed by sweat chloride testing. Sweat chloride concentration can be difficult to interpret in the initial 6 months of life.

ENDO

E 031   Which of the following medicines may cause hyperglycemia?

    A. Prednisone
    B. Niacin
    C. Naproxen
    D. Pravastatin
    E. Diltiazem

Answer: A and B
A is correct because prednisone causes hyperglycemia by increasing gluconeogenesis and by inhibiting glycogen storage. B is correct because niacin induces insulin resistance causing the patient to become hyperglycemic.

■ **You should know:**

1. Niacin causes hyperglycemia, increases serum uric acid (even precipitating acute gout), may cause hypotension when used in conjunction with vasodilators, and may exacerbate ischemic symptoms in the patient with unstable angina pectoris.

2. Additional side effects of prednisone include osteoporosis, peptic ulcer, cataracts, and skin thinning with purpura.

3. Hypercortisolism of any etiology, including prednisone therapy, Cushing's disease, and cortisol-producing adrenal adenoma or carcinoma, can be associated with these adverse effects.

4. In an effort to prevent glucocorticoid-induced osteoporosis, the following recommendations are appropriate:
   - All patients who are to be on glucocorticoid therapy longer than 3 months should take supplemental calcium and vitamin D.
   - All men and postmenopausal women in whom glucocorticoid therapy is initiated should take a bisphosphonate in an effort to prevent osteoporosis. The clinician will exercise judgment based upon the expected duration of glucocorticoid therapy.

DERM, ENDO, GI/N

E 032   Which of the following conditions is associated with acanthosis nigricans?

    A. Obesity
    B. Diabetes mellitus
    C. Gastrointestinal cancer
    D. Cushing's syndrome
    E. Systemic lupus erythematosus

Answer: A, B, C, and D
A, B, and D are correct because the common denominator in all nonmalignancy-associated cases of acanthosis nigricans is insulin resistance. Therefore, there is an association of this skin disorder with diabetes mellitus, obesity, and Cushing's syndrome. C is correct because gastric and hepatocellular cancer and, less frequently, lung cancer are particularly associated with acanthosis nigricans.

Essentials is designed to promote critical thinking and enrich your knowledge base.
Therefore, many questions will have more than one correct answer.

■ **You should know:**

1. Acanthosis nigricans (AN) lesions are gray-brown to black, are rough, and have prominent skin lines. They most commonly occur in the axillae, back and sides of neck, and inguinal creases.

2. The classic rash associated with systemic lupus erythematosus (SLE) is the "butterfly" rash in the malar area of the face. The facial rash may be erythema lasting a few days or inflammatory discoid scarring that is permanent.

3. The classic clinical presentation of SLE is pain caused by antinuclear antibody–induced inflammation of serosal membranes. Patients have pain caused by arthritis, pleuritis, or pericarditis. Anemia and leukopenia result from antibody damage to blood elements.

GU, GI/N, ENDO

E 033   Which of the following is a cause of hypokalemia?

A. Diarrhea
B. Primary hyperaldosteronism
C. Furosemide therapy
D. Aspirin poisoning
E. Acute renal failure

Answer: A, B, and C
A is correct because diarrheal stools contain considerable potassium and bicarbonate. Therefore, hypokalemia and metabolic acidosis may result, particularly with chronic diarrhea. B is correct because primary hyperaldosteronism causes renal sodium retention in the kidney and increased potassium loss in the urine. C is correct because loop diuretics and thiazide diuretics increase potassium loss in the urine. Without potassium supplementation, hypokalemia may result.

■ **You should know:**

1. In a patient who takes digoxin, hypokalemia of any etiology predisposes to digoxin toxicity. Digoxin toxicity can be manifest as:
   • Ectopy, including ventricular premature beats, ventricular tachycardia, and atrial premature beats
   • Atrioventricular block, including 1st degree, 2nd degree (Mobitz I, also called Wenckebach), and 3rd degree

2. Acute and chronic renal failure cause hyperkalemia due to the kidney's inability to excrete this electrolyte.

3. Medicines that increase serum potassium concentration include potassium-sparing diuretics, angiotensin-converting enzyme inhibitors (ACEIs), angiotensin-receptor blockers (ARBs), NSAIDs, and pentamidine. The hyperkalemia is caused by reduced urinary excretion of potassium.

GU, PUL

E 034   Which of the following is a therapeutic intervention in the treatment of hyperkalemia?

     A. Administration of intravenous calcium
     B. Administration of intravenous sodium bicarbonate
     C. Hemodialysis
     D. Administration of intravenous hypertonic saline
     E. Administration of inhaled albuterol

Answer: A, B, C, and E
A is correct because calcium antagonizes the electrophysiologic effects of potassium. B is correct because bicarbonate causes potassium to leave the serum and enter cells. C is correct because dialysis can rapidly remove potassium from the circulation. E is correct because beta$_2$-adrenergic agonists drive potassium from the serum into cells.

You should know:

1. Intravenous calcium is indicated in those patients with severe hyperkalemia who have marked electrocardiographic abnormalities, including loss of P waves and widening of the QRS complex. Calcium should not be given when digoxin toxicity is suspected because calcium can worsen the effect of the digoxin.

2. Medications given to emergently lower the serum potassium include inhaled albuterol, intravenous glucose with added insulin, and intravenous sodium bicarbonate.

3. Inhaled albuterol promotes potassium entry into cells and begins to lower serum potassium in 15 to 30 minutes. This effect lasts approximately 2 hours.

4. The combination of intravenous glucose and insulin drives potassium into the cells. The effect begins in approximately 30 to 60 minutes and lasts 4 to 6 hours.

5. Sodium bicarbonate begins to lower serum potassium in 15 to 30 minutes, and its effect lasts 1 to 2 hours.

6. Sodium polystyrene sulfonate, a cation exchange resin, may be given orally or as an enema in less emergent cases. Potassium levels begin to decrease in 1 to 2 hours.

7. Hemodialysis may be employed when conservative measures are ineffective or in cases of marked tissue breakdown.

ID, NEURO, HEME, CV

E 035   Which of the following is a complication of infectious mononucleosis?

     A. Aseptic meningitis
     B. Bell's palsy
     C. Hemolytic anemia
     D. Pericarditis
     E. Nephrotic syndrome

Essentials is designed to promote critical thinking and enrich your knowledge base.
Therefore, many questions will have more than one correct answer.

Answer: A, B, C, and D

A and B are correct because neurologic complications of mononucleosis include aseptic meningitis, Bell's palsy, and Guillain-Barré syndrome. C is correct because hemolytic anemia, thrombocytopenia, and neutropenia are recognized hematologic complications. D is correct because acute pericarditis is an uncommon cardiac complication.

▓ **You should know:**

1. Diagnosis of infectious mononucleosis (IM) is most commonly based upon presence of heterophile antibodies including the Monospot test.

2. The presence of atypical lymphocytes on peripheral blood smear is a very common hematologic finding but may not be seen until the third week of illness.

3. IM, most commonly related to Ebstein-Barr virus infection, is manifest as fever, sore throat, malaise, and lymphadenopathy. The presence of posterior cervical adenopathy should suggest the diagnosis. The clinician must recognize that nearly one third of IM patients have coexisting streptococcal pharyngitis.

4. Adults older than 35 years of age who have IM have an atypical presentation with pharyngitis and myalgia as prominent symptoms. Lymphadenopathy is less frequently noted in the adult patient who has IM.

5. Other known causes of Bell's palsy include Lyme disease and sarcoidosis. Half of the cases are of unknown etiology but are thought to be related to viral infection, notably herpes simplex or zoster.

EENT

E 036   Which of the following is a complication of contact lens wear?

A. *Acanthamoeba* keratitis
B. Chalazion
C. Blepharitis
D. Corneal abrasion
E. Keratoconjunctivitis sicca

Answer: A and D

A is correct because amebas may infect the eye, especially in patients who wear contact lens and who are not careful in cleaning and storage of the lens. D is correct because corneal abrasion or ulceration is the major complication of contact lens wear. Soft lens appear to be the primary hazard, especially with extended wear.

▓ **You Should Know**

1. Amebas are found in soil and in chlorinated swimming pools.

2. Fluorescein dye application in the eye is used in diagnosis of corneal abrasion.

3. Corneal abrasions that damage the corneal epithelium increase the risk of infection of the cornea, called keratitis. Keratitis is characterized by waxing and waning ocular pain, blurred vision, and conjunctival erythema.

4. Abrasions are treated with discontinuation of lens wear; prophylactic antibiotics, including ofloxacin, ciprofloxacin, or tobramycin; cold compresses; and oral NSAIDs. Patching of the eye should be *avoided*.

E 037   Which of the following is a maneuver that tests function of cranial nerve VII?

A. Move eyes in vertical gaze
B. Frown
C. Curl tongue
D. Raise shoulders against resistance
E. Rapid repetition of a three-word phrase

Answer: B

B is correct because cranial nerve VII (facial nerve) is a motor nerve to the face, thus being responsible for facial expressions.

■ **You should know:**

1. Cranial nerve VII activation causes the patient to close the eyes, frown, wrinkle the forehead, and smile. Important: The forehead receives bilateral innervation; thus, in peripheral nerve palsy (Bell's palsy), the patient is unable to wrinkle the forehead on the affected side. In central VII nerve palsy, there is drooping of the face and inability to tightly close the eyes, but the patient can wrinkle the forehead.

2. Cranial nerve VII also contains the following nerves:
   • parasympathetic nerves to the salivary glands
   • afferent fibers that relate to taste on the anterior two thirds of the tongue
   • somatic sensory fibers to the external ear

3. Cranial nerve V (trigeminal) has both motor and sensory function in the face. Motor function can be tested by closing the jaw against resistance or by moving the chin from side to side.

4. Cranial nerves III, IV, and VI innervate eye muscles and are responsible for extraocular muscle movements.

5. Pupil size is related to smooth muscle function. Myasthenia gravis is an autoimmune disease that affects only skeletal muscle. Extraocular muscles are skeletal muscles. Therefore, in myasthenia gravis, abnormal extraocular muscle movements and ptosis are *intermittently* noted, but pupil size is *always* normal.

6. Cranial nerve III (oculomotor nerve) palsy causes both extraocular muscle abnormalities and a dilated pupil because this nerve carries parasympathetic nerve fibers. An important clinical point: Diabetes mellitus is a common cause of cranial nerve III palsy. However, in the majority of cases, the pupil size is *normal* in the diabetic.

7. Lyme disease is a common cause of facial nerve paralysis, at times causing bilateral Bell's palsy. The preferred initial diagnostic study is an ELISA test. Lyme disease is typically associated with headache, arthralgia or arthritis, and erythema migrans, a flat or slightly raised red lesion with central clearing and a necrotic center.

Essentials is designed to promote critical thinking and enrich your knowledge base.
Therefore, many questions will have more than one correct answer.

E 038   Which of the following serum laboratory values is typically elevated in the tumor lysis syndrome?

    A. Potassium
    B. Sodium
    C. Uric acid
    D. Norepinephrine
    E. 5-Hydroxyindoleacetic acid

Answer: A and C
A is correct because rapid tumor cell death leads to release of potassium from cells. C is correct because nucleic acids released from dying tumor cells are converted to uric acid causing hyperuricemia.

■ **You should know:**

1. Tumor lysis syndrome (TLS) occurs in patients who have rapidly proliferating malignancies that are very sensitive to chemotherapy (e.g., acute leukemia and lymphoma).

2. Chemotherapy causes rapid tumor cell death. As a result, intracellular products spill into the blood causing hyperkalemia, hyperphosphatemia, and hyperuricemia. Tumor lysis syndrome (TLS) may result in acute renal failure requiring hemodialysis.

3. Efforts to prevent tumor lysis syndrome (TLS) include prophylactic administration of oral allopurinol and vigorous volume expansion.

4. Carcinoid tumors are found primarily in the gastrointestinal tract and bronchi. These tumors release humoral factors causing carcinoid syndrome, which is characterized by flushing, diarrhea, and wheezing. Tricuspid or pulmonary valve disease may develop. The diagnosis of carcinoid syndrome is based upon increased urinary excretion of 5-hydroxyindoleacetic acid (5-HIAA).

E 039   An increased serum level of which of the following is consistent with a diagnosis of sarcoidosis?

    A. Calcium
    B. Immunoglobulin A
    C. Antiphospholipid antibodies
    D. Angiotensin-converting enzyme
    E. Creatine kinase

Answer: A and D
A and D are correct because serum angiotensin-converting enzyme is elevated in approximately 50% of sarcoidosis cases, and elevation of serum calcium is noted in 3% to 5%.

■ **You should know:**

1. Sarcoidosis is a disease of unknown etiology that commonly targets the lungs, skin, heart, eyes, liver, and kidney. Lymphadenopathy and parotid gland enlargement are also frequently noted.

2. Pulmonary involvement typically starts with bilateral hilar enlargement (similar to Hodgkin's disease). Later in the disease course, the hilar adenopathy recedes, and pulmonary fibrosis (interstitial fibrosis) develops and can cause restrictive pulmonary abnormalities to be manifest.

3. Restrictive pulmonary abnormalities include increased stiffness of the lungs, hyperventilation, and reduced oxygen diffusion across the alveolar-capillary membrane but not with outflow air obstruction. As a result, the systemic arterial blood gas determination in the restrictive disease patient shows respiratory alkalosis, *hypoxemia* (low Pao_2), and *hypocapnia* (low $Paco_2$).

4. Pulmonary function tests in any patient who has restrictive lung disease show reduced total lung capacity and decreased carbon monoxide (CO) diffusing capacity, but forced expiratory volume 1 sec/forced vital capacity (FEV1 sec/FVC) ratio is normal or increased.

5. In contrast, in obstructive lung disease (e.g., asthma or chronic bronchitis), there is a decreased FEV1 sec/FVC ratio.

6. The normal FEV1 sec/FVC ratio is dependent upon the patient's age. In a patient who is 20 to 39 years of age, the normal ratio is 80%; the normal ratio drops to 70% in a patient who is 60 to 80 years.

EENT, NEURO

E 040   Which of the following disorders is a cause of diplopia?

    A. Cranial nerve III palsy
    B. Myasthenia gravis
    C. Bell's palsy
    D. Multiple sclerosis
    E. Trigeminal neuralgia

Answer: A, B, and D
A is correct because cranial nerve III palsy, which causes lateral deviation of the affected eye, results in diplopia. B is correct because myasthenia gravis causes intermittent weakness in the extraocular muscles (skeletal muscles) resulting in intermittent diplopia. D is correct because multiple sclerosis (MS) frequently is associated with diplopia caused by cranial nerve VI (abducens nerve) palsy.

▉ **You should know:**

1. Diplopia may be monocular or binocular.

2. Monocular diplopia (i.e., double vision with the fellow eye covered) is not due to serious systemic disease but rather is due to refractive error or cataract.

3. Binocular diplopia (i.e., double vision with both eyes uncovered) is due to malalignment of the two eyes.

4. Binocular diplopia, when secondary to inflammatory, neoplastic, metabolic, or vascular disease, typically is due to impaired function of the cranial nerves that innervate the extraocular muscles—namely, cranial nerves III, IV, and VI.

5. Cerebral aneurysms are an important cause of diplopia. Aneurysms may cause cranial nerve palsy, especially involving cranial nerve III. *Any patient who develops a cranial nerve palsy should be evaluated for cerebral aneurysm.*

6. Oculomotor (cranial nerve III) palsy is characterized by ptosis, lateral deviation of the eye, and dilated pupil.

7. An important exception: Diabetes mellitus is a common cause of cranial nerve III palsy, but *in 80% of cases the pupil size is normal.*

8. Wernicke's encephalopathy, associated with chronic alcohol abuse, is typically characterized by extraocular muscle dysfunction, nystagmus, and disorientation or inattentiveness.

9. Myasthenia gravis, an autoimmune disease in which antibodies to acetylcholine (ACH) receptors are present, causes diffuse, intermittent skeletal muscle weakness. Extraocular muscle weakness is intermittent; therefore, diplopia is intermittent. The pupil size is always normal in myasthenia because it is smooth muscle, not skeletal muscle, that influences pupil size.

10. Multiple sclerosis commonly causes optic neuritis, an inflammatory disease of the optic nerve causing eye pain with eye movement and diminished visual acuity. The eye movement disorder in multiple sclerosis (MS) is accompanied by nystagmus.

NEURO, CV, GU

E 041   Which of the following congenital disorders is associated with cerebral aneurysm?

A. Coarctation of the aorta
B. Polycystic kidney disease
C. Tetralogy of Fallot
D. Congenital adrenal hyperplasia
E. Ostium primum atrial septal defect

Answer: A and B
A and B are correct because 10% of coarctation patients and 5% to 20% (dependent upon patient's age) of polycystic kidney disease patients have congenital cerebral aneurysms.

You should know:

1. In most cases, coarctation patients have equal and bilateral hypertension in the arms, low blood pressure in the legs, and radial-femoral arterial pulse lag. A bicuspid aortic valve is found in approximately 70% of those with coarctation.

2. Cerebral aneurysms may rupture and cause subarachnoid hemorrhage, even years after surgical correction of the coarctation or treatment of the kidney disease.

3. Polycystic kidney disease, with autosomal dominant inheritance, is characterized by hematuria (microscopic or gross), hypertension, flank pain, progressive renal failure, and often nephrolithiasis.

CV

E 042 Which of the following is a complication of acute dissection of the thoracic aorta?

A. Pericardial tamponade
B. Left pleural effusion
C. Aortic valve regurgitation
D. Acute myocardial infarction
E. Papillary muscle rupture

Answer: A, B, C, and D
A is correct because the dissection may rupture into the pericardial sac causing tamponade. B is correct because the dissection may rupture into the left pleural space causing a left hemothorax. C and D are correct because the dissection may cause distortion of the proximal aorta causing occlusion of a coronary artery with resultant acute myocardial infarction or distortion of the aortic cusps causing acute aortic valve regurgitation.

■ **You should know:**

1. Acute thoracic aorta dissection causes tearing or ripping pain in the chest. The pain may be located in the anterior and/or posterior chest.

2. Pericardial tamponade is characterized by hypotension, tachycardia, elevated jugular venous pressure, and paradoxical pulse.

3. Transesophageal echocardiography (TEE), computed tomography (CT scan), and magnetic resonance imaging (MRI) are valuable in the diagnosis of dissection of the thoracic aorta.

4. Transesophageal echocardiography (TEE) is the preferred diagnostic modality in pericardial tamponade. Diastolic collapse of the right atrium or the right ventricle is found in tamponade.

5. In any patient who has chest pain and a new murmur of aortic valve regurgitation, aortic dissection must be the initial consideration.

6. The medical treatment of dissection includes an intravenous vasodilator (e.g., nitroprusside) to lower blood pressure in addition to a beta blocker, which decreases pulsatile flow.

7. Isolated use of a vasodilator such as diazoxide or hydralazine is contraindicated because these may increase shear stress on the aorta and propagate the dissection.

8. Selected patients with dissection require emergent surgical intervention.

GI/N, REPRO, CV

E 043 Which of the following must be considered in a 34-year-old woman who is to start tetracycline therapy?

A. Ingestion of milk
B. Concomitant intake of warfarin
C. Concomitant intake of oral contraceptives
D. Ingestion of aluminum-containing antacids
E. Concomitant intake of digoxin

Essentials is designed to promote critical thinking and enrich your knowledge base.
Therefore, many questions will have more than one correct answer.

Answer: A, B, C, and D
A and D are correct because aluminum-containing antacids and milk decrease the absorption of tetracycline (TCN). B is correct because tetracycline (TCN) increases the anticoagulant effect of warfarin. C is correct because tetracycline (TCN) decreases the effect of oral contraceptives.

▨ You should know:

1. Tetracycline (TCN) must be taken at least 2 hours apart from ingestion of milk and aluminum-containing antacids.

2. In the woman taking an oral contraceptive, an additional method of birth control (e.g., barrier method) should be used during tetracycline (TCN) therapy.

3. Tetracyclines (TCN) have broad-spectrum antimicrobial activity against many gram-positive and gram-negative bacteria. TCN have activity against *Chlamydia, Mycoplasma pneumoniae,* rickettsiae, and *Coxiella burnetii.*

4. Tetracyclines and fluoroquinolones are *not* recommended in the treatment of gonococcal urethritis because of the high incidence of resistance to these medications.

5. Ceftriaxone is the preferred antibiotic in treatment of gonococcal urethritis.

6. *All patients* who are treated for gonococcal urethritis should be treated for *Chlamydia* infection. Single-dose azithromycin or doxycycline taken for 7 days is effective therapy for infection caused by *Chlamydia.*

GI/N

E 044   Which of the following suggests an esophageal motility disorder as the etiology of dysphagia?
A. Presence of anemia
B. Dysphagia in conjunction with heartburn
C. Occurrence of hematemesis
D. Dysphagia to solids and liquids at onset of symptoms
E. Dysphagia to liquids prior to solids

Answer: D
D is correct because dysphagia to both solids and liquids at the onset of symptoms suggests a motility disorder, in contrast to dysphagia to solids that later involves liquids, which suggests mechanical esophageal obstruction.

▨ You should know:

1. Stricture of the esophagus is a common complication of gastroesophageal reflux disease (GERD).

2. Cancer of the esophagus typically causes dysphagia in the presence of weight loss and anorexia.

3. Barrett's esophagus, another complication of GERD, is characterized by a change in the microscopic appearance of the esophageal mucosa, specifically from squamous to columnar epithelium.

4. Barrett's esophagus markedly increases the risk of esophageal adenocarcinoma.

5. Dysphagia to solids and liquids is common in scleroderma. In addition to esophageal involvement, patients who have scleroderma commonly have the following medical complications:
   - Raynaud's phenomenon, in which emotional stress or exposure to cold (e.g., a frozen food package) will cause intense cutaneous vasoconstriction, usually in the fingers and hands, manifest by pallor or cyanosis. The vasoconstriction is followed by a recovery period of hyperemia manifest by rubor of the affected area.
   - Pulmonary disease manifest by interstitial pulmonary fibrosis or pulmonary vascular disease, both of which can cause pulmonary hypertension and right heart failure (cor pulmonale).
   - Heart disease manifest as acute pericarditis or myocardial fibrosis. The myocardial fibrosis may lead to development of diastolic heart failure or, less commonly, systolic failure.
   - Kidney disease manifest by proteinuria, renal insufficiency, and hypertension.

6. Scleroderma patients produce a number of autoantibodies, most commonly antinuclear antibodies (90%). There is no autoantibody that is specific for scleroderma.

CV

E 045   In a patient who has an acute myocardial infarction complicated by pulmonary edema, which of the following medications is contraindicated?
   A. Streptokinase
   B. Nitroglycerin
   C. Aspirin
   D. Metoprolol
   E. Heparin

Answer: D
D is correct because beta-adrenergic blockers are contraindicated in acute heart failure because they have a negative inotropic effect.

▧ **You should know:**

1. Beta-adrenergic blockers are *indicated* in treatment of chronic systolic heart failure (SHF).

2. When given to the patient with chronic SHF, beta blockers are part of polypharmacy therapy, including angiotensin-converting enzyme inhibitors (or receptor blockers) and loop diuretics. Nitrates and digoxin may be added in selected patients.

3. Systolic heart failure is characterized by left ventricular dilation (increased preload), reduced power of ventricular contraction, reduced ejection fraction, and reduced cardiac output. The primary symptoms of SHF are fatigue, weakness, and mental obtundation.

Essentials is designed to promote critical thinking and enrich your knowledge base.
Therefore, many questions will have more than one correct answer.

CV

E 046   In a patient who has an acute myocardial infarction complicated by hypertension and pulmonary edema, which of the following medications is the preferred therapy?
  A. Intravenous nitroglycerin
  B. Intravenous diazoxide
  C. Intravenous labetalol
  D. Sublingual captopril
  E. Oral ingestion of liquid nifedipine

Answer: A
A is correct because intravenous nitroglycerin lowers blood pressure (decreasing after-load) and causes venodilation (reducing preload), both of which are indicated in the patient whose myocardial infarction is complicated by heart failure and hypertension.

■ **You should know:**

  1. Beta-adrenergic blockers are *contraindicated* in the acute heart failure patient.

  2. Nifedipine, verapamil, and diltiazem reduce ventricular contractility and therefore should not be given to the patient who is in systolic heart failure.

  3. There is no calcium channel blocker that reduces mortality in acute myocardial infarction (AMI). In fact, mortality is increased when nifedipine, verapamil, or diltiazem is given to the patient with an AMI that is complicated by systolic dysfunction or atrioventricular block.

CV, GU

E 047   Which of the following increases the risk of toxicity in a patient taking digoxin?
  A. Hypomagnesemia
  B. Hypokalemia
  C. Iron deficiency anemia
  D. Hypo-osmolar serum
  E. Hypernatremia

Answer: A and B
A and B are correct because hypomagnesemia and hypokalemia increase myocardial sensitivity to digoxin, thus making digoxin toxicity more likely.

■ **You should know:**

  1. Digoxin toxicity is manifest as:
     • Ectopy, both ventricular (ventricular premature beats, ventricular tachycardia) and supraventricular (atrial premature beats, atrial tachycardia)
     • Atrioventricular block (1st, 2nd, and 3rd degree)

  2. In the patient who takes digoxin, hypokalemia of any etiology predisposes to toxicity. The two most common causes of hypokalemia are:
     • Thiazide and loop diuretic therapy causing loss of potassium in the urine
     • Diarrhea causing loss of potassium and bicarbonate in stool

  3. Hypomagnesemia, even in the absence of hypokalemia, predisposes to digoxin toxicity. The two most common causes of this electrolyte abnormality are:
     • Thiazide and loop diuretic therapy causing loss of magnesium in the urine
     • Chronic alcohol abuse, which causes a reversible renal tubular defect that results in increased urinary excretion of the ion

4. Hypomagnesemia causes prolongation of the QT interval on the electrocardiogram. Other causes of acquired long QT syndrome are hypocalcemia and medicines (e.g., phenothiazines, haloperidol, risperidone, tricyclic antidepressants, and the antihistamines terfenadine and astemizole). A long QT interval increases the risk of the patient developing polymorphic ventricular tachycardia (torsades de pointes).

5. Long QT syndrome may also be congenital. Torsade ventricular tachycardia commonly occurs in these children during times of sympathetic nervous system activity (e.g., during exercise or emotional stress).

CV, NEURO

E 048   Which of the following is an indication for verapamil therapy?

A. Variant angina pectoris
B. Migraine headaches
C. Ventricular ectopic beats
D. Hypertension
E. Hypertrophic obstructive cardiomyopathy

Answer: A, B, D, and E
A and D are correct because verapamil is a smooth muscle dilator. Thus, verapamil reverses coronary artery spasm, which is the mechanism producing variant angina pectoris. Dilatation of the smooth muscle in arterioles makes verapamil effective in treatment of hypertension. B is correct because verapamil reduces frequency of migraine attacks, although its mechanism of action is unknown. E is correct because verapamil slows heart rate and has a negative inotropic effect, thus making it beneficial in the patient with hypertrophic obstructive cardiomyopathy.

▨ **You should know:**

1. Verapamil is effective in therapy of variant angina pectoris that is due to coronary artery vasospasm. This medicine both relieves the acute vascular constriction and also can be used as a preventive medication.

2. Verapamil is effective in the patient who has chronic stable angina pectoris even when spasm is not an influencing factor. Verapamil is particularly suited for the anginal patient who concomitantly has migraine headaches or esophageal spasm.

3. In the anginal patient who also has obstructive lung disease or claudication, verapamil is preferred in comparison to beta-adrenergic blockers. Beta blockers increase outflow air obstruction and worsen arterial claudication symptoms.

4. Verapamil is effective in terminating paroxysmal supraventricular tachycardia (PSVT), particularly when adenosine is contraindicated or ineffective. In addition, this medication may be prescribed to prevent recurrent episodes of PSVT. An important clinical point: Adenosine may worsen bronchospasm in the patient who has obstructive lung disease.

5. Verapamil slows atrioventricular conduction and therefore is effective in slowing the ventricular rate in the atrial fibrillation (AF) patient. Caution: Verapamil reduces ventricular contractility. Consequently, in the patient with atrial fibrillation who is in systolic heart failure, verapamil may worsen

the heart failure. In this patient, digoxin alone or in combination with a beta-adrenergic blocker is the preferred therapy to slow the ventricular rate.

GU, HEME

E 049   Which of the following conditions is associated with hematuria?

A. Acute glomerulonephritis
B. Renal cell carcinoma
C. Cystitis
D. Henoch-Schönlein purpura
E. Polycystic kidney disease

Answer: A, B, C, D, and E
A and D are correct because dysmorphic (abnormal-shaped) erythrocytes, red blood cell casts in the urine, and proteinuria suggest glomerular disease (acute glomerulonephritis and Henoch-Schönlein purpura). B and E are correct because these disorders are associated with red blood cells leaking into the urine. C is correct because the inflamed urinary bladder wall in the cystitis patient will cause hematuria.

▉ **You should know:**

1. Henoch-Schönlein purpura is the most common vasculitis in children, but it does affect adults as well. This disease commonly follows an upper respiratory infection. In addition to the renal manifestation, rash (palpable purpura), arthritis, and abdominal pain are frequent features of this illness.

2. Henoch-Schönlein purpura may produce an acute glomerulonephritis that is identical to IgA nephropathy. IgA is deposited in the glomerular mesangium, the phagocytic cells between capillaries in the glomerulus. The clinical expression of the nephritis is variable, including asymptomatic hematuria, nephrotic syndrome, or nephritic syndrome.

3. Cystitis, renal cell carcinoma, and polycystic kidney disease (PCKD) are common causes of hematuria. These diseases may cause microscopic or gross hematuria.

4. Red blood cell casts are diagnostic of glomerular disease. They will not be seen in the urine of patients with cystitis, renal cell carcinoma, or polycystic kidney disease.

5. The autosomal-dominant inherited PCKD is typically associated with hypertension, progressive renal failure, flank pain, and often nephrolithiasis. Patients with PCKD, similar to patients with coarctation of the aorta, have an increased incidence of congenital cerebral aneurysm. Rupture of these aneurysms causes acute subarachnoid hemorrhage.

6. Cerebral aneurysm formation, *not associated with congenital disease,* is increased in patients who smoke or have hypertension or hypercholesterolemia.

HEME, GI/N, ENDO

E 050   Which of the following is a cause of macrocytosis?

A. Alcohol ingestion
B. Liver disease
C. Hypothyroidism
D. Chronic adrenal insufficiency
E. Bronchiectasis

Answer: A, B, and C

A is correct because alcohol ingestion may cause macrocytosis unrelated to folic acid metabolism. B is correct because liver disease is a common cause of macrocytosis. C is correct because hypothyroidism alone occasionally causes macrocytosis. In each of these cases, the mechanism producing macrocytosis is unknown.

■ **You should know:**

1. Megaloblastic anemia is associated with macrocytosis, but not all macrocytosis is related to a megaloblastic bone marrow.

2. Alcohol ingestion causes macrocytosis even before anemia occurs and even when body stores of folate and vitamin B_{12} are adequate.

3. Hypothyroidism is associated with an increased risk of the patient developing pernicious anemia. A patient who has Hashimoto's hypothyroidism is at increased risk of developing pernicious anemia.

4. Vitamin B_{12} deficiency anemia causes development of a megaloblastic bone marrow, macrocytosis, and hypersegmented neutrophils (more than six segments). Remember that vitamin B_{12} deficiency may result from an autoimmune disease (pernicious anemia) or may be unrelated to antibody formation. Nonautoimmune vitamin B_{12} deficiency may be related to dietary intake of the vitamin, gastrectomy, bacterial overgrowth in the intestinal tract, or inflammatory bowel disease.

5. Patients who have one autoimmune disease are likely to develop another autoimmune disease. Children and adolescents with type 1 diabetes mellitus are at increased risk for developing autoimmune thyroiditis or celiac disease. Up to 20% of these diabetic patients have positive anti–thyroid peroxidase or antithyroglobulin antibodies. All children with type 1 diabetes should be screened regularly for the presence of thyroid antibodies. Similarly, 5% of type 1 diabetics develop celiac disease. The clinician must recognize that gastrointestinal symptoms are *minimal or not present* in these patients. Rather, the diabetic child who has celiac disease will manifest *poor glycemic control or growth failure* as the manifestation of celiac disease.

6. Pernicious anemia develops in 10% of patients who have Hashimoto's autoimmune hypothyroidism. Patients who have Graves disease have an increased risk of developing myasthenia gravis.

HEME, GI/N

E 051   Which of the following is a cause of vitamin B_{12} deficiency?

   A. Pernicious anemia
   B. Strict vegan diet
   C. Crohn's disease
   D. Hypertriglyceridemia
   E. Sulfonylurea medication

Answer: A, B, and C

A is correct because there is impaired intestinal absorption of vitamin B_{12} in the patient with pernicious anemia. B is correct because vitamin B_{12} is found in food of animal origin. Therefore, patients who follow a strict vegan diet will develop vitamin B_{12} deficiency. C is correct because inflammation in the terminal ileum in patients with

Essentials is designed to promote critical thinking and enrich your knowledge base. Therefore, many questions will have more than one correct answer.

Crohn's disease will cause vitamin B_{12} malabsorption that may lead to megaloblastic anemia. Vitamin B_{12} therapy must be considered in all patients who have Crohn's disease with involvement of the terminal ileum.

▦ **You should know:**

1. Intrinsic factor is essential for vitamin B_{12} to be absorbed in the distal ileum.

2. Pernicious anemia (PA) is associated with the presence of anti–intrinsic factor antibodies and anti–parietal cell antibodies. The anti–intrinsic factor antibodies prevent absorption of vitamin B_{12}. PA patients have achlorhydria.

3. Persons who follow a strict vegan diet without intake of dairy products, meat, and fish will develop vitamin B_{12} deficiency.

4. Gastrectomy will lead to deficiency of vitamin B_{12} because the stomach is the source of intrinsic factor production.

5. Vitamin B_{12} deficiency megaloblastic anemia may cause the patient to complain of paresthesias, ataxia, and sore tongue. Typical neurologic abnormalities include loss of proprioception and position sense.

6. Patients with vitamin B_{12} deficiency anemia have increased serum levels of methylmalonic acid. The serum level of methylmalonic acid should be determined when pernicious anemia is suspected and the serum vitamin B_{12} level is borderline low.

7. Folic acid deficiency anemia does not cause neurologic impairment.

8. In a patient with vitamin B_{12} deficiency anemia, dietary folate will reverse the anemia but will not reverse the neurologic impairment.

9. Peripheral blood examination in the patient who has vitamin B_{12} deficiency or folic acid deficiency will show macrocytosis and hypersegmented neutrophils.

NEURO, ENDO

E 052   Which of the following diseases is associated with the presence of antibodies in the serum?

A. Myasthenia gravis
B. Graves disease
C. Hashimoto's disease
D. Systemic lupus erythematosus
E. Sarcoidosis

Answer: A, B, C, and D
A is correct because acetylcholine receptor antibodies are found in patients with myasthenia gravis, a disease that affects skeletal muscle. B is correct because Graves disease patients typically have thyroid-stimulating hormone (TSH) receptor antibodies in the serum. C is correct because nearly all patients with Hashimoto's disease have antibodies to thyroglobulin and thyroid peroxidase. D is correct because systemic lupus erythematosus (SLE) patients typically have serum antinuclear antibodies. Antibodies to double-stranded (ds) DNA and anti-Smith (anti-Sm) antibodies are specific for SLE but are not sensitive.

▦ **You should know:**

1. Myasthenia gravis is a disease of skeletal muscle; it does not affect smooth muscle.

2. Graves disease patients, in contrast to patients with hyperthyroidism of other etiology, may have exophthalmos, pretibial myxedema, and periorbital and conjunctival edema.

3. Systemic lupus erythematosus (SLE) is much more common in women. Frequent symptoms include arthralgia or arthritis and chest pain due to pleuritis or pericarditis. Pericarditis may be the initial manifestation of the disease. SLE must be considered in any female who has acute pericarditis.

4. Patients with SLE often have a malar rash or a rash in sun-exposed areas. Patients should try to avoid high sun exposure, and they should use sunscreen.

5. Neurologic complications of SLE include seizures, psychosis, and delirium.

6. Seventy-five percent of patients with untreated sarcoidosis have elevated serum levels of angiotensin-converting enzyme. The earliest radiographic chest abnormality in sarcoidosis is bilateral hilar adenopathy. Over time, the hilar adenopathy recedes, and reticular and nodular infiltrates appear resulting in the functional abnormalities of restrictive lung disease.

EENT

E 053   Eosinophils are found in the nasal secretions in which of the following disorders?
A. Allergic rhinitis
B. Nasal polyposis
C. Viral rhinitis
D. Rhinitis medicamentosa
E. Bacterial sinusitis

Answer: A and B
A and B are correct because eosinophils are typically found in atopic tissues (tissues affected by an allergic process).

■ **You should know:**

1. The nasal mucosa in allergic rhinitis may be pale or may be violaceous.

2. Nasal polyposis is a potential complication of chronic allergic rhinitis.

3. The asthmatic patient who has nasal polyps should not take aspirin or traditional nonsteroidal anti-inflammatory medicines. A cyclooxygenase inhibitor medicine (COX-2 inhibitor) might be safely taken but only after successful challenge by an allergist.

4. Intranasal corticosteroid sprays are the most effective agents in the treatment of allergic rhinitis.

5. Rhinitis medicamentosa (RM) is a condition in which the nasal mucosa is inflamed from overzealous use of sympathomimetic decongestants. Patients should be counseled not to use decongestants more than 3 or 4 days consecutively in order to prevent RM. The treatment of RM is zealous avoidance of decongestants, an intranasal corticosteroid or anticholinergic agent, or a short, tapering course of oral glucocorticoid.

CV

E 054   Which of the following medications may cause orthostatic hypotension?

A. Hydralazine
B. Isosorbide dinitrate
C. Niacin
D. Risperidone
E. Diltiazem

Answer: A, B, C, and E
A, B, C, and E are correct because hydralazine, nitrates (including isosorbide dinitrate), niacin, and calcium channel blockers are all smooth muscle dilators and can cause orthostatic hypotension.

You should know:

1. Niacin is most likely to cause hypotension when taken with other vasodilators.

2. The normal response of the body to assumption of the upright position is characterized by the following sequence: (a) decreased venous return to the right atrium; (b) decreased arterial blood pressure; (c) stimulation of the baroreceptor reflex; and (d) increase in sympathetic nervous system tone resulting in an increase in heart rate and systemic vascular resistance. Thus, with assumption of the upright position, the normal response is a small decrease in systolic pressure (5 to 10 mm Hg), an increase in diastolic pressure (5 to 10 mm Hg), and an increase in heart rate (10 to 20 beats/min). The change in heart rate as the blood pressure falls is an important clinical sign (see following item 5).

3. Orthostatic hypotension is characterized by a drop in both systolic and diastolic blood pressure, typically considered to be a 20-mm Hg drop in systolic pressure and a 10-mm Hg drop in diastolic pressure in association with symptoms of decreased cerebral blood flow—namely, lightheadedness, visual blurring or darkening of the visual fields, or syncope.

4. The most common causes of orthostatic hypotension are medicines, hypovolemia, and autonomic insufficiency (sympathetic nervous system dysfunction). Medicines that commonly provoke orthostatic hypotension include hydralazine, angiotensin-converting enzyme inhibitors, nitrates, calcium channel blockers, tricyclic antidepressants, phenothiazines, and diuretics.

5. A patient who has orthostatic hypotension due to hypovolemia (e.g., blood loss or hypovolemia due to excessive diuresis or adrenal insufficiency) will have a compensatory increase in heart rate when the blood pressure decreases in the standing position. In contrast, the patient who has orthostatic hypotension due to autonomic insufficiency (as commonly occurs in patients with diabetes mellitus) will have a significant decrease in blood pressure when assuming the standing position *without a compensatory increase in heart rate*. Again, the heart rate response to the decrease in blood pressure helps differentiate between hypovolemia and autonomic insufficiency as the underlying cause.

E 055 In which of the following diseases are petechiae typically found on physical examination?

A. Aplastic anemia
B. Meningococcemia
C. Endocarditis
D. Rocky Mountain spotted fever
E. Polycythemia rubra vera

Answer: A, B, C, and D
A, B, and D are correct because each of these conditions is characterized by thrombocytopenia. The low platelet count results in a petechial rash. C is correct because endocarditis is associated with circulating immune complexes that damage capillaries resulting in petechiae formation.

■ **You should know:**

1. Petechiae may appear in several unrelated disorders, including thrombocytopenia of any etiology, vasculitis (Henoch-Schönlein purpura, rheumatoid arthritis), infectious emboli (meningococcemia), immune complex deposition on capillary walls (endocarditis), and cholesterol emboli to the toes ("blue toe syndrome").

2. Petechiae are very tiny (pinhead) accumulations of blood that have leaked out of capillaries. They are nontender and do not blanch upon pressure.

3. Petechiae are noted on the physical examination of patients with thrombocytopenia and with certain infectious diseases in which the platelet count is normal.

4. In any disease manifest by a reduced platelet count petechiae may be found. The thrombocytopenia may be due to bone marrow disease with decreased platelet production. Alternatively, the low platelet count may be due to immunologic peripheral destruction of platelets.

5. Immunologic destruction is found in patients with idiopathic thrombocytopenic purpura and some patients with systemic lupus erythematosus.

6. In addition, thrombocytopenia may result from antibody formation against platelets in patients who take the following medicines:
   • Heparin (thrombocytopenia peaks at 5 to 10 days of therapy)
   • Sulfonamides
   • Quinine
   • Thiazides
   • Cimetidine
   • Gold

7. Glycoprotein IIb/IIIa inhibitors can cause severe immune-mediated thrombocytopenia *minutes to hours* after initial administration. Treatment is immediate cessation of the medication and platelet transfusion.

8. Rocky Mountain spotted fever is a rickettsial disease. Patients have the sudden onset of fever, chills, myalgia, and headache. Typically, 2 days later,

a diffuse macular and petechial rash is noted, including on the soles and palms. The platelet count is reduced in this disease.

9. In meningococcemia, the number and extent of petechiae are proportional to the decrease in platelet count.

10. In endocarditis, petechiae may be noted while the platelet count is in the normal range.

11. Remember that endocarditis may be *acute,* as in the intravenous drug abuser who uses cocaine or heroin and develops tricuspid valve endocarditis from *Staphylococcus aureus* infection or the patient whose endocarditis is secondary to an indwelling intravascular catheter. These patients have high fever, are acutely ill, and may have associated pneumonia or heart failure.

12. Alternatively, endocarditis may be *subacute,* often related to viridans streptococcal infection, in which the patient has a more indolent course manifest by fatigue, arthralgia, and low-grade fever followed perhaps by symptoms related to valvular dysfunction.

13. All patients suspected of having endocarditis should have blood cultures drawn and an echocardiographic study, preferably transesophageal echocardiography (TEE).

EENT, PUL

E 056   Which of the following disorders may be complicated by the development of nasal polyps?
A. Chronic allergic rhinitis
B. Cystic fibrosis
C. Bronchiectasis
D. Rhinitis medicamentosa
E. Vasomotor rhinitis

Answer: A and B
A is correct because nasal polyps are often a complication of chronic allergic rhinitis. B is correct because the majority of cystic fibrosis (CF) patients develop sinus disease, and nasal polyps may be found in nearly one third of patients.

■ You should know:

1. Vasomotor rhinitis is manifest by rhinorrhea, sneezing, nasal congestion, and postnasal drip. It has no specific allergic, infectious, metabolic, or pharmacologic etiology. Symptoms are present all year long. Intranasal ipratropium appears to be the medication of choice in those patients who require therapy.

2. Allergic rhinitis may be seasonal or perennial.

3. Cystic fibrosis (CF) is an autosomal recessive disease with viscous secretions in ducts of the respiratory, gastrointestinal, and reproductive tracts. Respiratory involvement includes persistent cough progressing to chronic bronchitis, lung hyperinflation, bronchiectasis, and cor pulmonale. Pancreatic insufficiency and infertility are common. *Pseudomonas aeruginosa* infection is responsible for the death of the majority of CF patients.

4. In patients with nasal polyps and a history of asthma, intake of aspirin or other NSAIDs should be avoided because severe bronchospasm could result.

CV, ENDO

E 057   In a patient with newly diagnosed hypertension, which of the following suggests a secondary cause of the elevated blood pressure?

A. Radial-femoral arterial pulse lag
B. Rounded face and buffalo hump
C. Orthostatic hypotension
D. Nasal polyposis
E. Spooning of fingernails

Answer: A, B, and C

A is correct because coarctation of the aorta causes hypertension. A radial-femoral pulse lag is noted on physical examination. B is correct because hypertension is common in Cushing's syndrome. C is correct because pheochromocytoma may cause episodic or chronic hypertension. Those with chronic hypertension may have a low plasma volume that can cause orthostatic hypotension.

You should know:

1. Approximately 40% of patients who have coarctation of the aorta will have a bicuspid aortic valve. An apical ejection click is often the physical sign of the bicuspid valve. Coarctation patients also have an increased incidence (approximately 10%) of associated congenital cerebral aneurysms.

2. The pheochromocytoma patient who has *paroxysmal* hypertension (about half) classically has associated sweating and tachycardia.

3. In the patient who has *chronic hypertension with orthostatic hypotension* pheochromocytoma should be suspected.

4. A summary of the findings in all causes of hypercortisolism known as Cushing's syndrome (note: Cushing's *disease* is *one* cause of Cushing's *syndrome*):
   • Appearance: A rounded face; buffalo hump; truncal obesity; depressed abdominal purple striae; oily skin; hirsutism
   • Metabolic: Glucose intolerance, hyperglycemia; hypokalemia, notably with ectopic adrenocorticotropic hormone (ACTH) secretion; osteoporosis
   • Cardiovascular: Hypertension
   • Gynecologic: Oligomenorrhea or amenorrhea
   • Psychological: Depression; anxiety; irritability; panic disorder

5. Hypercortisolism may be due to the following conditions:
   • Exogenous intake of glucocorticoid medication
   • Functioning pituitary adenoma (Cushing's disease)
   • Adenoma, hyperplasia, or carcinoma of the adrenal gland
   • Ectopic adrenocorticotropic hormone (ACTH) secretion as in the patient who has small cell carcinoma of the lung

6. There are many similarities between hypercortisolism and polycystic ovary syndrome (PCOS). The following contrasts the two conditions:
   • *Both* are associated with menstrual irregularity—amenorrhea or oligomenorrhea.
   • *Both* are associated with androgen excess manifest by hirsutism.
   • *Both* are associated with emotional mood disorders.

Essentials is designed to promote critical thinking and enrich your knowledge base.
Therefore, many questions will have more than one correct answer.

- *Both* are associated with insulin resistance and hyperglycemia.
- *Both* are associated with obesity, with a truncal pattern in hypercortisolism.
- *Only hypercortisolism* is associated with hypertension and increased serum and urinary cortisol.

	Hypercortisolism	**PCOS**
Serum cortisol	Increased	Normal
Serum androgen	Increased	Increased
Luteinizing hormone hypersection	No	Yes, often
Ectopic ACTH production	Yes, small cell lung cancer	No

Of course, the underlying cause and pathology of the two conditions is different.

7. A patient born with a bicuspid aortic valve commonly will develop severe aortic valve stenosis or regurgitation in adulthood at approximately age 50 years.

PUL, CV

E 058   Which of the following disorders is associated with clubbing of the fingers and toes?

   A. Chronic obstructive pulmonary disease
   B. Metastatic cancer in the lung
   C. Cyanotic congenital heart disease
   D. Endocarditis
   E. Cystic fibrosis

Answer: **B, C, D, and E**
B is correct because both primary and metastatic lung cancer are associated with clubbing. C is correct because clubbing is noted in patients who have cyanotic congenital heart disease (e.g., tetralogy of Fallot). D is correct because clubbing may occur in left-sided endocarditis, though typically late in the course of the disease. E is correct because clubbing is common in patients with long-standing cystic fibrosis.

▌ **You should know:**

1. Clubbing is *not* a sign of chronic obstructive pulmonary disease (COPD). If a COPD patient has clubbing, *look for another cause,* particularly lung cancer.

2. Other causes of clubbing include lung mesothelioma, bronchiectasis, lung abscess, idiopathic pulmonary fibrosis, hepatic cirrhosis, and Crohn's disease.

3. Hypertrophic osteoarthropathy (HO) is found in patients when clubbing is due to lung cancer, mesothelioma, bronchiectasis, or cirrhosis. HO is a painful condition in which there is subperiosteal formation of new bone. This causes pain in the shoulders, knees, ankles, wrists, and elbows.

E 059   Which of the following is associated with an increased pulse pressure on physical examination?

A. Elderly age
B. Hyperthyroidism
C. Aortic valve regurgitation
D. Cushing's syndrome
E. Pulmonic stenosis

Answer: A, B, and C

A is correct because in the elderly the systolic blood pressure continues to increase. This is a result of reduced compliance (increased stiffness) of the large arteries. B is correct because hyperthyroidism is characterized by increased pulse pressure due to the increased stroke volume and reduced systemic vascular resistance found in this disease. C is correct because chronic aortic valve regurgitation has increased pulse pressure due to the increased stroke volume increasing systolic pressure and the diastolic regurgitant flow into the left ventricle decreasing the diastolic blood pressure.

You should know:

1. With increasing age, the systolic pressure increases, but diastolic blood pressure does not change or may decrease. Thus, in the elderly, isolated systolic hypertension (ISH) may result.

2. Isolated systolic hypertension (ISH) is not benign, for it is associated with an increased risk of heart failure, acute myocardial infarction, stroke, and cardiovascular mortality. It should be treated with medication.

3. The preferred initial treatment for isolated systolic hypertension (ISH) is a long-acting thiazide diuretic (e.g., chlorthalidone) or a long-acting dihydropyridine calcium channel blocker. However, an ACEI or ARB may be prescribed as initial therapy in selected patients.

4. In the older patient, the presentation of hyperthyroidism may be different from the younger patient. One third of elderly patients appear apathetic rather than demonstrating hyperactivity and tremor. Tachycardia may be absent. However, anorexia, weight loss, and atrial fibrillation are common in the elderly hyperthyroid patient. Hyperthyroidism should be considered in any patient who has atrial fibrillation, particularly one over the age of 60 years.

5. Chronic aortic valve regurgitation, with its increased left ventricular (LV) preload causing a dilated LV, may lead to development of systolic heart failure (SHF). *Remember that any cardiac condition associated with a dilated LV predisposes to the development of SHF.*

E 060   On physical examination, which of the following neurologic signs is most likely to be abnormal in a patient who has pernicious anemia?

A. Stereognosis
B. Extraocular muscle movements
C. Vibratory sensation
D. Proprioception sense
E. Romberg test

Essentials is designed to promote critical thinking and enrich your knowledge base. Therefore, many questions will have more than one correct answer.

Answer: C, D, and E
C and D are correct because pernicious anemia causes degeneration of dorsal (posterior) and lateral spinal columns. Loss of vibratory sensation and proprioception is noted on physical examination. E is correct because the Romberg test is abnormal when the patient's eyes are closed because balance is then dependent upon proprioception sense.

▨ **You should know:**

1. The earliest neurologic abnormalities in vitamin B_{12} deficiency anemia are loss of vibratory sensation and proprioception. As the disease progresses, ataxia and weakness are noted.

2. Remember, in vitamin B_{12} deficiency, neurologic signs, even including dementia, may be present while the hematocrit and red blood cell indices are normal. This may occur if the patient is ingesting enough folate to reverse or prevent the anemia. The folate will not, however, prevent the peripheral (spinal cord) and central (brain) neurologic pathology of vitamin B_{12} deficiency.

3. Dementia caused by vitamin B_{12} deficiency is potentially reversible if the patient receives supplemental vitamin B_{12} in a timely fashion.

NEURO, ID, ENDO

E 061   Which of the following disorders may cause cranial nerve palsy?
   A. Lyme disease
   B. Cerebral aneurysm
   C. Sarcoidosis
   D. Diabetes mellitus
   E. Myasthenia gravis

Answer: A, B, C, and D
A is correct because Lyme disease may affect any cranial nerve, but cranial nerve VII palsy is most common. B is correct because an unruptured cerebral aneurysm will most commonly cause cranial nerve III palsy. C is correct because 50% of sarcoidosis patients will develop cranial nerve VII palsy. D is correct because diabetes mellitus commonly causes palsy of cranial nerves III, IV, and VI, thus affecting extraocular muscle movement.

▨ **You should know:**

1. Bell's palsy caused by Lyme disease may be bilateral.

2. Sarcoidosis may be associated with multiple neurologic disorders. Cranial mononeuropathy (Bell's palsy), hypothalamic disease (central diabetes insipidus), or peripheral neuropathy (motor, sensory, or autonomic) may be noted.

3. Cranial nerve III palsy in the diabetic is often atypical because *pupil size often remains normal*, in contrast to the usual cranial nerve III palsy, in which the affected eye has a dilated pupil.

4. Diabetes mellitus often causes autonomic and peripheral neuropathy. Autonomic neuropathy may be manifest as orthostatic hypotension, gastroparesis, or retrograde ejaculation. Peripheral neuropathy is typically sensorimotor and is manifest by burning and paresthesias in the feet. Examination

shows loss of vibratory, proprioceptive, light touch, and temperature senses. Commonly, bilateral ankle and knee deep tendon reflexes are absent.

5. Myasthenia gravis is an autoimmune disease that affects skeletal muscle but not smooth muscle. Although ptosis is common, it is not due to a cranial nerve palsy.

6. An unruptured cerebral aneurysm may cause the patient to experience facial pain, headache, or visual acuity loss even if a cranial nerve palsy is not evident.

ENDO, PSY/LE, CV

E 062   Which of the following medications may cause the patient to become hypothyroid?

A. Radioactive iodine
B. Amiodarone
C. Lithium
D. Cholestyramine
E. Furosemide

Answer: A, B, and C
A is correct because the direct effect of radiation in the radioactive iodine used in treatment of the hyperthyroid patient can cause hypothyroidism to develop months or years later. B is correct because amiodarone is an iodine-containing antiarrhythmic medication that has a direct toxic effect on the thyroid gland. C is correct because lithium can cause goiter, hypothyroidism, and chronic immune thyroiditis due to its inhibition of thyroid hormone secretion.

■ **You should know:**

1. Hypothyroidism usually develops within the first 2 years of lithium therapy. Thyroid and kidney function should be checked every 3 to 4 months in patients receiving lithium.

2. The following medicines should not be given to a pregnant woman:
   • Lithium
   • An ACEI
   • An ARB
   • Carbamazepine
   • An HMG CoA reductase inhibitor (statin)
   • Trimethoprim (should be avoided, particularly in early pregnancy, because it is a folate antagonist)

3. Amiodarone therapy may result in either hypothyroidism or hyperthyroidism. Thyroid function should be checked every 4 months during therapy and for 2 years afterward.

GI/N, HEME, NEURO

E 063   Which of the following is a consequence of chronic alcohol abuse?

A. Hypomagnesemia
B. Folic acid deficiency
C. Wernicke's encephalopathy
D. Adenomatous polyps of the colon
E. Hypertrophic cardiomyopathy

Essentials is designed to promote critical thinking and enrich your knowledge base.
Therefore, many questions will have more than one correct answer.

Answer: A, B, and C
A is correct because hypomagnesemia in the patient with alcohol abuse is due to increased renal loss of magnesium and poor nutritional intake of this nutrient. B is correct because alcohol abuse can cause a sharp fall in body folate in 4 to 5 days. C is correct because chronic alcohol abuse with its associated thiamine deficiency may cause development of Wernicke's encephalopathy.

You should know:

1. Wernicke's encephalopathy typically has three manifestations: encephalopathy, with confusion; oculomotor abnormality, with multiple eye movement disorders including nystagmus; and ataxia due to peripheral neuropathy, cerebellar degeneration, and vestibular dysfunction.

2. Folate deficiency causes a megaloblastic anemia but does not cause the neuropathy seen in vitamin B_{12} deficiency megaloblastic anemia.

3. Chronic alcohol abuse may lead to congestive (dilated) cardiomyopathy with its associated atrial and ventricular arrhythmias and systolic heart failure.

4. Hypomagnesemia may be due to alcohol abuse or to diuretic (thiazide or loop) therapy.

CV

E 064   A child with congenital long QT interval is most likely to faint during which of the following activities?
A. Straining at stool
B. Arising quickly from bed
C. Gulping a very cold drink
D. Vomiting
E. Playing volleyball

Answer: E
E is correct because in congenital long QT interval syndrome syncope due to polymorphic ventricular tachycardia (torsades de pointes) commonly occurs during sympathetic nervous system activation, such as occurs during exercise or emotional upset.

You should know:

1. Patients with long QT interval syndrome, preexcitation syndrome, and hypertrophic obstructive cardiomyopathy are all at increased risk of syncope or sudden cardiac death.

2. When asymptomatic, the long QT interval syndrome patient has a normal cardiac examination because the heart is structurally normal.

3. When asymptomatic, the patient with preexcitation syndrome will have a normal cardiac examination because the heart is structurally normal.

4. In contrast, a child with hypertrophic obstructive cardiomyopathy who faints will typically have an abnormal cardiac examination when the patient is asymptomatic. The examination may show an apical lift related to left ventricular hypertrophy, a systolic ejection murmur near the apex, and a bisferiens carotid pulse.

E 065   Which of the following is associated with chronic primary adrenal insufficiency (Addison's disease)?

A. Weight loss
B. Nausea
C. Hyperpigmentation of the skin
D. Orthostatic dizziness
E. Weakness

Answer: A, B, C, D, and E

A is correct because chronic adrenal insufficiency is associated with anorexia resulting in weight loss. B is correct because nausea is common in this condition, though the reason for nausea is unknown. C is correct because hyperpigmentation in Addison's disease is due to the melanocyte-stimulating effect of increased plasma adrenocorticotropic hormone (ACTH) levels. D is correct because orthostatic dizziness is related to hypovolemia from aldosterone and cortisol depletion in adrenal cortical insufficiency. E is correct because weakness is a common presenting symptom related to hypovolemia and electrolyte imbalance.

■ **You should know:**

1. *Primary* adrenal insufficiency is most often due to autoimmune destruction of the adrenal cortex. Infectious etiologies include tuberculosis, HIV, and disseminated fungal infection.

2. Laboratory diagnosis of primary adrenal insufficiency includes low (subnormal) plasma cortisol and an elevated plasma adrenocorticotropic hormone (ACTH) level. The cosyntropin test is used in diagnosis of primary adrenal insufficiency.

3. Pigmentation in Addison's disease is most noticeable in palmar creases, friction areas, and sun-exposed areas of the skin.

4. Hyponatremia occurs in 90% and hyperkalemia in 65% of Addison's disease patients.

5. The hypovolemia, caused by the deficiency in mineralocorticoid secretion, is manifest as symptomatic orthostatic hypotension.

6. *Secondary* adrenal insufficiency may be due to pituitary tumor or postsurgical or postradiation effects. Hyperpigmentation does not occur in secondary insufficiency. Otherwise, symptoms are the same as in primary adrenal insufficiency. In the secondary form, plasma adrenocorticotropic hormone (ACTH) is low and hyperkalemia does not occur.

7. Patients who have adrenal insufficiency have a depletion of both glucocorticoid and mineralocorticoid hormones. In addition to taking the glucocorticoid prednisone, most patients who have chronic adrenal insufficiency require a mineralocorticoid medication in order to prevent hyperkalemia, intravascular volume depletion, and orthostatic hypotension. Fludrocortisone (9-alpha fluorohydrocortisone) is an oral mineralocorticoid that is commonly prescribed in adrenal insufficiency in order to increase circulating blood volume and to correct hyperkalemia.

E 066   A 70-year-old man has diffuse bone pain. Evaluation confirms the diagnosis of Paget's disease of bone. Which abnormal laboratory value is expected in this patient?

A. Hypercalcemia
B. Increased serum alkaline phosphatase level
C. Increased serum gamma-glutamyl transpeptidase level
D. Increased urinary hydroxyproline level
E. Increased hemoglobin level

Answer: B and D
B is correct because the increased serum alkaline phosphatase reflects the increased bone formation that occurs in Paget's disease. D is correct because the increased urinary hydroxyproline is a result of the accelerated bone resorption that is also present in this disease.

▓ **You should know:**

1. Paget's disease is often diagnosed because of asymptomatic elevation of serum alkaline phosphatase or radiologic findings that may include expanded bone that is denser than normal or has a "cotton wool" appearance.

2. Bone pain may occur in Paget's disease. The head often increases in size causing damage to cranial nerve VIII resulting in hearing loss.

3. In this disease, serum calcium and phosphorus are normal.

4. Bisphosphonates are used to treat Paget's disease.

5. Gamma-glutamyl transpeptidase (GGTP) is found *only in the liver*. Alkaline phosphatase is found in *liver and bone.*

6. Increased GGTP levels are found in patients who have disease of the liver, biliary tract, or pancreas but *not in bone disorders*. In contrast to the patient who has Paget's disease, patients with liver, biliary tract, and pancreatic disease have increased serum levels of both alkaline phosphatase and GGTP.

E 067   Which of the following medicines may cause peripheral edema?

A. Diltiazem
B. Ibuprofen
C. Captopril
D. Doxazosin
E. Aspirin

Answer: A and B
A is correct because calcium channel blockers increase capillary hydrostatic pressure. This causes fluid from the vascular space to move into the interstitium resulting in edema formation. B is correct because nonselective nonsteroidal anti-inflammatory drugs (NSAIDs) cause sodium and water retention via a kidney mechanism.

▓ **You should know:**

1. Verapamil appears to cause edema less frequently than other calcium channel blockers.

2. Other medicines that may be associated with edema formation include diazoxide, minoxidil, fludrocortisone, and estrogen.

E 068   A 72-year-old man has chronic stable angina pectoris. He received his only pneumococcal vaccination at age 69 years. Which of the following is the recommendation for this patient?

A. Revaccination at age 74 years
B. No need for revaccination
C. Revaccination only if patient develops pneumococcal pneumonia
D. Revaccination only if patient moves to an adult congregate facility
E. Revaccination based upon antibody titer to *Streptococcus pneumoniae*

Answer: B
B is correct because revaccination is indicated only if the patient was under the age
of 65 years at the time of initial pneumococcal vaccination and more than 5 years has
elapsed or the patient is in an immunocompromised state.

▨ **You should know:**

Pneumococcal vaccine:
1. Vaccination is recommended for all adults at or after age 65 years.

2. Vaccination is recommended for younger patients who have chronic cardiopulmonary disease, diabetes mellitus, chronic alcohol abuse, chronic
liver disease, or immunocompromised health status.

3. Immunocompromised patients would include those with HIV infection,
malignancy, chronic renal disease, those on chemotherapy or corticosteroid
medication, those who are asplenic (postsurgical splenectomy or autosplenectomy), and those after organ or bone marrow transplantation.
Autosplenectomy may occur in patients who have infarction of the spleen
(e.g., sickle cell anemia).

4. Finally, vaccination is recommended for those who, at any age, are residents
in special environments (e.g., nursing homes).

Meningococcal vaccine:
1. Meningococcal vaccine is recommended for college students who live in
dormitories.

Herpes zoster vaccine:
1. Herpes zoster vaccine is recommended for adults more than 60 years of
age. It is not recommended for patients with immunocompromised health
status.

E 069   A 79-year-old woman has a 1-week history of worsening dyspnea. She has smoked
cigarettes for many years and has a history of remote myocardial infarction. Which
of the following blood diagnostic studies is most appropriate to determine the cause
of the dyspnea?

A. Nt-BNP (brain natriuretic peptide)
B. Troponins
C. C-reactive protein
D. Systemic arterial P_{O_2} (Pa_{O_2})
E. Alpha-1 antitrypsin

Essentials is designed to promote critical thinking and enrich your knowledge base.
Therefore, many questions will have more than one correct answer.

Answer: A

A is correct because plasma Nt-BNP levels are used in the evaluation of dyspnea, particularly in differentiation of dyspnea due to heart failure from pulmonary dyspnea. Elevated plasma levels of Nt-BNP are found in heart failure patients.

■ **You should know:**

1. There are several natriuretic peptides. BNP and Nt-BNP are fragments of pro-B-type natriuretic peptide (BNP). The natriuretic hormones are released from atria and ventricles caused by *stretching of the ventricular walls.*

2. B-type natriuretic peptide (BNP) has multiple physiologic effects, including diuresis and natriuresis (loss of sodium in the urine); it also inhibits the vasoconstrictive effect of endothelin.

3. Nesiritide is a brain natriuretic peptide that is administered intravenously to selected patients who have acute pulmonary edema. Hypotension is an important adverse effect.

4. Normal values of B-type natriuretic peptide (BNP) depend upon a number of factors. One important factor is age; B-type natriuretic peptide (BNP) levels increase threefold between the ages of approximately 40 years and 80 years.

5. The greatest value of plasma Nt-BNP appears to be its negative predictive value. In other words, a *normal* plasma level of Nt-BNP is excellent in excluding heart failure.

6. Elevated plasma levels of Nt-BNP are found in heart failure patients. Again, the hormone level must be correlated with the patient's age, making interpretation more difficult. Thus, a normal Nt-BNP level (less than 125 pg/mL) is more valuable in *excluding the diagnosis of heart failure.*

CV

E 070   A 62-year-old healthy woman has newly diagnosed essential hypertension. Which of the following classes of medicines should not be initial monotherapy?

A. Angiotensin-receptor blocker
B. Angiotensin-converting enzyme inhibitor
C. Thiazide diuretic
D. Beta-adrenergic blocker
E. Calcium channel blocker

Answer: D

D is correct because therapy with a beta-adrenergic blocker as monotherapy in the healthy patient who is over 60 years of age is associated with increased risk of stroke. If the older patient with hypertension has another, specific indication for beta blocker therapy, then it is appropriate therapy.

■ **You should know:**

1. A thiazide diuretic, a long-acting dihydropyridine calcium channel blocker, an angiotensin-converting enzyme inhibitor (ACEI), or an angiotensin-receptor blocker (ARB) is equally effective as initial monotherapy in the healthy patient who has essential hypertension.

2. Thiazide diuretics lower urinary calcium excretion. Therefore, they are pre-ferred in patients who have recurrent urinary calcium stones. They have a beneficial effect in hypertensive patients who also have osteoporosis. Thiazides increase serum uric acid and should not be given to patients who have gout or hyperuricemia.

3. Chlorthalidone is the preferred thiazide diuretic because its duration of action is much longer than that of hydrochlorothiazide.

4. ACEIs are first-line agents in treatment of hypertensive patients who have heart failure, asymptomatic left ventricular dysfunction, history of ST segment elevation myocardial infarction, diabetes mellitus, or renal failure with accompanying proteinuria. ACEIs should *not* be given to a pregnant woman or to a woman who is likely to become pregnant.

5. An alpha-1-adrenergic blocker may be the preferred initial antihypertensive therapy in the male hypertensive who has symptomatic benign prostatic hyperplasia (BPH).

6. The alpha-2a-adrenergic receptor agonist clonidine should not be stopped suddenly. It should be withdrawn over 7 to 10 days to avoid an acute hypertensive reaction.

7. A beta-adrenergic blocker or a nondihydropyridine calcium channel blocker may be the preferred antihypertensive therapy in the patient who has angina pectoris or atrial fibrillation.

8. A beta-adrenergic blocker may worsen manifestations of depression.

GU, CV

E 071   Which of the following medicines is contraindicated in the man who takes sildenafil?

A. Isosorbide dinitrate
B. Doxazosin
C. Adenosine
D. Captopril
E. Verapamil

Answer: A
A is correct because isosorbide dinitrate in the man taking sildenafil may cause profound orthostatic hypotension.

■ **You should know:**

1. Sildenafil is a phosphodiesterase 5 inhibitor.

2. Sildenafil should not be taken by the male who is taking long-acting nitrates.

3. Sildenafil may be taken with caution by the man who also takes the alpha blocker doxazosin. It is recommended that the sildenafil be taken at least 4 hours after the last dose of the doxazosin.

4. Selective serotonin receptor inhibitors (SSRIs), thiazides, spironolactone, clonidine, ACEIs, and ARBs may cause sexual dysfunction in the male. Beta-adrenergic blockers *rarely* are causative. In addition, use of marijuana, cocaine, or heroin may cause sexual dysfunction in the male.

Essentials is designed to promote critical thinking and enrich your knowledge base.
Therefore, many questions will have more than one correct answer.

E 072   Which of the following skin disorders may have pustular lesions?

A. Rosacea
B. Tinea barbae
C. Impetigo
D. Lichen planus
E. Scabies

Answer: A, B, C, and E
A, B, C, and E are correct because bacterial and fungal infection, as well as mite infestation, can produce pustular lesions.

■ You should know:

1. Pustules are fluid collections of white blood cells and serous fluid.

2. Rosacea, a disorder of unknown etiology, is frequently found in the central face and neck. The pustules are associated with erythema and telangiectasia. Flushing episodes are common in rosacea patients. This disorder is exacerbated by alcohol and stress. Topical application of benzoyl peroxide or metronidazole is an appropriate initial treatment.

3. Tinea barbae is a fungal infection of the face. A potassium hydroxide (KOH) test done from material removed from the roof of the pustule or a plucked beard hair will show hyphae.

4. Impetigo is a staphylococcal or streptococcal folliculitis. The pustules may develop into honey-colored crusts. A razor blade can spread the bacteria on the face. Gram stain and culture confirm the diagnosis.

5. Scabies due to mite infestation can produce pruritic pustules, papules, and vesicles. Lesions typically involve the finger webs, flexor aspects of the wrists, and male genitalia. Scrapings from the pustules, when viewed under light microscopy, may show mites, eggs, or fecal material. Treatment includes bagging of recently worn clothes in a plastic bag for at least 3 days, then machine washing and hot drying. Topical application of permethrin or ivermectin is preferred therapy. Systemic antibiotics may be necessary. At the minimum, all *infected* family members should be treated; some recommend that all family members be treated.

6. Lichen planus is a violaceous papular rash with fine white streaks on the skin and mucous membranes. Buccal involvement may be painful. The etiology is unknown. Many medicines, including NSAIDs and ACEIs, have been associated with lichen planus.

E 073   Which of the following is the primary pathophysiologic abnormality in cor pulmonale?

A. Decreased right ventricular afterload
B. Increased left atrial pressure
C. Hypercarbia
D. Respiratory alkalosis
E. Pulmonary hypertension

Answer: E

E is correct because pulmonary hypertension due to lung disease increases right ventricular afterload that, in turn, can cause development of right heart failure.

■ **You should know:**

1. *Cor pulmonale is heart disease secondary to lung disease.* The lung disease may be vascular (e.g., multiple pulmonary emboli) or parenchymal (e.g., chronic bronchitis, pulmonary fibrosis, or pneumoconiosis). Pickwickian syndrome patients, with massive obesity and hypoventilation, may also develop cor pulmonale.

2. *The common denominator in cor pulmonale is pulmonary hypertension (PH)* that leads to right ventricular heart failure. PH is due to the combination of vascular and parenchymal lung damage plus, in some lung disorders, alveolar hypoxia that causes pulmonary arteriolar constriction further elevating the pulmonary artery pressure.

3. Signs of cor pulmonale include left parasternal lift, elevated jugular venous pressure, congestive hepatomegaly, ascites, and peripheral edema.

4. Chronic bronchitis (CB) is much more likely than emphysema to cause cor pulmonale. Chronic bronchitis is associated with pulmonary hypertension in contrast to a normal or near-normal pulmonary artery pressure in the patient with emphysema. Therefore, CB is associated with cor pulmonale and emphysema is not.

5. Alveolar ventilation provides fresh air in the gas exchange areas of the lung where air is in proximity to blood in the pulmonary capillaries. The partial pressure of carbon dioxide in systemic arterial blood ($Paco_2$) relates to *alveolar ventilation*. Alveolar hypoventilation of any etiology causes hypercarbia (elevated $Paco_2$) and respiratory acidosis.

6. Alveolar hypoventilation may occur in many disorders including drug intoxication, chronic obstructive lung disease, neoplasm or disease of the brainstem respiratory center (e.g., meningitis, encephalitis, and infarction), massive obesity, and neuromuscular diseases (e.g., myasthenia gravis).

7. In contrast, patients who have restrictive lung disease may have hypoxemia, but the $Paco_2$ is typically low because the small, stiff lungs cause the patients to *hyperventilate*.

PSY/LE

E 074 Which of the following psychotropic medicines may cause an extrapyramidal adverse effect?

A. Haloperidol (Haldol)
B. Thiothixene (Navane)
C. Fluphenazine (Prolixin)
D. Diazepam
E. Sertraline (Zoloft)

Answer: A, B, and C

Although haloperidol appears to have a greater likelihood to produce extrapyramidal signs (EPS), EPS are common in patients who take thiothixene or fluphenazine.

Essentials is designed to promote critical thinking and enrich your knowledge base. Therefore, many questions will have more than one correct answer.

■ **You should know:**

1. Extrapyramidal signs (EPS) include dystonia (abnormal movements or postures), akathisia (a desire to be in constant motion), and parkinsonism.

2. Side effects of benzodiazepine antianxiety medicines are typically dose dependent. They may include ataxia, dysarthria, and poor judgment. In addition, agitation, psychosis, and confusion may occur.

3. Sertraline is a selective serotonin reuptake inhibitor (SSRI) antidepressant that may cause somnolence, dizziness, and gastrointestinal symptoms.

4. *Serotonin has central and peripheral nervous system effects.* Centrally, it modulates attention and behavior. Peripherally, it influences intestinal motility, vasoconstriction, uterine contraction, and bronchoconstriction.

5. "Serotonin syndrome" is a potentially life-threatening condition most frequently related to either a high dose of the selective serotonin reuptake inhibitor (SSRI) or to a drug interaction. Drug interactions may include the selective serotonin reuptake inhibitor (SSRI) plus one of the following: amphetamine (or other adrenergic-stimulating agent), meperidine, St. John's wort, sumatriptan, and lithium.

6. Serotonin syndrome is typically manifest as agitation, delirium, vomiting, diarrhea, and sweating. Physical signs include dilated pupils, flushed skin, tachycardia, and fluctuating hypertension.

CV, GI/N, GU

E 075   Which of the following is a potential adverse effect of nonaspirin, nonselective, nonsteroidal anti-inflammatory drugs (NSAIDs)?

A. Heart failure
B. Peptic ulcer
C. Azotemia
D. Hypernatremia
E. Increased anion gap metabolic acidosis

Answer: A, B, and C
A, B, and C are correct because nonsteroidal anti-inflammatory drugs (NSAIDs) may produce gastritis or peptic ulcer. The gastric mucosal injury is thought to be related to the effect of NSAIDs on cyclooxygenase activity in the mucosa. Further, they may cause interstitial nephritis and acute renal failure. NSAIDs may precipitate heart failure due to hypertension from systemic vasoconstriction and the sodium and water retention promoted by these agents.

■ **You should know:**

1. Renal effects of NSAIDs are more common in the elderly and those taking diuretics.

2. NSAIDs do not alter disease progression in rheumatoid arthritis, but do ease pain and inflammation.

3. Hemorrhagic colitis from NSAIDs is most common in elderly patients or in those who take these agents for extended periods of time.

E 076   A patient who takes methotrexate for treatment of malignant disease should be counseled to do which of the following?

   A. Take daily supplement of colchicine
   B. Take daily supplement of folic acid
   C. Drink 24 ounces (3 glasses) of milk daily
   D. Avoid intake of plain fat-free yogurt
   E. Take a daily supplement of omega-3 fish oil

Answer: B

B is correct because methotrexate is an antimetabolite that interferes with cellular utilization of folic acid.

   ▪ **You should know:**

   1. Milk reduces gastrointestinal absorption of methotrexate.

   2. Methotrexate is usually the agent of choice for rheumatoid arthritis patients who do not respond to NSAIDs. This medicine is also used in treatment of selected patients who have ectopic pregnancy, psoriasis, hematologic malignancies, and solid malignant neoplasms.

   3. Patients taking this medication should have liver function tests performed every 4 to 8 weeks. Folic acid supplement ingestion reduces the risk of hepatotoxicity.

   4. Patients with liver disease should not take methotrexate. Further, patients on this medication should be strongly cautioned to avoid alcohol ingestion because this increases the risk of medicine-induced hepatotoxicity.

E 077   The risk of acetaminophen toxicity is increased in the patient who is characterized by which of the following?

   A. Has chronic alcohol abuse
   B. Takes cyclophosphamide (Cytoxan)
   C. Takes isoniazid (INH)
   D. Takes captopril
   E. Is older than 80 years of age

Answer: A, C, and E

A, C, and E are correct because patients suffering from chronic alcohol abuse or those taking medicines that increase P450 enzyme activity (e.g., isoniazid) are at increased risk of acetaminophen toxicity. Elderly patients are at increased risk for acetaminophen toxicity, although the reason is not clear.

   ▪ **You should know:**

   1. The initial manifestations of acetaminophen toxicity are nonspecific, including nausea, vomiting, diaphoresis, and pallor. At 24 to 72 hours after ingestion, hepatotoxicity is evident.

   2. The specific antidote to acetaminophen is *N*-acetylcysteine. This may be given orally or intravenously to the patient.

Essentials is designed to promote critical thinking and enrich your knowledge base.
Therefore, many questions will have more than one correct answer.

3. Specific indications for treatment of the patient suffering from acetaminophen toxicity are outlined in a published nomogram.

MS

E 078   After an evening of excessive beer intake, a 59-year-old man suddenly awakens with severe pain at the base of the left great toe. The joint is swollen and exquisitely tender. Which of the following is the preferred initial therapy?

A. Aspirin
B. Acetaminophen
C. Indomethacin
D. Probenecid
E. Allopurinol

Answer: C

C is correct because alcohol ingestion increases serum uric acid levels and may precipitate acute gout. NSAIDs are the treatment of choice for acute gout.

■ **You should know:**

1. 80% of primary gout patients are male.

2. Hyperuricemia in gout is due to either overproduction or underexcretion of uric acid and sometimes both.

3. Primary gout is metabolic; secondary gout is acquired and may be due to medicines (e.g., thiazide or loop diuretics, low-dose aspirin, and niacin) or to myeloproliferative diseases.

4. Early in its course, gout is intermittent and monoarticular. Later, it may become polyarticular.

5. Presence of synovial urate crystals is diagnostic. These crystals are negatively birefringent.

6. The kidney is the primary organ for uric acid excretion. To avoid uric acid–induced renal damage, the hyperuricemic patient must avoid intake of food and medicines that increase serum uric acid level, exercise aggressive hydration, and take medicine to reduce the elevated serum uric acid level. Ingestion of meat and seafood increases the serum uric acid level. Milk products reduce the risk of recurrent gouty attacks.

7. NSAIDs are the treatment of choice for acute gout. The patient typically has a dramatic response to these agents. They should be continued for 5 to 10 days until all symptoms have resolved.

8. In a patient who has recurrent attacks of acute gout, a uricosuric agent (e.g., probenecid or sulfinpyrazone) is given if 24-hour urinary uric acid is less than 800 mg/day. Patients taking a uricosuric agent should take an agent to alkalinize the urine (e.g., potassium chloride).

9. If the gouty patient's urinary uric acid excretion is greater than 800 mg/day, allopurinol therapy is initiated.

10. Pseudogout, also characterized by acute arthritis, is associated with positively birefringent calcium pyrophosphate crystals in the joint. Radiography

may show chondrocalcinosis of the joints even when the pseudogout patient is asymptomatic.

CV, ID

E 079   A 50-year-old man has a mechanical prosthetic heart valve. Endocarditis prophylaxis is recommended if the patient is to undergo which of the following procedures?

A. Dental extraction
B. Transurethral resection of the prostate
C. Endoscopic retrograde cholangiography
D. Percutaneous balloon angioplasty
E. Endodontic root canal

Answer: A, B, and C

A, B, and C are correct because antibiotic prophylaxis is recommended when a procedure is associated with a significant risk of bacteremia.

▌**You should know:**

1. In 2007, the American Heart Association made major revisions in its guidelines for the prevention of infective endocarditis.

2. The recommendation for antimicrobial prophylaxis is now limited to those patients with cardiac conditions with the highest risk of adverse outcome from infective endocarditis.

3. Patients at the highest risk include the following:
   • Prosthetic heart valves
   • A prior history of endocarditis
   • Unrepaired cyanotic congenital heart disease
   • Repaired congenital heart defects with prosthetic material or device during the first 6 months after the procedure
   • Repaired congenital heart disease with residual defects at or adjacent to the site of the prosthetic device
   • Cardiac valvulopathy (i.e., leaflet pathology with regurgitation) in a transplanted heart

4. Antimicrobial prophylaxis is no longer recommended for the patient who has the following disorders:
   • Bicuspid aortic valve
   • Acquired mitral or aortic valve disease, including patients who have undergone valve repair
   • Hypertrophic cardiomyopathy

5. For dental, upper respiratory, or oral procedures, patients requiring endocarditis prophylaxis should take oral amoxicillin 30 minutes to 1 hour prior to the procedure. Penicillin-allergic patients may take clarithromycin, azithromycin, or cephalexin.

6. For gastrointestinal or genitourinary procedures, endocarditis prophylaxis would include ampicillin or amoxicillin or vancomycin.

7. Prophylaxis is not recommended for heart catheterization including balloon angioplasty, endotracheal intubation, or endodontic treatment.

Essentials is designed to promote critical thinking and enrich your knowledge base.
Therefore, many questions will have more than one correct answer.

E 080   A 17-year-old woman has a 2-day history of fever, sore throat, myalgia, and fatigue. Examination shows diffuse, symmetrical lymphadenopathy, inflamed tonsils with exudates, and palatal petechiae. Which of the following is the most likely diagnosis?

    A. Hodgkin's disease
    B. Infectious mononucleosis
    C. Sarcoidosis
    D. Tonsillar abscess
    E. Angioneurotic edema

Answer: B
B is correct because patients with infectious mononucleosis due to Epstein-Barr virus type 1 (EBV-1) have pharyngitis, often with tonsillar exudates, palatal petechiae, and diffuse adenopathy.

▪ **You should know:**

    1. Posterior cervical adenopathy is highly suggestive of mononucleosis.

    2. Saliva may remain infectious for 6 months from onset of symptoms. Patients should avoid contact sports for 4 weeks even if splenomegaly has not been present.

    3. Positive heterophile agglutination or elevated anti-EBV titer is confirmatory. These tests usually become abnormal 3 to 4 weeks after symptom onset. EBV-specific antibody titers are indicated when Epstein-Barr infection is strongly suspected and the heterophile agglutination test is negative.

    4. One third of mononucleosis patients have superimposed streptococcal tonsillitis requiring treatment with penicillin or erythromycin. Avoid amoxicillin and ampicillin because they commonly cause a rash in these patients.

    5. Atypical lymphocytes appear approximately 1 week after symptom onset. Hemolytic anemia and/or thrombocytopenia may occur.

    6. Uncomplicated mononucleosis cases are treated with saline gargles, acetaminophen, or NSAIDs.

E 081   Which of the following is characterized by annular lesions?

    A. Psoriasis
    B. Secondary syphilis
    C. Tinea versicolor
    D. Tinea corporis
    E. Henoch-Schönlein purpura

Answer: A, B, and D
A, B, and D are correct because annular lesions may occur in fungal and bacterial diseases as well as in psoriasis.

▪ **You should know:**

    1. *Trichophyton rubrum* is the most common organism causing tinea corporis. Lesions tend to be few in number and are erythematous rings with central clearing. Potassium hydroxide (KOH) preparation of scales taken from lesions shows hyphae.

2. Tinea corporis may be treated with miconazole, clotrimazole, econazole, sulconazole, terbinafine, naftifine, or butenafine. Betamethasone dipropionate with clotrimazole (Lotrisone) is not recommended.

3. Competitive athletes (e.g., wrestlers) who have tinea corporis can easily infect the second athlete. Therefore, it is recommended that such athletes take an oral systemic preparation and not practice or compete for 2 weeks.

4. Secondary syphilis, caused by infection with the spirochete *Treponema pallidum*, is associated with diffuse annular lesions that typically involve the palms and soles. Another specific lesion in secondary syphilis is condyloma lata characterized by raised white lesions involving mucous membranes and moist areas in the perineum. Condyloma lata is highly infectious.

5. Condyloma lata must be distinguished from condyloma acuminata, which are anogenital warts caused by human papillomavirus infection.

6. Psoriasis typically causes lesions on knees, elbows, and scalp. Lesions on the penis and vulva are common. The intergluteal fold may be red. Fingernails may be pitted (stippled). Pitting of the nails is highly suggestive of psoriasis, but it is not specific. Pitting may also be seen in the patient who has reactive arthritis.

DERM

E 082   A 26-year-old man has pruritic lesions on his elbows, knees, and glans penis. There are annular red plaques with silvery scales. No lymphadenopathy is noted. The palms are not affected. Which of the following is the most likely diagnosis?

A. Psoriasis
B. Secondary syphilis
C. Drug eruption
D. Erythema migrans
E. Kaposi sarcoma

Answer: A
A is correct because psoriasis typically is associated with plaques having overlying silvery scales.

■ **You should know:**

1. Chloroquine, lithium, and beta-adrenergic blockers may cause a psoriasislike rash.

2. 15% of psoriasis patients develop some type of arthritis, often distal and affecting few joints (oligoarticular). Radiographic imaging generally shows marginal erosion of bone and involvement of the phalanges with a "sharpened pencil" appearance. It should be noted, however, that psoriatic arthritis may take many clinical and radiographic forms.

3. In contrast, radiographic changes in rheumatoid arthritis tend to occur initially in the wrists or feet. Soft tissue swelling and demineralization are early signs.

4. In the patient who has psoriasis, treatment with beta-adrenergic blockers, lithium, antimalarials, and HMG-CoA reductase inhibitors ("statins") may worsen the rash. This can be an important consideration in the psoriasis patient who has a coexisting cardiovascular disease.

Essentials is designed to promote critical thinking and enrich your knowledge base.
Therefore, many questions will have more than one correct answer.

5. Pitting of nails is an important diagnostic sign of psoriasis. In addition, a tan-brown discoloration of the nails may occur.

I/N, ID, REPRO, GU

E 083   Which of the following is associated with an elevated serum amylase level?

A. Acute pancreatitis
B. Mumps
C. Mesenteric infarction
D. Ruptured ectopic pregnancy
E. Renal failure

Answer: A, B, C, D, and E
A, B, C, D, and E are correct because an elevated serum amylase level is of nonspecific origin and may be due to gastrointestinal, renal, or reproductive diseases.

▮ **You should know:**

1. Serum amylase and lipase are elevated in patients who have renal failure due to reduced clearance of the enzymes.

2. Patients with acute pancreatitis precipitated by alcohol ingestion or by elevated plasma triglycerides commonly have normal serum amylase at the onset of symptoms. The serum amylase level rises in 6 to 12 hours and, in uncomplicated cases, returns to normal in 3 to 5 days.

3. The usual serum amylase determination by the laboratory does not differentiate between salivary and pancreatic origin.

4. Many medicines may elevate serum amylase levels. Examples include aspirin, codeine, estrogens, metronidazole, thiazides, and iodine-containing contrast media.

5. Several medical conditions are associated with elevated serum amylase levels. These include mesenteric infarction, ruptured ectopic pregnancy, multiple myeloma, cystic fibrosis, obstructed or perforated bowel, and pelvic inflammatory disease.

GI/N

E 084   An 83-year-old man with chronic systolic heart failure has a blood urea nitrogen (BUN) value of 41 mg/dL and a serum creatinine of 1.4 mg/dL. Which of the following is the most likely cause of the elevated BUN/creatinine ratio?

A. Acute tubular necrosis
B. Bilateral ureteral obstruction
C. Renal hypoperfusion
D. Decreased muscle mass
E. Iron deficiency anemia

Answer: B and C
B is correct because bilateral ureteral obstruction or prostatic hyperplasia can cause an increased blood urea nitrogen (BUN)/creatinine ratio ("postrenal" disease). C is correct because decreased renal perfusion associated with the low cardiac output state of chronic systolic failure ("prerenal" disease) increases the ratio.

■ **You should know:**

1. A brief physiology note: Urea is reabsorbed in the tubules of the nephron. The amount of urea reabsorbed is *inversely related* to urine flow. Decreased urine flow is associated with greater urea reabsorption and the BUN level increases. Serum creatinine is not related to urine flow. Therefore, in conditions in which there is reduced urine flow, the BUN/creatinine ratio increases.

2. Decreased urine flow occurs in both prerenal and postrenal disease. As a result, the BUN/creatinine ratio is increased in both.

3. The *upper limit of normal* for the blood urea nitrogen (BUN)/creatinine ratio is 20:1.

4. The two most common causes of acute renal failure are:
   • Acute tubular necrosis secondary to ischemia (e.g., hemodynamic shock, sepsis, or cardiac arrest) or nephrotoxins (e.g., aminoglycosides, radiographic contrast media, myoglobinuria, or uric acid)
   • Prerenal disease with decreased renal perfusion (heart failure, hypovolemia)

5. In acute tubular necrosis, the ratio is normal in contrast to "prerenal" and "postrenal" azotemia.

6. Importantly, the blood urea nitrogen (BUN)/creatinine ratio is also increased in patients who:
   • Have gastrointestinal bleeding
   • Take medicines that interfere with protein anabolism (e.g., tetracycline or corticosteroids)
   • Are chronically ill with loss of muscle mass

7. An increased ratio is more important clinically than a normal ratio.

8. A *low* blood urea nitrogen (BUN)/creatinine ratio is found in patients who have severe liver disease because of an impaired hepatic production of urea.

ENDO

E 085   In addition to a deficiency in islet cell response to glucagon, which of the following is the pathophysiologic abnormality in type 2 diabetes mellitus?

A. Tissue resistance to insulin
B. Increased hepatic gluconeogenesis
C. Deficient level of glucose-6-phosphate dehydrogenase
D. Autoimmune destruction of B pancreatic cells
E. Defect in oxidative metabolism

Answer: A
A is correct because type 2 diabetes mellitus is due to a combination of tissue resistance to insulin (insensitivity to endogenous insulin) and a deficiency in response of pancreatic islet cells to glucose.

■ **You should know:**

1. *Type 1* diabetes mellitus is due to autoimmune destruction of pancreatic B (islet) cells. Circulating insulin is nearly absent, but plasma glucagon is elevated. Ninety-five percent of patients have HLA-DR3 or HLA-DR4 genes.

Essentials is designed to promote critical thinking and enrich your knowledge base.
Therefore, many questions will have more than one correct answer.

2. Early in the natural history of *type* 2 diabetes, hyperplasia of pancreatic B cells often occurs explaining the fasting hyperinsulinism and exaggerated insulin response to a glucose load. Later in the disease, the hyperinsulinism does not typically occur.

3. A waist-to-hip fat ratio of greater than 0.9 is a sign of increased insulin resistance and indicative of an increased risk of diabetes mellitus.

CV, ENDO, REPRO

E 086   A 32-year-old obese, sedentary woman has hypertension, fasting plasma triglyceride of 400 mg/dL, serum uric acid of 8.1 mg/dL, and fasting plasma glucose of 114 mg/dL. Her menstrual cycles are regular. Examination shows normal hair distribution. Which of the following is the most likely diagnosis?

A. Cushing's syndrome
B. Metabolic syndrome
C. Polycystic ovary syndrome
D. Resorptive hypercalciuria
E. Type 2 diabetes mellitus

Answer: B
B is correct because the metabolic syndrome is found in nondiabetic patients who typically have abdominal obesity and a combination of metabolic abnormalities, including insulin resistance, elevated plasma triglycerides, low serum HDL cholesterol, hypertension, and hyperuricemia.

▓ **You should know:**

1. Metabolic syndrome patients are at significantly increased risk for atherosclerotic disease.

2. In these patients, it may be preferable to avoid thiazide or beta-adrenergic blocker therapy in hypertension due to their potential to worsen the dyslipidemia. Further, niacin therapy for the lipid disorder may significantly increase plasma glucose.

3. Polycystic ovary syndrome (PCOS) patients exhibit biochemical evidence of elevated testosterone, luteinizing hormone, and prolactin. These patients frequently have amenorrhea or abnormal uterine bleeding. They show insulin resistance and hyperinsulinemia placing them at risk for type 2 diabetes. Polycystic ovary syndrome (PCOS) patients are most often hirsute with a male hair distribution pattern.

4. The treatment of PCOS is variable, depending upon the patient's age and desire for pregnancy. Succinctly, the principles of treatment and treatment are the following:

Principle	Treatment
Endometrial protection	Oral contraceptives
Induction of ovulation	Clomiphene; metformin
Reduction of insulin resistance	Weight loss; metformin; thiazolidinediones
Reduction of androgen excess	Oral contraceptives; spironolactone

E 087   In a patient who has new-onset hypertension, verapamil is preferred therapy over hydrochlorothiazide if the patient has which of the following?

A. Claudication of the legs
B. Gout
C. Chronic obstructive lung disease
D. Tachy-brady syndrome (sick sinus)
E. Cholelithiasis

Answer: B

B is correct because thiazide diuretics increase serum uric acid levels and therefore should not be given to the patient who has a history of gout or who has asymptomatic hyperuricemia.

■ **You should know:**

1. Verapamil is particularly valuable in the patient who has hypertension in association with angina pectoris or atrial fibrillation.

2. Verapamil, diltiazem, digoxin, and beta-adrenergic blockers may worsen patients who have tachy-brady syndrome (sick sinus syndrome). All of these medicines slow depolarization of the sinoatrial node, slow the sinus heart rate, and slow atrioventricular conduction. They may precipitate 1st degree, 2nd degree, and even 3rd degree atrioventricular block.

3. Beta-adrenergic blockers appear to worsen leg claudication via a decrease in cardiac output and inhibition of beta-2 receptor–mediated vasodilation. This appears to be most significant in the patient with moderate to severe claudication.

4. Nonelective beta-adrenergic blockers increase airway resistance by inhibiting beta-2–induced bronchodilation. Beta-1 blockers appear to cause less bronchoconstriction.

E 088   Several days after an upper respiratory infection, a healthy 4-year-old girl has community-acquired pneumonia. Which of the following is the most likely infecting organism?

A. Respiratory syncytial virus
B. *Streptococcus pneumoniae*
C. *Chlamydia pneumoniae*
D. Hantavirus
E. Varicella

Answer: A

A is correct because respiratory syncytial virus is the most common infecting organism causing community-acquired pneumonia (CAP) in a child under 5 years of age.

■ **You should know:**

1. Viruses cause community-acquired pneumonia (CAP) in approximately 20% of adults, but in children under age 5 years, viruses are the most common etiology of CAP.

Essentials is designed to promote critical thinking and enrich your knowledge base. Therefore, many questions will have more than one correct answer.

2. The child (not infant) who is thought to have viral CAP (i.e., one with the gradual onset of symptoms, preceding upper respiratory infection, and diffuse auscultatory findings [rales, rhonchi]) should not receive antibiotics as long as the patient is not toxic.

GI/N

E 089   Which of the following is a risk factor for gastric adenocarcinoma?

A. *Helicobacter pylori* gastritis
B. Pernicious anemia
C. Candidal esophagitis
D. Gastroesophageal reflux
E. Billroth I gastroduodenostomy

Answer: A and B
A and B are correct because chronic gastric infection and achlorhydria increase risk of gastric cancer.

■ **You should know:**

1. Chronic *Helicobacter pylori* is a strong risk factor, increasing risk of gastric cancer 5 to 20 times.

2. Upper endoscopy should be performed in all patients greater than 55 years who have new epigastric symptoms and anyone whose symptoms fail to respond to a short course of antisecretory medicines.

3. Achlorhydria of any etiology (e.g., pernicious anemia) leads to a compensatory increase in serum gastrin, a potent inducer of gastric epithelial cell proliferation. This may be the mechanism by which pernicious anemia increases the risk of gastric cancer.

4. Prior *Billroth II gastrojejunostomy* is considered to be a risk factor as well.

ID

E 090   Which of the following is considered to be a high-risk infectious disease from a bioterrorist attack?

A. Plague
B. Lassa fever
C. Tularemia
D. Dengue fever
E. Anthrax

Answer: A, C, and E
A, C, and E are correct because plague, anthrax, and tularemia are easily transmitted to humans and may have high mortality.

■ **You should know:**

1. Anthrax produces a black eschar on exposed skin with surrounding vesicles. Inhaled spores of the gram-positive aerobic bacillus can cause pneumonia complicated by hemodynamic shock. Anthrax, naturally, is a disease of cattle, sheep, and swine. It has been used to infect humans in a purposeful (i.e., terrorist) manner.

2. Tularemia is a disease of rabbits and rodents that appears to be acquired from contact with animal tissue or aerosol inhalation. A papular lesion may be noted at the site of skin contact. Pneumonia may occur from inhalation and abdominal pain from ingestion of the organism.

3. Plague, a natural disease of rodents, is due to a gram-negative organism that may manifest as pneumonia, meningitis, or septicemia, the last causing purpura, giving the historic name, "black death." If the infection occurs through the skin, then buboes may be noted. A bubo is an extremely painful inflammation of a lymph node with overlying skin edema.

CV, GU

E 091　A 42-year-old woman is transported to the emergency department after having suffered extensive hemorrhaging in a vehicular accident. Blood pressure is 70/40 mm Hg; pulse, 140/min; and respirations, 29/min. Infusion of which of the following is the preferred initial therapy?

A. Normal saline
B. Half-normal saline
C. Dextrose 5% in water
D. Dextrose 5% in half-normal saline
E. Dextrose 5% with added dopamine

Answer: A
A is correct because an isotonic crystalloid solution (e.g., normal saline) will have the greatest portion of infused volume staying in the intravascular space, thus increasing blood pressure and tissue perfusion.

■ **You should know:**

1. Vasopressors will not correct hypovolemia and may further reduce perfusion.

2. Infusion of hypotonic solutions (e.g., dextrose 5% in water or half-normal saline) will result in rapid movement of fluid from vascular to interstitial space.

3. Blood products will be started as soon as possible in the hemorrhagic patient.

4. There does not appear to be any clear advantage of colloid solutions (e.g., albumin or hetastarch) over isotonic saline.

5. "Third spacing" is an important cause of hypovolemia and reduction in circulating blood volume that may occur within the body, as blood or serum moves quickly from the vascular bed into a "third space." The "third space" is a nonvascular compartment that could be the abdominal cavity, retroperitoneal area, or joint space. These patients may present clinically with prerenal azotemia, shock, or acute tubular necrosis.

6. Examples of disorders that are associated with "third spacing" include major fractures (e.g., hip), severe pancreatitis, peritonitis, bowel obstruction, and crush injuries.

CV

E 092 A 66-year-old man has acute, severe hypovolemia related to gastrointestinal bleeding. Which of the following is an expected sign on examination?
   A. Elevated jugular venous pressure
   B. Orthostatic hypotension
   C. Loud first heart sound (S1)
   D. Warm, moist skin
   E. Flushing

Answer: **B**
B is correct because blood pressure in the *recumbent* position may be near normal in the hypovolemic patient, but orthostatic hypotension is characteristically noted.

■ **You should know:**

1. Hypovolemia excites the sympathetic nervous system, resulting in arteriolar and venous constriction and decreased renal blood flow. The skin is typically cool and often moist from sweating. Oliguria results from decreased renal blood flow and the avid sodium and water retention by the kidney.

2. When the jugular venous pressure (JVP) is 0, marked hypovolemia is present. Otherwise, JVP is not a good indicator of hypovolemia.

3. Reduced skin turgor is noted in the hypovolemic patient when the skin of the thigh is pinched.

4. Hypovolemia is one of the causes of an increased blood urea nitrogen/serum creatinine ratio. The upper limit of normal of the ratio is 20:1. (Please refer to E 084 You Should Know.)

5. Elevated JVP is noted in right heart failure, constrictive pericarditis, superior vena cava syndrome, and pericardial tamponade.

PSY/LE

E 093 A 20-year-old woman is diagnosed as having panic disorder. Which of the following is a clinical manifestation of this condition?
   A. Panic episodes are typically unrelated to menses
   B. Tends to be familial
   C. Increased risk of suicide
   D. Onset usually under age 25 years
   E. Increased association with obsessive-compulsive disorder

Answer: **B, C, D, and E**
B, C, D, and E are correct because panic disorder typically is associated with increased frequency of episodes in the premenstrual period and is related to other psychiatric disorders.

■ **You should know:**

1. Panic disorder is manifest by recurrent, brief episodes of intense fear or terror occurring with physiologic manifestations (e.g., sweating and palpitations). Chest pain, smothering sensation, abdominal pain, and paresthesias are common somatic complaints.

2. 25% of patients have concurrent obsessive-compulsive disorder.

3. It is common for these patients to develop depression with increased suicide risk.

4. Benzodiazepine medications may be given sublingually, orally, or intravenously.

E 094   Which of the following is associated with ascites formation?

A. Cirrhosis
B. Left heart failure
C. Peritoneal carcinomatosis
D. Cholecystitis
E. Polycystic ovary syndrome

Answer: A and C
A and C are correct because cirrhosis, with associated portal hypertension and hypoalbuminemia, is the most common cause of ascites. In addition, ascites will occur in abdominal or pelvic malignancy that has peritoneal seeding.

■ **You should know:**

1. It is suggested that the two most important tests on ascites fluid are (1) serum to ascites albumin gradient (SAAG) and (2) culture and sensitivity.

2. A SAAG gradient equal to or greater than 1.1 g/dL indicates portal hypertension. A gradient less than 1.1 g/dL indicates absence of portal hypertension.

3. Culture is indicated in patients with new-onset ascites and those with ascites who have fever, abdominal pain, azotemia, acidosis, or confusion. These are signs of *spontaneous bacterial* peritonitis (SBP).

4. SBP must be differentiated from *secondary bacterial* peritonitis (e.g., peritonitis from a perforation in peptic ulcer or colonic diverticulitis).

5. Constrictive pericarditis (CP) is always associated with ascites. Left heart failure does not cause congestive hepatomegaly or ascites. Right heart failure is always associated with peripheral edema. Ascites is present but is less prominent than in CP.

6. Hepatocellular carcinoma and lymphoma may cause ascites without peritoneal seeding.

E 095   Which of the following suggests that a diabetic patient has developed gastroparesis?

A. Poor glycemic control despite vigorous measures
B. Nocturnal wheezing attacks
C. Hematemesis
D. Vomiting of bile-stained material
E. Residual food in stomach after overnight fast

Answer: A and E
A and E are correct because delayed emptying of the stomach may result in slow absorption of an oral hypoglycemic medication or, in the insulin-dependent patient, a temporal imbalance between food digestion and insulin administration. Specifically,

Essentials is designed to promote critical thinking and enrich your knowledge base.
Therefore, many questions will have more than one correct answer.

the patient with gastroparesis may administer insulin just before a meal. However, the delay in the food leaving the stomach causes the insulin to exert its hypoglycemic effect before the food enters the intestine for digestion. In both cases, the diabetic patient will appear to have lost proper control of blood sugar levels.

You should know:

1. Gastroparesis and nocturnal diarrhea are gastrointestinal manifestations of diabetic neuropathy.

2. Gastroparesis is delayed emptying of the stomach. The patient may experience nausea, vomiting, or bloating.

3. In gastroparesis, upper endoscopy typically is normal except for the presence of residual food after an overnight fast. Gastric scintigraphy, with ingestion of a radioactive-labeled meal, is considered the optimal test for evaluating stomach emptying.

4. A succinct review of diabetic autonomic neuropathy:
   - Cardiovascular: Orthostatic hypotension
   - Gastrointestinal: Gastroparesis; nocturnal diarrhea
   - Genitourinary: Incontinence; erectile dysfunction; retrograde ejaculation
   - Peripheral: Callus formation; loss of nails

CV, HEME

E 096   Which of the following is the pathophysiologic mechanism by which cyclooxygenase-2 (COX-2) inhibitors increase the risk of arterial thrombosis?

A. Increased effect of prostacyclin
B. Increased marrow production of platelets
C. Increased presence of factor V Leiden
D. Production of antiphospholipid antibodies
E. Unopposed effect of thromboxane

Answer: E
E is correct because a cyclooxygenase-2 enzyme (COX-2) inhibitor medication inhibits the vasodilation and antiplatelet aggregation effects of prostacyclin, leaving an unopposed COX-1 effect of thromboxane-induced platelet aggregation and vasoconstriction.

You should know:

1. COX enzymes produce prostaglandins, prostacyclin, and thromboxane. Prostacyclin and thromboxane have *opposing effects in the arterial circulation*.

2. COX-1 enzyme is responsible for *platelet* production of thromboxane and mucosal integrity of the stomach. Remember, COX-1 relates to platelets producing thromboxane that causes vasoconstriction and *increased* platelet aggregation.

3. COX-2 enzyme is responsible for the *endothelium* of blood vessels producing prostacyclin. Further, COX-2 activity is increased in inflammatory states. Remember, COX-2 relates to endothelium producing prostacyclin that causes vasodilation and *inhibition* of platelet aggregation.

4. Intake of a COX-2 inhibitor reduces the vasodilation in the coronary circulation and increases platelet agglutination. As a result, COX-2 inhibitor medicines

produce an exaggerated thromboxane effect that results in an increased incidence of arterial thrombosis, myocardial infarction, and stroke.

5. COX enzyme inhibition is a key mechanism of action of aspirin and NSAIDs. Aspirin and nonsalicylate NSAIDs inhibit *both COX-1 and COX-2* enzymes. Aspirin inhibits COX-1 to a greater degree than COX-2.

CV, NEURO

E 097   Which of the following is an absolute contraindication to thrombolytic therapy?

A. Active internal bleeding
B. Blood pressure 230/120 mm Hg
C. Trauma causing loss of consciousness within 4 weeks
D. Previous hemorrhagic stroke
E. Intracranial malignant neoplasm

Answer: A, B, C, D, and E

A, B, C, D, and E are correct because the risk of adverse effects from thrombolytic therapy is increased in patients with intracranial malignant neoplasm, uncontrolled hypertension, recent significant head or facial trauma, previous hemorrhagic stroke, active internal bleeding, previous ischemic stroke within 3 months, and dissection of the aorta.

You should know:

1. Thrombolytic therapy is effective in selected patients with *acute ischemic stroke* when administered within 3 hours of onset of symptoms.

2. The mechanism of action of thrombolytic medicine is to activate plasminogen resulting in degradation of fibrin in the thrombotic clot.

3. Thrombolytic therapy has an increased risk of intracerebral bleeding in the ischemic stroke patient, especially in the elderly patient. However, the benefit of therapy outweighs the relative increase in bleeding risk in this group. Those patients who have an intracranial neoplasm have increased risk of bleeding into the tumor. In this latter group, the thrombolytic agent should not be administered.

4. The thrombolytic agent may be started in the markedly hypertensive patient when the blood pressure is less than 170/110 mm Hg and there are no other contraindications.

5. In both acute ischemic stroke and acute myocardial infarction, patients older than age 80 years have an increased risk of intracerebral bleeding from thrombolytic agents. It is important to note, however, that the benefit of therapy outweighs the added risk.

DERM

E 098   Which of the following is characteristic of uncomplicated herpes zoster infection?

A. Pain may precede rash
B. Rash is unilateral
C. Rash is macular eruption
D. Only occurs in immunocompromised persons
E. Rash occurs along course of a nerve

Essentials is designed to promote critical thinking and enrich your knowledge base.
Therefore, many questions will have more than one correct answer.

Answer: A, B, and E

A, B, and E are correct because the pain of zoster may precede the rash for 24 to 48 hours, and infection in uncomplicated cases affects a single, unilateral dermatome.

You should know:

1. HIV-infected patients are much more likely to develop zoster, and in these patients the infection is often generalized.

2. Zoster affecting a single dermatome does not imply an immunocompromised state or an internal malignancy.

3. Therapy early in the disease course with acyclovir, famciclovir, or valacyclovir reduces the incidence and severity of postherpetic neuralgia.

4. Corticosteroid therapy may increase the risk of herpes zoster dissemination in an immunocompromised host.

5. Pleurodynia is a coxsackievirus infection that causes pleuritic pain in the area of the diaphragm. Patients may have headache, fever, and nausea. The length of illness is approximately 5 to 7 days.

MS, ID

E 099   An increased risk for which of the following is the basis for not recommending fluoroquinolones to a patient who is under 18 years of age?

A. Uveitis
B. Erosion of joint cartilage
C. Allergic pneumonitis
D. Chemical hepatitis
E. Aseptic necrosis

Answer: B

B is correct because fluoroquinolones are not recommended in patients under 18 years of age because they may cause erosion of cartilage in weight-bearing joints.

You should know:

1. Fluoroquinolones are generally more effective against gram-negative than gram-positive organisms.

2. They are generally very effective against *Escherichia coli, Moraxella, Haemophilus,* and *Campylobacter*.

3. Fluoroquinolones are used to treat epididymitis caused by enteric organisms or with negative gonococcal culture.

4. Fluoroquinolones are no longer recommended for the treatment of gonococcal infections and associated conditions (e.g., pelvic inflammatory disease) because of increasing resistance. Similarly, penicillin G and tetracycline are associated with widespread resistant strains and are no longer recommended agents.

5. For gonococcal urethritis or cervicitis, intramuscular ceftriaxone is the preferred therapy. Alternatively, parenteral cefixime, ceftizoxime, cefotaxime, or cefoxitin may be given. Oral azithromycin is an appropriate therapy in the penicillin-allergic patient. Spectinomycin is not presently available in the United States.

6. For oral gonococcal infection, only ceftriaxone is recommended.

7. It is cost-effective to treat for coexistent *Chlamydia* infection without screening for *Chlamydia trachomatis*. Doxycycline or azithromycin may be prescribed.

8. Females should be tested for pregnancy before any tetracycline is given.

ENDO, GI/N

E 100   A 57-year-old man follows a Mediterranean diet. Which of the following is an expected result?

A. Reduced low-density lipoprotein (LDL) cholesterol
B. Reduced insulin resistance
C. Reduced C-reactive protein
D. Increased platelet agglutination
E. Reduced prostaglandin activity

Answer: A, B, and C
A, B, and C are correct because the Mediterranean diet reduces LDL cholesterol in addition to decreasing insulin resistance and decreasing inflammatory markers (e.g., C-reactive protein).

■ **You should know:**

1. The Mediterranean diet is high in unsaturated oils (canola, olive), peanuts, and avocados.

PUL

E 101   A 62-year-old woman has a nonproductive cough for the past 2 weeks. Which of the following medicines may be the causative factor?

A. Diltiazem
B. Doxazosin
C. Hydrochlorothiazide
D. Clonidine
E. Captopril

Answer: E
E is correct because 10% to 20% of patients taking an angiotensin-converting enzyme inhibitor (ACEI) develop a nonproductive cough.

■ **You should know:**

1. Angiotensin-receptor blockers are much less likely than ACEIs to produce a cough.

2. ACEI-induced cough generally starts within 1 week of initiation of therapy, but the onset may be delayed up to 6 months.

3. After cessation of the ACEI, resolution of the cough typically occurs in 1 week but may take up to 1 month after cessation of the medication.

4. The medication-induced cough is *not more common* in the asthmatic patient. Further, the ACEI does not exacerbate airflow obstruction in the asthmatic.

5. The heart failure patient in whom ACEI therapy is initiated and then develops a cough represents an important clinical problem. The ACEI may be causing the cough, but worsening heart failure itself may produce a cough

due to pulmonary congestion. The clinician must use such factors as weight gain (or loss), presence (or absence) of pulmonary rales, and presence (or absence) of gallop rhythm in determining the etiology of the cough.

PUL, ID

E 102   The primary goal of Pneumonia Patient Outcomes Research Team (PORT) is which of the following?

A. Define the specific antibiotic for treatment of pneumonia
B. Select patients requiring intensive care unit
C. Identify patients requiring pneumococcal vaccine
D. Select low-risk patients for outpatient treatment
E. Identify patients requiring intubation

Answer: D

D is correct because PORT score is based upon the patient's age, comorbid conditions (e.g., heart failure, liver or renal disease), physical examination, and laboratory and radiographic findings. The total point sum recommends the site of patient care.

You should know:

1. The causative organism is not identified in nearly half of adult patients who develop community-acquired pneumonia (CAP). However, *Streptococcus pneumoniae* is the most common identified infecting organism.

2. Other bacteria that commonly cause community-acquired pneumonia (CAP) include *Haemophilus influenzae, Mycoplasma pneumoniae,* and *Chlamydia pneumoniae.* Common viral pathogens include influenza virus, respiratory syncytial virus, and adenovirus.

3. Sputum Gram stain should be performed in the patient whose sputum is purulent.

4. Outpatient treatment of CAP may include macrolides (clarithromycin, azithromycin), doxycycline, or fluoroquinolones. These antibiotics are preferred over penicillin because penicillin is not effective against *Mycoplasma* and *Chlamydia.*

5. Pneumonias that may be complicated by cavitation and lung abscess include those caused by *Staphylococcus aureus, Klebsiella pneumoniae, Pseudomonas aeruginosa,* and *Legionella pneumophila.* In aspiration pneumonia, the lung abscess is typically related to infection by anaerobic organisms including *Peptostreptococcus, Fusobacterium,* and *Bacteroides.*

6. Gram-negative *Pseudomonas* is an important infecting organism, for it is a common cause of nosocomial pneumonia, urinary tract infection, surgical site infection, and bacteremia. Cystic fibrosis patients are particularly prone to infection from *Pseudomonas* and *Staphylococcus.*

7. The patient who has diabetes mellitus and the patient suffering from chronic alcohol abuse are at increased risk *of Klebsiella pneumoniae.*

8. In most cases, Legionnaires' disease is transmitted to humans by inhalation of the infecting organism. Showers, mist machines, and whirlpool spas have been identified as sources of infected aerosols. Patients with chronic lung disease, smokers, and immunocompromised patients are at highest risk for

developing Legionnaires' disease. Patients may be toxic with high fever, pleurisy, and cavitary pneumonia. Azithromycin, clarithromycin, or a fluoroquinolone is appropriate therapy.

9. In a patient who has pneumonia, do not await test results before starting an antibiotic.

CV, ENDO, GU, REPRO

E 103   A patient who has which of the following diseases should be treated with an angiotensin-converting enzyme inhibitor (ACEI)?

A. Acute anterior wall myocardial infarction
B. Diabetic nephropathy
C. Hypertension and diabetes without nephropathy
D. Amyloidosis
E. Hypertensive heart disease

Answer: A, B, C, and E
A, B, C, and E are correct because patients with proteinuria, both diabetic and non-diabetic, have reduced *progression* of glomerular disease when taking an angiotensin-converting enzyme inhibitor (ACEI). There is no evidence that an ACEI or an ARB is effective in primary prevention of diabetic nephropathy, that is, *preventing* the onset of microalbuminuria. An ACEI should be given early and continued indefinitely in the patient who has had an ST elevation myocardial infarction (STEMI) regardless of the left ventricular ejection fraction unless a contraindication exists.

■ **You should know:**

1. In patients who have had ST elevation myocardial infarction (STEMI), beta-adrenergic blockers added to ACEIs further improve survival.

2. In patients with hypertensive heart disease, ACEIs promote regression of hypertrophy. Their use in other patients who have pure *diastolic* heart failure (i.e., without concomitant systolic failure) is unclear.

3. Adverse effects of ACEIs include hypotension, renal failure (especially in patients who have bilateral renal stenosis), cough, and hyperkalemia. Hyperkalemia is more common in the elderly and in those taking potassium-sparing diuretics or NSAIDs.

4. ACEIs are contraindicated in the pregnant woman.

PUL

E 104   A 64-year-old man with a long history of smoking has a 3-month history of progressive weakness and increasing cough. In the past week, he has twice coughed up a teaspoonful of red blood. Examination shows a wasted man with a firm right supraclavicular node, decreased tactile fremitus, and absent breath sounds over the lower half of the right posterior chest. Which of the following is the most likely diagnosis?

A. Squamous cell carcinoma of lung with effusion
B. Adenocarcinoma of lung with effusion
C. Atelectasis of right lower lobe
D. Bronchiectasis of right lower lobe
E. Right pneumothorax

Essentials is designed to promote critical thinking and enrich your knowledge base. Therefore, many questions will have more than one correct answer.

Answer: A

A is correct because squamous cell carcinoma of the lung commonly metastasizes to regional lymph nodes and causes development of pleural effusion.

▓ You should know:

1. The typical signs of pleural effusion are decreased tactile fremitus, dullness to percussion, and decreased breath sounds in the area overlying the effusion.

2. Pleural fluid samples should be examined for glucose, lactate dehydrogenase (LDH), protein, amylase, and differential white blood cell count.

3. An *exudative* pleural effusion is caused by pleural and lung inflammation or from movement of fluid from the peritoneal into the pleural space. An exudate has one or more of these features:
   - Pleural fluid protein/serum protein ratio greater than 0.5
   - Pleural fluid lactate dehydrogenase (LDH)/serum LDH ratio greater than 0.6
   - Pleural fluid lactate dehydrogenase (LDH) greater than two thirds of upper limit of normal of serum lactate dehydrogenase (LDH)
   - A pleural fluid lactate dehydrogenase (LDH) greater than 1,000 IU/L is typically found in the patient with empyema

4. A *transudative* effusion occurs in the absence of pleural disease. Pleural fluid glucose is equal to plasma glucose. The white blood cell count in the pleural fluid is less than 1,000/microL and predominantly mononuclear. Total fluid protein is usually less than 3.0 g/dL.

5. Causes of transudative pleural effusion include heart failure, hypoalbuminemia (cirrhosis, nephrotic syndrome), hypothyroidism, and pulmonary embolism.

6. Causes of an exudative effusion include pneumonic effusions (bacterial, fungal, and viral), malignant effusions, tuberculosis, sarcoidosis, pulmonary embolism, and abdominal inflammation (e.g., abscess, pancreatitis) or abdominal malignancy. Note that pulmonary embolism may cause transductive or exudative effusion.

7. A low pleural fluid glucose occurs in exudative effusions, most commonly due to pneumonia or malignancy.

8. A pleural fluid amylase level greater than the upper limit of normal of serum amylase suggests acute pancreatitis, esophageal rupture, or lung cancer.

9. In consolidation of the lung, as in lobar pneumonia due to *Streptococcus pneumoniae*, physical signs include increased tactile fremitus and bronchial (tubular) breath sounds.

10. Paraneoplastic syndromes occur in about 15% of lung cancer patients. *Small cell* lung cancer may be associated with:
    - Inappropriate secretion of antidiuretic hormone (SIADH) producing hyponatremia and low serum osmolality
    - Ectopic adrenocorticotropic hormone (ACTH) production

11. *Squamous cell* carcinoma of the lung may be associated with a paraneoplastic syndrome causing hypercalcemia due to secretion of parathyroid hormone–related protein.

12. Remember, hypercalcemia in malignancy is most often due to osteolytic metastases, especially from breast cancer and non–small cell cancer of the lung.

PUL

E 105   A 54-year-old healthy woman is receiving heparin for treatment of deep vein thrombosis caused by trauma to her lower right leg. A normal value of which of the following is considered to be most specific in excluding a complicating pulmonary embolism?

A. Serum brain natriuretic peptide
B. Systemic arterial P_{CO_2} (Pa_{CO_2})
C. Serum D-dimer
D. Systemic arterial P_{O_2} (Pa_{O_2})
E. Right ventricular chamber volume on echocardiography

Answer: C
C is correct because a normal serum value of D-dimer less than 500 ng/mL by ELISA is sufficient to exclude pulmonary embolism in a patient with a low or moderate pretest probability of pulmonary embolism.

▪ **You should know:**

1. Deep vein thrombosis (DVT) and pulmonary embolism (PE) may be considered as two manifestations of the same disorder—venous thromboembolism. Therefore, a combination of clinical algorithms and objective diagnostic tests is used in an effort to more accurately diagnose these conditions.

2. In determining the probability of DVT, Wells criteria are used to determine which patients should undergo testing (e.g., ultrasonography). Wells criteria for the probability of DVT include the following:
   • Recent orthopedic casting or paralysis/paresis
   • Recent bed confinement longer than 3 days or major surgery within the past month
   • Swelling of the entire leg
   • Calf swelling
   • Pitting edema
   • Collateral nonvaricose veins
   • Active cancer or cancer treated within 6 months
   • An alternative diagnosis is more likely

3. In summary, the evaluation of the patient *suspected of having DVT* includes history, physical examination, Wells probability score, D-dimer testing, and, if indicated, compression ultrasonography or impedance plethysmography.

4. The evaluation of the patient *suspected of having PE* includes history, physical examination, a *modified Wells probability score,* D-dimer testing, and, if indicated, helical (spiral) CT scanning with radiographic contrast or pulmonary angiography.

5. D-dimer, a degradation product of fibrin, is elevated in the presence of thrombus.

6. A serum level greater than 500 ng/mL is abnormal.

Essentials is designed to promote critical thinking and enrich your knowledge base.
Therefore, many questions will have more than one correct answer.

7. Use of D-dimer in diagnosis of pulmonary embolism reveals good sensitivity but poor specificity. D-dimer values are abnormal in 95% of patients who have pulmonary embolism.

8. D-dimer measurement is of greater clinical value when the serum level is normal. If the D-dimer, measured by ELISA, is less than 500 ng/mL, embolism can be excluded with 95% accuracy *in patients considered to have low or moderate probability of pulmonary embolism based on the Wells probability criteria.*

MS, ENDO

E 106   Three days after hitting her right calf against a coffee table, a 57-year-old diabetic woman has aching pain in the affected calf. Examination shows erythema and a palpable linear venous cord in the right calf. No edema is present. Which of the following is the most likely diagnosis?

A. Superficial phlebitis
B. Deep vein thrombosis
C. Cellulitis
D. Erythema nodosum
E. Necrobiosis lipoidica diabeticorum

Answer: A
A is correct because superficial phlebitis causes pain in the area of the inflamed vein. Induration, redness, and a palpable venous cord are typically present.

■ **You should know:**

1. Superficial phlebitis may extend into the deep venous system, resulting in deep vein thrombosis with its potential complication of pulmonary embolism.

2. Treatment of superficial phlebitis includes NSAIDs, local heat, and elevation. Anticoagulants are indicated when there is concomitant deep vein involvement, especially involving the deep femoral vein.

3. Superficial phlebitis arising from the presence of indwelling catheters requires removal of the catheter and antibiotic administration.

4. *Migratory* phlebitis should arouse suspicion of an underlying malignant disease.

5. Chills and fever suggest an infected (suppurative) phlebitis.

6. Necrobiosis lesions are asymptomatic, typically oval yellowish plaques on the anterior leg and ankle areas. This is one dermatologic disorder associated with diabetes mellitus; another is acanthosis nigricans.

CV, ENDO, MS

E 107   Which of the following may be associated with high cardiac output heart failure?

A. Arteriovenous fistula
B. Hyperthyroidism
C. Paget's disease of bone
D. Beriberi
E. Aortic valve regurgitation

Answer: A, B, C, and D

A, B, C, and D are correct because high cardiac output heart failure is of diverse origin, including thiamine vitamin deficiency, hyperthyroid state, arteriovenous fistula, and Paget's disease of bone.

You should know:

1. High-output heart failure is characterized by ventricular performance that is greater than normal yet inadequate to meet the metabolic needs of the body. Symptoms include dyspnea and edema. Signs typically include tachycardia, bounding pulses, increased pulse pressure, rales, peripheral edema, and gallop rhythm.

2. Arteriovenous fistulas may be congenital or acquired. Acquired fistulas are usually the result of penetrating trauma (e.g., bullet wound). The direct communication between artery and vein arises as part of the healing process. The onset of high-output failure from such a wound occurs about 2 years after the injury but may occur as early as 6 months.

3. Hyperthyroidism increases the metabolic rate, which in turn causes a reduction in systemic vascular resistance with subsequent increase in cardiac output. Hyperthyroidism is a common cause of atrial fibrillation, especially in the elderly patient.

4. Beriberi, resulting from thiamine vitamin deficiency, may produce high-output heart failure.

5. Paget's disease of bone results in formation of arteriovenous fistulas within bone that may cause high-output failure. Patients with Paget's disease of bone have elevated serum alkaline phosphatase, normal serum calcium and gamma glutamyl transpeptidase (GGTP), and increased urinary excretion of hydroxyproline. Bone radiography may show radiolucent areas or a "cotton wool" appearance. Bone scan is diagnostic of Paget's showing "hot spots" in affected bone areas.

GU, CV, ENDO, GI/N

E 108 In a patient who has metabolic acidosis, which of the following is the most important laboratory determination to be made?

A. Osmolal gap
B. Auscultatory gap
C. Systemic arterial carboxyhemoglobin
D. Anion gap
E. Left ventricular end-diastolic pressure

Answer: D

D is correct because the anion gap helps define the underlying cause of the metabolic acidosis.

You should know:

1. Metabolic acidosis (MA) is characterized by low pH and low bicarbonate concentration.

2. Metabolic acidosis (MA) may be due to increased acid production in the body (lactic acidosis or diabetic ketoacidosis), to loss of bicarbonate (severe

diarrhea), or, less frequently, to diminished ability of the kidney to excrete acid.

3. A patient with MA has a compensatory increase in ventilation. This reduces $Paco_2$ in an attempt to normalize pH. Kussmaul breathing in the patient with diabetic ketoacidosis is an example of increased compensatory ventilation.

4. Every patient with metabolic acidosis (MA) should have an anion gap calculation in order to determine the etiology of the acidosis.

5. Anion gap = Na − (Cl + HCO$_3$). Generally, the normal anion gap is 7 to 12 mEq/L.

6. Causes of *increased anion gap metabolic acidosis (MA)* include:
   • Lactic acidosis due to reduced systemic perfusion and tissue hypoxia
   • Diabetic ketoacidosis
   • Renal failure (occurs in most renal failure patients)
   • Toxic agent ingestion (e.g., ethylene glycol, methanol, or overdose of aspirin)

7. *Normal anion gap metabolic acidosis (MA)* is most commonly noted in the patient who has severe diarrhea causing marked bicarbonate loss.

8. Treatment of metabolic acidosis (MA) includes, in addition to treatment of the underlying disorder, administration of intravenous sodium bicarbonate.

MS, REPRO, ENDO

E 109   Which of the following conditions may be complicated by carpal tunnel syndrome affecting both hands and wrists?

A. Acromegaly
B. Hypothyroidism
C. Rheumatoid arthritis
D. Amyloidosis
E. Pregnancy

Answer: A, B, C, D, and E

A, B, C, D, and E are correct because carpal tunnel syndrome (CTS) is common in systemic disorders. These include rheumatoid arthritis, hypothyroidism, diabetes mellitus, acromegaly, and amyloidosis as well as the patient on long-term hemodialysis. Systemic disorders cause bilateral carpal tunnel syndrome with both wrists and hands involved over a short time period. Carpal tunnel syndrome (CTS) is very common during pregnancy. The symptoms disappear promptly after delivery.

▌ **You should know:**

1. Symptoms include pain, burning, and tingling in the first 2½ fingers and the palmar aspect of the thumb. Symptoms are *typically worse at night.*

2. Examination shows decreased sensation in the median nerve distribution. Muscle weakness and thenar atrophy appear later.

3. Tinel's sign and Phelan's sign are typically positive in carpal tunnel syndrome (CTS).

4. Treatment of the underlying disorder is the first consideration. Carpal tunnel syndrome (CTS) is treated with wrist splinting, corticosteroid injection into the tunnel, nonsteroidal anti-inflammatory drugs (NSAIDs), or surgical decompression.

5. In addition to systemic disorders, carpal tunnel syndrome (CTS) occurs in those with repetitive use of the wrists.

ID, REPRO, ENDO

E 110   In which of the following patients is live attenuated influenza vaccine recommended?

A. Chronic obstructive lung disease
B. Diabetes mellitus
C. 48-year-old healthy woman
D. Pregnant woman
E. Person with egg allergy

Answer: C
C is correct because the live vaccine is recommended for healthy persons between ages 2 and 49 years.

▪ **You should know:**

1. There are two influenza vaccines in the United States: trivalent, *inactivated* vaccine and the intranasally administered trivalent *live-attenuated* vaccine.

2. Adults who receive the live-attenuated vaccine should be given one dose. Healthy children between ages 2 and 8 years who have never received any influenza vaccine should receive two doses of live vaccine, separated by at least 4 weeks.

3. *Contraindications to live, intranasal vaccine:*
   • Immunocompromised patients or contacts with these patients
   • Pregnant women
   • Patients with diabetes mellitus and chronic lung or heart disease
   • Persons who are allergic to eggs
   • Persons with a history of Guillain-Barré syndrome

4. Recommendations for *inactive* vaccine:
   • Persons 50 years of age and older
   • Residents of long-term care facilities
   • Patients with chronic lung and heart disease
   • Patients with chronic metabolic disorders (e.g., diabetes mellitus, renal disease, immunosuppressed states)
   • Women who will become pregnant during the flu season
   • Health-care workers and contacts of high-risk patients

5. The antibody response to influenza vaccine in the HIV-infected patient is related to the CD4 counts and viral load. Vaccine is recommended for all these patients.

6. The clinician should know that *both inactivated and live intranasal* influenza vaccines contain egg protein. Careful assessment of risk must be considered before administering either vaccine to a patient who is allergic to eggs.

Essentials is designed to promote critical thinking and enrich your knowledge base.
Therefore, many questions will have more than one correct answer.

7. All children with cystic fibrosis (CF) should receive pneumococcal vaccine. CF patients older than 6 months should receive inactive, not live, influenza vaccine.

8. Please refer to three Recommended Immunization Schedules, CDC, U.S. 2012: For Ages 0 through 6 Years; 7 Years through 18 Years; and Adult Immunization Schedule. The CDC schedules delineate the proper form of vaccine to be administered to specific patient populations.

ENDO, CV, EENT, REPRO

E 111   A 41-year-old woman has a 3-week history of insomnia, increased warmth, tremulousness, and palpitations. Blood pressure is 160/60 mm Hg; pulse, 122/min; and respirations, 19/min. Examination shows lid lag and exophthalmos. Which of the following is the most likely diagnosis?

A. Toxic adenoma of the thyroid
B. Factitious hyperthyroidism
C. Graves disease
D. Thyrotropin-secreting pituitary tumor
E. Thyroiditis

Answer: C
C is correct because Graves disease is the only hyperthyroid condition that is associated with exophthalmos.

▓ You should know:

1. The hyperthyroid state is caused by the following disorders:
   • Graves disease, an autoimmune disease characterized by presence of anti–thyroid-stimulating hormone (TSH) receptor antibodies; only Graves disease patients may exhibit exophthalmos and pretibial myxedema
   • Toxic adenomas, either single or multiple
   • Excessive exogenous thyroid hormone ingestion
   • Thyroiditis, causing transient hyperthyroidism

2. Atrial fibrillation is associated with any cause of hyperthyroidism and is more frequent in the elderly patient.

3. A suppressed serum TSH level is the best test for hyperthyroidism. Only in the *rare* cases of a TSH-secreting pituitary tumor is the serum TSH elevated.

4. Propranolol reduces tremor, sweating, and palpitations in the hyperthyroid patient.

5. Thiourea medications (propylthiouracil [PTU] and methimazole) may be given for 12 to 24 months in young adults. Propylthiouracil (PTU) is preferred in pregnant patients or those who are breastfeeding. Thiourea agents are used to prepare patients for thyroid surgery and for selected patients, usually elderly or cardiac patients, who are to receive radioactive iodine (RAI) treatment.

6. Agranulocytosis may occur from thiourea agents. It tends to occur in the first 2 months of therapy. A sore throat in the patient often heralds the onset of this blood disorder.

7. Radioactive iodine (RAI) should not be given to pregnant women. Patients given radioactive iodine (RAI) must be followed serially for the development of hypothyroidism.

8. Subacute thyroiditis (de Quervain's) is of suspected viral etiology. It is most common in young women. It is associated with painful enlargement of the thyroid, often associated with dysphagia and fever. A hyperthyroid state occurs in half of these patients and is transitory, lasting several weeks. Ultimately, most of these patients regain euthyroid status.

9. Serum TSH is considered to be the most sensitive test to diagnose hyperthyroidism and *primary* hypothyroidism.

10. In the patient with primary hypothyroidism, monitoring of serum TSH level and assessment of the clinical response are used to determine optimal dosing of thyroid medication.

11. The clinician should be aware that many medicines will influence levothyroxine dosage by one of the following mechanisms:
    • Increased liver metabolism of the medication
    • Inhibition of gastrointestinal absorption of thyroxine related to gastric acidity or coexisting gastrointestinal disorders (e.g., inflammatory bowel disease, celiac disease, and *H. pylori* gastritis)

NEUR, ID

E 112 Suspicion of which of the following is an indication for performing lumbar puncture?
  A. Meningitis
  B. Subarachnoid hemorrhage
  C. Multiple sclerosis
  D. Guillain-Barré syndrome
  E. Lewy body dementia

Answer: A, B, C, and D
A is correct because lumbar puncture (LP) is indicated in the patient with fever, headache, and altered mental status. The lumbar puncture may help to differentiate bacterial from viral meningitis. B is correct because lumbar puncture is important in the patient with suspected subarachnoid hemorrhage when CT imaging is negative. C is correct because the cerebrospinal fluid (CSF) in multiple sclerosis (MS) often shows lymphocytosis and slightly increased protein level. Elevated level of IgG in the cerebrospinal fluid (CSF) is noted in many MS patients. D is correct because the Guillain-Barré patient has an increased protein level but a normal cell count in the CSF.

You should know:

1. The finding of xanthochromic CSF is an important indicator of earlier bleeding as opposed to a traumatic tap causing red cells in the cerebrospinal fluid.

2. Complications of a lumbar puncture include headache, infection, bleeding, and cerebral herniation. Headache typically occurs 24 to 48 hours after the procedure and may be frontal or occipital. Headache is increased in the upright and lessened in the recumbent position. These patients may also have nausea, vomiting, dizziness, and visual symptoms.

Essentials is designed to promote critical thinking and enrich your knowledge base. Therefore, many questions will have more than one correct answer.

3. Treatment of the LP-related headache includes epidural blood patch, bed rest, and analgesics.

4. Herniation due to increased intracranial pressure is the most serious complication. Those at greatest risk are patients with focal neurologic signs or papilledema.

5. Preferably, CT imaging is performed before a lumbar puncture. However, neurologists may opt to perform LP without prior CT imaging in selected patients who are suspected of having bacterial meningitis.

6. Contraindications to lumbar puncture include the following:
   - Increased intracranial pressure
   - Bleeding diathesis (e.g., thrombocytopenia)
   - Spinal epidural abscess

7. In a succinct review, the following table compares cerebrospinal fluid (CSF) findings in aseptic (viral) and purulent (bacterial meningitis):

	Cells/microL	Glucose (mg/dL)	Protein (mg/dL)	Pressure (mm H_2O)
Bacterial	200–20,000 neutrophils	Low, less than 45	High, greater than 50	Increased
Viral	25–2,000 lymphocytes	NL or low	High, greater than 50	Increased

(NL = normal)

8. In suspected meningitis the following studies should be performed on CSF:
   - Gram stain
   - Culture and sensitivity
   - Polymerase chain reaction if herpes simplex or varicella infection is suspected

9. Up to 40% of asymptomatic persons are carriers of *Neisseria meningitidis*, the infecting bacteria in meningococcal meningitis.

10. Meningococcal meningitis occurs in children, adolescents, and adults. In addition to the classic signs and symptoms of meningitis, including fever, headache, nausea, and vomiting, patients who have meningococcal meningitis will have a petechial or purpuric rash.

11. Meningococcal vaccine is recommended for college freshmen (particularly those who live in a dormitory), military recruits, and asplenic patients (surgical splenectomy or autosplenectomy). Asplenic patients are at markedly increased risk of infection from encapsulated bacteria (*N. meningitidis*, *H. influenzae*, *S. pneumoniae*). Asplenic patients should also receive pneumococcal and *H. influenzae* vaccines.

12. In an outbreak of meningococcal meningitis antibiotic therapy is indicated to eradicate nasal carriage in asymptomatic persons. Prophylactic antibiotics are also given to "close contacts" of patients, meaning those who were within 3 feet of patients or spent more than 8 hours with the patient just before onset of symptoms.

13. With few exceptions, patients who have pneumococcal meningitis do not have a rash. Chemoprophylaxis is not given to persons in contact with patients.

14. Guillain-Barré syndrome (GBS) is an ascending inflammatory disease of the nervous system. *Campylobacter infection is the most common precipitant of GBS.* The patient typically has symmetrical neurologic symptoms including paresthesias of the feet and weakness of the legs. The weakness may proceed in a cephalad direction. Loss of deep tendon reflexes is typical. GBS may be treated with either plasma exchange or infusion of intravenous immune globulin (IVIG).

15. A summary of *Campylobacter*-related diseases is appropriate. *Both GBS and reactive arthritis are associated with Campylobacter infection.* However, reactive arthritis is also associated with other infecting organisms—namely, enteric infection by *Salmonella, Shigella, Yersinia,* and *Clostridium difficile.* Further, reactive arthritis is associated with the genital pathogen *Chlamydia trachomatis.* Therefore, in a patient who has reactive arthritis, stool culture and urinary DNA amplification for *Chlamydia* should be performed.

ID, GI/N

E 113 Which of the following is an organism that causes an infectious, noninflammatory diarrhea?

A. Norovirus
B. Rotavirus
C. Enterotoxigenic *Escherichia coli*
D. *Staphylococcus aureus*
E. *Giardia*

Answer: A, B, C, D, and E
A, B, C, D, and E are correct because norovirus, rotavirus, *Giardia*, enterotoxic *Escherichia coli,* and *Staphylococcus aureus* enterotoxin cause infectious, noninflammatory diarrhea.

■ **You should know:**

1. Acute infectious diarrhea is divided into two categories:
   • Noninflammatory, with symptoms related to the small bowel (i.e., cramps and nonbloody diarrhea)
     (1) Organisms include norovirus, rotavirus, *Giardia, Cryptosporidium, Staphylococcus aureus* enterotoxin, and enterotoxigenic *Escherichia coli*
   • Inflammatory, with symptoms related to the colon (i.e., bloody diarrhea)
     (1) Invasive organisms include *Entamoeba histolytica, Shigella, Campylobacter, Salmonella,* and *Yersinia*

2. Outbreaks of diarrhea at a common location (e.g., cruise ship or school) suggest viral infection or toxic food source. Norovirus affects all age groups and is a major cause of epidemic diarrhea. This is the primary etiology of nonbacterial gastroenteritis in the United States. Restaurants, long-term care facilities, cruise ships, and day-care centers are frequent venues of infection. Fecal-oral route is the primary route of infection.

3. Unpurified water exposure suggests *Giardia* or *Cryptosporidium* infection. *Giardia* infection is commonly due to drinking mountain water when camping or swimming. *Giardia* is primarily water borne but may be food borne when contaminated, uncooked food is eaten. Patients with giardiasis may be asymptomatic or have diarrhea. Stool microscopy looking for cysts

and trophozoites is performed. Stool immunoassay techniques are utilized in addition to microscopy. Metronidazole is the preferred therapy.

4. *Cryptosporidium* infection, causing noninflammatory diarrhea, is considered the leading cause of recreational water-associated outbreaks of diarrhea.

5. Recent travel suggests travelers' diarrhea. This is most commonly due to bacterial infection, frequently with enterotoxigenic *Escherichia coli, Shigella* species, or *Campylobacter jejuni,* although other organisms may be causative. This is usually benign and self-limited. Typically, stools are loose and the patient has cramps and occasionally vomiting. Fever is rare.

6. Watery, nonbloody diarrhea with cramps, nausea, or vomiting suggests a small bowel source caused by a toxin (*Staphylococcus aureus* or enterotoxigenic *Escherichia coli*), viral infection, or *Giardia.* Tissue invasion does not occur; therefore, leukocytes are not found in the feces.

7. AIDS patients commonly have enterocolitis related to bacteria (e.g., *Campylobacter, Shigella, Salmonella*), viruses, and protozoa (e.g., *Cryptosporidium, Entamoeba histolytica, Giardia*). HIV patients are likely to demonstrate more serious symptoms including bacteremia.

8. *Campylobacter* enterocolitis, in contrast to *Giardia,* is frequently associated with high fever and chills. Note that *Campylobacter* may be associated with benign travelers' diarrhea or with a much more toxic state, enteritis. In enteritis, fever is present. (*Campylobacter* infection is noted to be an antecedent infection in patients who develop Guillain-Barré syndrome.)

9. For those patients traveling to high-risk areas, *prophylaxis* is recommended for those who have irritable bowel syndrome, AIDS, diabetes mellitus, or are taking immunosuppressive medication. Norfloxacin, ciprofloxacin, ofloxacin, or trimethoprim-sulfamethoxazole may be taken. For healthy patients, prophylaxis against travelers' diarrhea is not recommended. However, patients may be given a supply of antimicrobial medication to be taken if needed.

10. *Treatment* of mild to moderate travelers' diarrhea includes the following:
    - Oral fluid replacement with broth, fruit juice, or electrolyte solutions
    - Antibiotics for more than four unformed stools per day, fever, blood, pus, or mucus in stool
      (1) Fluoroquinolones for 2 or 3 days; azithromycin or rifaximin may be prescribed
      (2) Fluoroquinolones are contraindicated in pregnancy
    - Antimotility agents
      (1) Use in conjunction with antibiotics

11. Clearly, protozoans are a common cause of infectious diarrhea. Therefore, a brief summary of the efficacy of metronidazole is appropriate.
    - Metronidazole is used *orally* in the treatment of the following:
      (1) Protozoans: *Giardia, Balantidium, Entamoeba* (amebiasis), *Trichomonas*
      (2) Anaerobic bacteria: *Bacteroides,* anaerobic streptococci, *Clostridium difficile* (antibiotic-related diarrhea), *Gardnerella* (bacterial vaginosis), *Helicobacter pylori* (microaerophilic)
    - Metronidazole is used *topically* in the treatment of rosacea.

GI/N

E 114 Which of the following is a typical manifestation of ulcerative colitis?

A. Bloody diarrhea
B. Abscess formation
C. Fecal urgency
D. Megaloblastic anemia
E. Malabsorption syndrome

Answer: A and C
A is correct because bloody diarrhea is the key manifestation of ulcerative colitis. C is correct because rectal inflammation causes the patient to experience fecal urgency.

■ **You should know:**

1. Ulcerative colitis (UC), a disease of unknown cause, is characterized by intermittent flare-ups and remissions.

2. Extent of colonic involvement in ulcerative colitis (UC) is variable, including limited proctitis, proctosigmoiditis, left-sided colitis, or generalized colon inflammation.

3. Diagnosis is established by sigmoidoscopy.

4. Colonoscopy should not be performed in patients with severe disease because of risk of perforation or inducing megacolon.

5. Patients with proctitis may be treated with mesalamine suppositories or hydrocortisone foam.

6. Patients with proctosigmoiditis may be treated with 5-aminosalicylate or hydrocortisone enemas.

7. The treatment of patients having more extensive involvement is variable, dependent upon extent and toxicity of disease. Some are treated with sulfasalazine or mesalamine tablets or balsalazide. Corticosteroids and tumor necrosis factor agents are reserved for those suffering from severe disease.

8. Relapses are common. Therefore, long-term therapy with sulfasalazine or olsalazine or mesalamine is recommended. Selected patients may require an anti-TNF (tissue necrosis factor) agent or an immunosuppressive medication.

9. Extraintestinal complications include uveitis, skin disorders (e.g., erythema nodosum or pyoderma gangrenosum), large joint arthritis, and cholangitis.

10. Ulcerative colitis patients have an increased risk of colon cancer.

11. Nonaspirin, nonselective NSAIDs can produce a hemorrhagic diarrhea that is similar to ulcerative colitis.

GI/N, EENT, PUL

E 115   Which of the following is a symptom that may be related to gastroesophageal reflux?

A. Hoarseness
B. Wheezing
C. Water brash
D. Diarrhea
E. Loss of taste

Answer: A, B, and C

A, B, and C are correct because, in addition to the classic symptom of heartburn, gastroesophageal reflux can cause hoarseness, water brash, and wheezing.

■ **You should know:**

1. The classic symptom of gastroesophageal reflux is heartburn, most frequently occurring about an hour after meals and also during recumbency. Other symptoms include water brash (hypersalivation, "foaming"), sour taste in the mouth, dysphagia, hoarseness, wheezing, sore throat, and chest pain. Laryngitis and hoarseness are related to gastric contents in contact with the pharynx.

2. Upper endoscopy is normal in half of patients who have reflux. In selected patients, ambulatory esophageal pH monitoring is performed. This is considered the best procedure to document reflux.

3. Some patients with chronic reflux will develop Barrett's esophagus in which the squamous epithelium of the esophagus is replaced by columnar epithelium. Barrett's esophagus may lead to stricture or, more seriously, adenocarcinoma.

4. Many patients can be treated empirically. If the patient does not properly respond, further investigation is warranted.

5. Principles of general medical treatment of reflux:
   • Do not lie down for at least 2 hours after a meal
   • Elevate head of bed
   • Avoid acidic foods (e.g., colas, red wine, orange juice)
   • Avoid fatty foods, peppermint, chocolate
   • Avoid alcohol intake and smoking

6. Medicinal treatment:
   • For occasional symptoms: H2-receptor antagonists (e.g., cimetidine, ranitidine, nizatidine)
   • For reflux-causing symptoms several times per week: the above H2-receptor antagonists or proton pump inhibitors (e.g., omeprazole, rabeprazole, esomeprazole)

7. Reflux is a trigger of asthma. Some of these patients may not have reflux symptoms. In addition, aspiration may cause acute wheezing in the nonallergic patient.

8. Other patients with reflux may have persistent cough. Again, some of these patients with reflux may have cough without associated heartburn or sour taste in the mouth.

PUL, CV

E 116   A 67-year-old man is receiving external radiation therapy for squamous cell carcinoma of the lung. He now has a 2-day history of aching discomfort in the left calf with associated edema in the affected calf and left ankle. The calf discomfort increases with walking, particularly when ascending stairs. Examination shows mild erythema and edema of the left calf and ankle. The affected calf is warm. No inguinal lymph nodes are felt. Which of the following is the most likely diagnosis?

A. Metastatic carcinoma to left tibia
B. Superficial phlebitis
C. Deep vein thrombosis
D. Paraneoplastic syndrome
E. Cellulitis

Answer: C
C is correct because malignancy, especially lung, pancreas, prostate, kidney, and colon, is a risk factor for deep vein thrombosis.

◼ **You should know:**

1. In 80% of cases, deep vein thrombosis (DVT) is thought to arise in the veins of the calf. Half of these patients may have no symptoms or signs. Others may show evidence of tenderness, overlying erythema, and a palpable venous cord.

2. In addition to trauma and surgery (especially orthopedic, major vascular, and cancer surgery), malignancy is a risk factor for DVT.

3. In addition, inherited hypercoagulable disorders increase risk of DVT. These include the following:
   • Factor V Leiden mutation
   • Deficiency in protein C, protein S, or antithrombin
   • Prothrombin gene mutation

4. Duplex ultrasonography is the preferred initial diagnostic test. (Please see E 105.)

5. Initial medicinal treatment of DVT includes the following:
   • Unfractionated heparin
   • Low molecular weight heparin
   • Fondaparinux

6. For the first episode of uncomplicated DVT the initial treatment is followed by warfarin for 3 to 6 months.

7. Indefinite warfarin therapy is recommended for those with recurrent DVT or a hypercoagulable state.

8. In a patient who has had a *pulmonary embolism,* duration of warfarin anticoagulation depends upon whether this is a first or recurrent embolus and whether an identifiable risk factor, reversible or irreversible, has been identified.

9. Oral contraceptive agents should not be given to women who smoke because of increased risk of venous thrombosis.

10. Venous thrombosis in a patient who has experienced recurrent spontaneous abortions suggests antiphospholipid syndrome.

Essentials is designed to promote critical thinking and enrich your knowledge base. Therefore, many questions will have more than one correct answer.

CV

E 117   A 43-year-old obese man has 30 minutes of diffuse anterior chest pain that is associated with sweating. Vital signs are normal. The patient is not cyanotic. Lungs are clear to auscultation. Heart tones are distant, but no murmur, gallop, or friction rub is heard. No peripheral edema is present. Homans' sign is negative. The patient's electrocardiogram is shown. Which of the following is the most likely diagnosis?

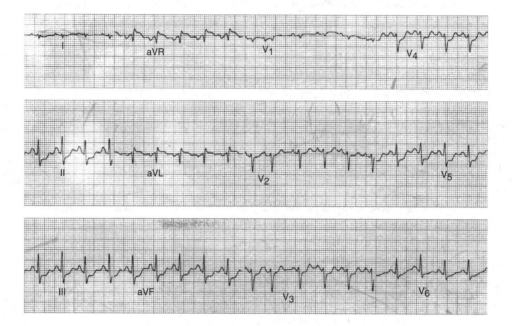

A. Acute pericarditis
B. Pleurodynia
C. Dissection of the aorta
D. Acute coronary syndrome
E. Acute pulmonary embolism

Answer: D
D is correct because *horizontal* ST segment depression is probably the most specific sign of subendocardial myocardial ischemia.

▇ **You should know:**

1. It is the subendocardial layer of the myocardium that is most susceptible to insufficient perfusion (ischemia). Subendocardial ischemia (SEI) is characterized on the electrocardiogram by horizontal ST segment depression or by downward sloping (toward the end) of the ST segment. The T waves may remain positive or may become negative.

2. J point depression followed by an upsloping ST segment may represent subendocardial ischemia but is nonspecific.

3. Changes in T waves are an unreliable indicator of myocardial ischemia. Subendocardial ischemia may be associated with symmetrical T wave inversion, usually in association with ST segment depression. However, T wave inversion is less sensitive and less specific than ST segment depression.

4. Nonspecific ST-T electrocardiographic abnormalities (NSSTTA) relate to slight ST segment depression or T wave inversion or T wave flattening that occurs

without evident cause. NSSTTA may occur in healthy persons, especially shortly after eating, in patients who have either acidosis or alkalosis, in patients who are febrile or anemic, in those who are in a state of heightened adrenergic tone, or in patients who have myocarditis or pulmonary embolism.

REPRO

E 118   Which of the following is a risk factor for a pregnant woman to develop preeclampsia?

A. Cigarette smoking
B. Past history of preeclampsia
C. Family history of preeclampsia
D. First pregnancy
E. Antiphospholipid antibodies

Answer: B, C, D, and E
B and D are correct, but the reason is unclear. C is correct because genetic factors are thought to play a role in susceptibility to preeclampsia. E is correct because antiphospholipid antibodies produce a hypercoagulable state that causes development of preeclampsia.

■ **You should know:**

1. There are four defined hypertensive disorders in pregnancy:
   • Preeclampsia
   • Preexisting hypertension (chronic hypertension)
   • Preeclampsia superimposed upon preexisting hypertension
   • Gestational hypertension

2. Preeclampsia is defined as new-onset hypertension and proteinuria after 20 weeks of gestation in a woman who was previously normotensive.

3. Other risk factors for preeclampsia include pregestational diabetes mellitus, multiple gestation, obesity, preexisting hypertension, collagen vascular disease, and renal disease.

4. Severe preeclampsia is characterized by the presence of central nervous system symptoms (e.g., blurred vision or severe headache), hepatocellular injury, and thrombocytopenia, superimposed upon the hypertension and proteinuria of mild preeclampsia.

5. Eclampsia refers to the onset of grand mal seizures in the woman with preeclampsia.

6. Generalized endothelial dysfunction in the pregnant woman is considered to be the pathophysiologic abnormality accounting for the clinical features of preeclampsia and eclampsia.

7. The definitive treatment of preeclampsia is delivery of the infant because this condition is reversible after delivery.

8. Gestational hypertension is new-onset hypertension developing after the 20th week of gestation and not associated with proteinuria. Blood pressure typically returns to normal by the 12th week postpartum. Antihypertensive therapy in gestational hypertension is reserved for those patients whose systolic blood pressure is 160 mm Hg or higher or whose diastolic pressure is 105 mm Hg or higher. Methyldopa, labetalol, or nifedipine may be prescribed.

Essentials is designed to promote critical thinking and enrich your knowledge base.
Therefore, many questions will have more than one correct answer.

9. Antiphospholipid antibody syndrome is characterized by a hypercoagulable state predisposing to arterial and venous thrombosis. Recurrent fetal loss after the 1st trimester is common. Antiphospholipid antibody syndrome (APS) may be primary or related to systemic lupus erythematosus.

REPRO

E 119   Seven weeks after her last menstrual period, a 32-year-old woman has amenorrhea, abdominal pain, and vaginal bleeding. In addition to serum human chorionic gonadotropin concentration, which of the following is the preferred test to diagnose ectopic pregnancy?

A. MRI scan of the pelvis
B. Culdocentesis
C. Curettage
D. Serum progesterone level
E. Transvaginal ultrasonography

Answer: E
E is correct because transvaginal ultrasonography is valuable in detecting the presence of a gestational sac. Ultrasonography is preferred to MRI scans, culdocentesis, laparoscopy, and curettage.

▓ **You should know:**

1. The diagnosis of ectopic pregnancy is based upon quantitative assay for human chorionic gonadotropin (hCG) and findings on transvaginal ultrasonography.

2. Clinical manifestations of ectopic pregnancy, occurring 6 to 8 weeks after the last menstrual period, are amenorrhea, vaginal bleeding, and abdominal pain.

3. However, these three manifestations are also common in threatened abortion. Transvaginal ultrasonography imaging is the most important diagnostic modality in differentiating ectopic pregnancy from threatened abortion.

4. Signs of ectopic pregnancy are highly variable. Therefore, the diagnosis is based upon human chorionic gonadotropin concentration and imaging study.

5. Risk factors for ectopic pregnancy include:
   • Previous ectopic pregnancy
   • Previous tubal pregnancy
   • History of bilateral coagulation sterilization
   • Current intrauterine device usage
   • In utero estrogen exposure
   • Pelvic inflammatory disease with salpingitis

6. Treatment of ectopic pregnancy includes surgical removal or, in selected cases, administration of methotrexate.

ID, GI/N

E 120   A 34-year-old man has the following hepatitis B serologic markers: HBsAg positive; IgM-anti-HBc positive. Which of the following is the most likely status of the patient?

A. Susceptible to hepatitis B infection
B. Immune to natural infection
C. Immune due to hepatitis B immunization
D. Chronic hepatitis B infection
E. Acute hepatitis B infection

Answer E

E is correct because HBsAg appears in serum 1 to 10 weeks after exposure to the virus and an IgM antibody is present during acute infection.

■ **You should know:**

1. Serologic markers for hepatitis B virus infection (HBV) include:
   - Hepatitis B surface antigen (HBsAg) that is detected by radioimmunoassay (RIA) or enzyme immunoassay (EIA). This marker is no longer detectable after 4 to 6 months in those who recover. Persistence of HBsAg after 6 months indicates chronic infection.
   - Hepatitis B surface antibody (anti-HBs). This persists for life, thus conferring long-term immunity. In hepatitis B infection, anti-HBs appears after disappearance of HBsAg.
   - Hepatitis B core antibody (anti-HBc). This is primarily an IgM antibody present during acute infection. Anti-HBc may persist in the serum for 2 years after acute infection.

2. Hepatitis B core antigen (HBcAg) is not detectable in serum. It is an intracellular antigen in infected liver cells.

3. A template of selected hepatitis B panels is shown.

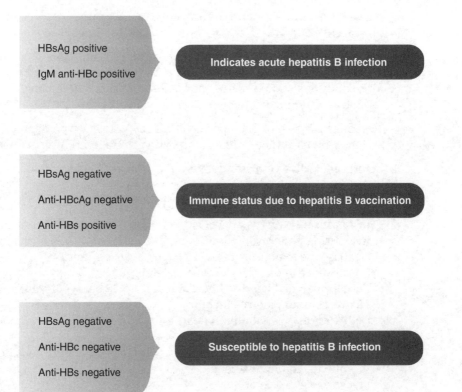

HBsAg positive

IgM anti-HBc positive

Indicates acute hepatitis B infection

HBsAg negative

Anti-HBcAg negative

Anti-HBs positive

Immune status due to hepatitis B vaccination

HBsAg negative

Anti-HBc negative

Anti-HBs negative

Susceptible to hepatitis B infection

Essentials is designed to promote critical thinking and enrich your knowledge base. Therefore, many questions will have more than one correct answer.

E 121   Which of the following is considered to be the least important indication for cesarean delivery?

A. Failure to progress in labor
B. Nonreassuring fetal status
C. Previous cesarean delivery
D. Breech lie
E. Under 1,500 g birth weight baby

Answer: E
E is correct because a low-birth-weight baby is considered a very controversial indication for cesarean delivery.

You should know:

1. Those considered to be the most important indications for cesarean delivery include the following:
   - Failure to progress in labor
   - Nonreassuring fetal status
   - Previous cesarean delivery or hysterotomy
   - Fetal malpresentation (breech or transverse lie)

2. Neural tube defects and hydrocephalus are other very controversial indications.

3. Relaxation of the lower esophageal sphincter and the increased intra-abdominal pressure of pregnancy predispose to gastric aspiration. Therefore, solid food should not be ingested for at least 6 hours and clear liquids for at least 2 hours before elective cesarean delivery.

4. To reduce the risk of postoperative infection, a single preoperative dose of an intravenous antibiotic (e.g., ampicillin or cefazolin) is recommended.

5. Before an elective cesarean delivery the following are indicated:
   - Assessment of fetal lung maturity
   - Maternal blood type and antibody screen

6. Fetal heart rate patterns are considered reassuring or nonreassuring.
   - Reassuring patterns include:
     (1) Baseline fetal heart rate (110 to 160 beats per min)
     (2) Absence of fetal heart rate decelerations
     (3) Normal fetal heart rate variability (6 to 25 beats per min)
   - Nonreassuring patterns include:
     (1) Abnormal variability in heart rate
     (2) Late decelerations
     (3) Sinusoidal heart rate (a pattern of regular variability considered to be due to fetal hypoxemia)
     (4) Variable decelerations

7. Nonreassuring heart rate patterns must be promptly addressed and a determination whether operative intervention in the pregnancy is indicated.

GI/N

E 122   A 49-year-old man has acute, severe, right-upper-quadrant abdominal pain, fever with chills, and jaundice. Blood pressure is 106/72 mm Hg; pulse, 120/min; and axillary temperature, 102°F. White blood cell count is 29,200/microL; hemoglobin, 13.1 g/dL. Which of the following is the preferred initial diagnostic test?

A. Transhepatic cholangiogram
B. Endoscopic retrograde cholangiography
C. Hepatic iminodiacetic acid (HIDA) scan
D. Intravenous cholangiogram
E. Percutaneous liver biopsy

Answer: B

B is correct because endoscopic retrograde cholangiography permits stone extraction or stent placement in the common bile duct in this patient who has cholangitis. Patients with cholangitis have an obstruction in the common bile duct, most commonly by stones, less frequently by benign stricture or malignancy.

■ **You should know:**

1. The clinical picture of right upper quadrant or epigastric pain, fever with chills, and jaundice suggests cholangitis.

2. Many antibiotic regimens appear to be effective. They include the following:
   • Fluoroquinolones
   • Ampicillin-sulbactam
   • Metronidazole-ceftriaxone

3. In evaluation of the patient with jaundice, first determine whether the hyperbilirubinemia is associated with normal or abnormal liver enzymes.

4. Jaundice with normal liver enzymes:
   • Elevated unconjugated ("indirect"): Think of hemolysis, resorption of a hematoma, Gilbert's syndrome
   • Elevated conjugated ("direct"): Think of Dubin-Johnson syndrome

5. Jaundice with abnormal liver enzymes is due to elevated serum conjugated bilirubin concentration. The abnormal liver enzymes may indicate hepatocellular, cholestatic, or infiltrative disease or mechanical biliary obstruction.

6. In hepatocellular disease elevation of serum alanine aminotransferase (ALT) and aspartate aminotransferase (AST) is disproportionate to increases in serum alkaline phosphatase and gamma-glutamyl peptidase (GGTP). Hepatocellular disease may be due to infection, alcohol, toxins (e.g., medicines, illicit drugs, herbal preparations), or autoimmune disease. In alcoholic hepatitis the AST/ALT ratio is often greater than 2:1.

7. Cholestatic jaundice is characterized by disproportionate increase in serum alkaline phosphatase and gamma-glutamyl peptidase (GGTP) compared to aminotransferases. Cholestasis may be intrahepatic as seen in primary biliary cirrhosis or due to medicines (e.g., acetaminophen, penicillins, chlorpromazine, rifampin, trimethoprim-sulfamethoxazole, anabolic and estrogenic steroids) or in primary sclerosing cholangitis that is associated with inflammatory bowel disease. Intrahepatic cholestasis is also present in infiltrative disease of the liver (e.g., due to the granulomatous diseases tuberculosis and sarcoidosis).

Essentials is designed to promote critical thinking and enrich your knowledge base. Therefore, many questions will have more than one correct answer.

8. Mechanical biliary obstruction may be due to benign disease (e.g., stone), parasitic disease (e.g., ascariasis), or malignancy (e.g., carcinoma of the pancreas or gallbladder, ampullary carcinoma, or cholangiocarcinoma).

9. Antimitochondrial antibody testing is highly sensitive and specific for primary biliary cirrhosis. This diagnosis should be suspected in the woman who has fatigue, hyperpigmentation, and itching in addition to cholestatic liver function abnormalities. The skin changes are due to melanin deposition, not jaundice.

10. Anti–smooth muscle antibodies, antinuclear antibodies, and elevated serum globulins are commonly found in patients with autoimmune hepatitis. The clinical presentation varies from an asymptomatic state to acute liver failure. This disease usually occurs in young to middle-aged women. This disease is more frequently noted in patients who have other autoimmune diseases (e.g., type 1 diabetes mellitus, celiac disease, thyroiditis, and idiopathic thrombocytopenic purpura).

GU/REPRO

E 123   Which of the following is the primary pathophysiologic mechanism that is associated with primary dysmenorrhea?
A. Impaired release of nitric oxide from arcuate arteries
B. Decreased estrogen stimulation of the endometrium
C. Heightened progestin stimulation of the endometrium
D. Increased secretion of luteinizing hormone
E. Prostaglandin induction of uterine contraction

Answer: E
E is correct because prostaglandin F 2-alpha (PGF2) and prostaglandin E 2 (PGE2) stimulation of uterine contraction causes uterine ischemia. This is considered to be the cause of the abdominal cramping that typically occurs just before or with onset of menstrual bleeding.

You should know:

1. Dysmenorrhea is characterized as primary or secondary. Primary dysmenorrhea is characterized by menstrual pain in the absence of pelvic disease.

2. Secondary dysmenorrhea may be due to causes including endometriosis, adenomyosis, or leiomyomata of the uterus and pelvic inflammatory disease.

3. Primary dysmenorrhea only occurs during ovulatory cycles.

4. Treatment of primary dysmenorrhea includes application of heat to the lower abdomen, physical exercise, and NSAIDs. Mefenamic acid, meclofenamate, or ibuprofen is commonly prescribed. To those desiring contraception, a combination estrogen-progestin is indicated.

5. Clinical guidelines suggest that routine *Chlamydia* testing be performed in those patients who have dysmenorrhea and who are under the age of 25 years and are sexually active. Transvaginal sonography is generally not considered as part of the initial evaluation of the woman who has dysmenorrhea and a normal gynecologic examination.

PSY/LE, GU

E 124   A 32-year-old woman has premenstrual dysphoric disorder. Her usual activity is impaired by which of the following?

A. Bloating
B. Hopelessness
C. Anger
D. Peripheral edema
E. Mood lability

Answer: B, C, and E

B, C, and E are correct because premenstrual dysphoric disorder is characterized by affective symptoms, including hopelessness, lability of mood, and anger. It is considered to be a more severe form of premenstrual syndrome (PMS).

■ You should know:

1. *Premenstrual syndrome* (PMS) is manifest by repetitive physical and behavioral symptoms that occur in the second half (luteal phase) of the menstrual cycle. PMS symptoms are multitudinous and include fatigue, bloating, edema, irritability, and inability to concentrate.

2. In addition to nonpharmacologic measures, medicinal therapy of both PMS and premenstrual dysphoric disorder includes the following:
   • Selective serotonin receptor inhibitors (SSRIs)
   • Leuprolide, a gonadotropin releasing hormone (GnRH) agonist
   • Danazol, a testosterone derivative (that may cause masculinizing side effects)
   • Alprazolam
   • Spironolactone

GI/N, ID

E 125   A 36-year-old man has active upper gastrointestinal bleeding requiring transfusion. Which of the following is the preferred diagnostic test for diagnosis of *Helicobacter pylori* infection?

A. Fecal antigen immunoassay
B. Gastric biopsy
C. ELISA serology
D. Blood culture
E. Urea breath test

Answer: B

B is correct because histologic analysis for *Helicobacter pylori* is preferred in patients who have active gastrointestinal bleeding.

■ You should know:

1. Serologic tests are less frequently used in the diagnosis of *Helicobacter pylori* infection because they are less accurate than a fecal antigen immunoassay and a C13 urea breath test.

2. Proton pump inhibitors significantly reduce the sensitivity of urea breath tests and fecal antigen assay. These medicines may cause false-negative results. Therefore, they should be discontinued 10 to 14 days before testing. However, these medicines do not affect serologic tests.

Essentials is designed to promote critical thinking and enrich your knowledge base. Therefore, many questions will have more than one correct answer.

3. The diagnosis of *H. pylori* during endoscopy can be made by one of three methods:
   - Urease test of biopsy specimen
   - Histology
   - Bacterial culture

4. Confirmation of *Helicobacter pylori* eradication can be done using either the urea breath test or stool antigen testing. The breath test or stool antigen immunoassay should be performed at least 4 weeks after termination of treatment.

GI/N, ID

E 126   Active *Helicobacter pylori* gastritis is diagnosed in a 51-year-old woman who has recurrent epigastric pain. Which of the following agents is not used in therapy?

A. Clarithromycin
B. Amoxicillin
C. Bismuth subsalicylate
D. Metronidazole
E. Ceftriaxone

Answer: E
E is correct because ceftriaxone is a third-generation cephalosporin that is not appropriate therapy for *Helicobacter pylori*. Ceftriaxone is the treatment of choice for penicillin-resistant gonococcal infections and meningitis due to ampicillin-resistant *Haemophilus influenzae*.

■ **You should know:**

1. *Helicobacter pylori* is a gram-negative rod that resides in the submucosal layer of the stomach causing gastritis. This infection also is present in the majority of non–NSAID-induced duodenal ulcers.

2. There are many treatment options for *H. pylori* ulcers; none has been proven to be optimal. Recommended therapeutic regimens include the following:
   - Proton pump inhibitor, clarithromycin, and amoxicillin
     - (1) In a patient allergic to penicillin, metronidazole may be substituted for amoxicillin
   - Proton pump inhibitor, bismuth subsalicylate, tetracycline, and metronidazole

(Please refer to E 125.)

ENDO, CV, GU

E 127   A 27-year-old man is in diabetic ketoacidosis. Blood pressure is 72/58 mm Hg; pulse, 146/min; respiratory rate, 36/min. Examination shows dry oral mucosa and poor turgor. Plasma glucose is 642 mg/dL; serum potassium, 3.2 mEq/L; and systemic arterial pH, 6.8. Which of the following is the preferred initial intravenous solution to be infused?

A. 0.9% saline
B. 0.45% saline
C. Ringer's lactate
D. 2½% dextrose in normal saline
E. 3% saline

Answer: A

A is correct because infused 0.9% saline (normal saline) remains in the extravascular space thus increasing circulating plasma volume and blood pressure. Sodium does not enter cells. It is the osmotic effect of the sodium that keeps water in the extravascular space.

■ **You should know:**

1. Normal saline (or Ringer's lactate in the patient *not in acidosis*) should be the initial treatment of hypovolemic shock not due to anemia or hemorrhage.

2. In the patient being treated for diabetic acidosis: When dehydration has been corrected with normal saline infusion, evaluate serum sodium concentration. If sodium is high, change the infusion to 0.45% saline (half-normal); if sodium is low, continue normal saline.

3. Insulin therapy in ketoacidosis: Regular insulin administration by continuous intravenous infusion is the treatment of choice. Insulin therapy may be delayed if the initial serum potassium concentration is less than 3.3 mEq/L until replenishment elevates the potassium level to greater than 3.3 mEq/L.

4. Patients with diabetic ketoacidosis need potassium replacement because of high urinary potassium losses during polyuria. Serial serum potassium values should be determined every 2 hours. If the arterial pH is less than 6.9, sodium bicarbonate in water may be given intravenously.

5. Hyperglycemic hyperosmolar state (HHS) is characterized by hyperglycemia (greater than 600 mg/dL), serum osmolality greater than 310 mOsm/kg but with a normal anion gap, and normal systemic arterial pH. Serum bicarbonate is generally in the 15 to 20 mEq/L range. Prerenal azotemia due to severe hypovolemia may occur in these patients causing development of severe azotemia with blood urea nitrogen levels nearly 100 mg/dL.

6. Hyperglycemic hyperosmolar state is most frequently noted in middle-aged and elderly patients with mild diabetes mellitus. It is frequently precipitated by infection (pulmonary or urinary), acute myocardial infarction, stroke, or recent surgery. Patients typically present with polyuria, polydipsia, and weakness. Confusion and coma may occur.

7. The therapy protocol of HHS therapy is the same as the therapy for diabetic ketoacidosis—namely, insulin to lower blood sugar, intravenous fluid administration to reverse hypovolemia and the hyperosmolar state, and replacement of electrolyte loss, particularly potassium.

8. In the HHS treatment plan, initiation of insulin therapy begins when the serum potassium is greater than 3.3 mEq/L. Intravenous administration of serum potassium replacement is dependent upon serum potassium concentration.

ENDO

E 128 A 52-year-old obese man has newly diagnosed type 2 diabetes mellitus. Which of the following is the preferred initial therapy?

A. Metformin
B. Rosiglitazone
C. Miglitol
D. Nateglinide
E. Glipizide

Essentials is designed to promote critical thinking and enrich your knowledge base.
Therefore, many questions will have more than one correct answer.

Answer: A

A is correct because metformin tends to cause less weight gain than other hypo-glycemic agents and thus is preferred therapy in the obese type 2 diabetic patient.

You should know:

1. Principles of treatment of type 2 diabetes include the following:
   - Education on diet, lifestyle, and hygiene
   - Normalization of hyperglycemia
   - Determination of whether diabetic complications exist
   - Assessment of long-term risk
   - Avoid medication that adversely affects plasma glucose or lipid status

2. Glycemic control in the patient who has type 2 diabetes mellitus reduces the risk of *microvascular* complications; it is not known whether *macrovascular* risk is decreased with improved glycemic control.

3. Metformin often leads to modest weight loss or, at least, stabilization. Hypo-glycemia is unlikely with metformin monotherapy. Gastrointestinal side effects are common.

4. Avoid metformin therapy when the patient has a disorder that predis-poses to lactic acidosis. Conditions predisposing to lactic acidosis include the following:
   - Serum creatinine concentration greater than 1.4 mg/dL in women or greater than 1.5 mg/dL in men
   - Decompensated heart failure or hemodynamic instability
   - Liver failure
   - Heavy alcohol intake

5. A patient receiving metformin therapy should not take the medication on the day an intravenous radiocontrast agent is received and for at least 2 days thereafter. Serum creatinine level should be determined 2 to 3 days after ra-diocontrast administration. This is to avoid lactic acidosis if renal insuffi-ciency occurs.

6. If metformin is ineffective or a contraindication to its use is present, a short-acting sulfonylurea (e.g., glipizide or gliclazide) is appropriate therapy. Sul-fonylureas are more likely than metformin to cause hypoglycemia and they tend to cause weight gain.

7. Hemoglobin A1C levels should be determined at 3- to 4-month intervals.

8. Type 2 diabetes mellitus patients who have hypertension must be aggres-sively treated. Blood pressure target is less than 130/80 mm Hg.

9. The "dawn phenomenon" is associated with rapidly rising plasma glucose levels between 3 a.m. and 8 a.m. It occurs in type 1 diabetes patients when the plasma insulin level is low due to complete absorption of the prior evening's insulin dose at the time (early morning) when there is an increased need for insulin (due to morning release of growth hormone, which antago-nizes the action of insulin).

ID, PUL

E 129   In the midst of a recognized influenza outbreak, a 34-year-old woman has fever, chills, sore throat, muscle aching, and cough productive of mucoid sputum. Which of the following should not be prescribed?

   A. Ibuprofen
   B. Oseltamivir
   C. Acetaminophen
   D. Iodopropylidine glycerol
   E. Amantadine

Answer: E
E is correct because amantadine is not recommended therapy due to the high number of resistant influenza viral strains.

■ **You should know:**

1. Influenza A and B produce the same clinical symptoms. Therapy with oseltamivir or zanamivir is of value when started within 48 hours of symptom onset.

2. Acute bronchitis in healthy persons is usually due to viral infection. The bronchitis due to influenza typically is associated with constitutional symptoms (e.g., fever, myalgia, prostration).

3. Viral bronchitis due to such organisms as coronavirus, rhinovirus, and respiratory syncytial virus typically do not have associated constitutional symptoms. Much less frequently, acute bronchitis is due to *Chlamydia*, *Mycoplasma*, or *Bordetella*.

4. Treatment of acute viral bronchitis in the adult includes an analgesic (NSAID, aspirin, acetaminophen), decongestants, bronchodilators, increased fluid intake, and occasionally a cough suppressant. Antibiotics are not recommended as routine treatment of acute bronchitis.

5. Amantadine is prescribed in patients who have Parkinson's disease manifest by mild rigidity or bradykinesia.

GU

E 130   Which of the following conditions is associated with hypokalemia?

   A. Pheochromocytoma
   B. Loop diuretic therapy
   C. Lidocaine therapy
   D. Angiotensin-converting enzyme inhibitor therapy
   E. Alkalosis

Answer: B and E
B is correct because loop diuretics and thiazide diuretics may cause hypokalemia due to increased urinary potassium excretion. E is correct because alkalosis of any etiology causes hydrogen ions to come out of cells into the blood. As a result, potassium moves from serum into cells resulting in hypokalemia.

Essentials is designed to promote critical thinking and enrich your knowledge base. Therefore, many questions will have more than one correct answer.

🔲 **You should know:**

1. Common symptoms associated with hypokalemia include weakness, muscle cramps, and fatigue.

2. The electrocardiographic manifestations of hypokalemia are flattening of the T wave, prominence of the U wave, and ST segment depression.

3. Beta 2-adrenergic agonists promote cellular uptake of potassium. Therefore, nebulized albuterol is a treatment for hyperkalemia. Other treatment options for hyperkalemia include intravenous calcium gluconate, intravenous insulin in glucose solution, and sodium bicarbonate.

4. Angiotensin-converting enzyme inhibitor therapy tends to increase serum potassium due to reduced aldosterone secretion. (With reduced aldosterone secretion, the kidney excretes more sodium and *retains more potassium*.) Patients at increased risk of hyperkalemia from ACEI therapy include those with diabetes mellitus, renal insufficiency, hypovolemia, or those with concurrent intake of potassium-sparing diuretics or NSAIDs.

5. Intravenous lidocaine is used to treat ventricular ectopy in the setting of acute myocardial infarction. Neurologic toxicity is the most common adverse effect of the medicine; the symptoms always resolve with discontinuation of the drug. Side effects include tremor, insomnia or drowsiness, slurred speech, change in sensorium, and hallucinations. Generalized seizures may occur. Lidocaine side effects are more common in the elderly and in those with heart failure or liver impairment.

NEURO

E 131   Antibodies to acetylcholine receptors are typically found in a patient who has which of the following conditions?

A. Myasthenia gravis
B. Multiple sclerosis
C. Amyotrophic lateral sclerosis
D. Guillain-Barré syndrome
E. Hashimoto's disease

Answer: A
A is correct because patients with myasthenia gravis typically have one of several subtypes of antibodies to acetylcholine receptors.

🔲 **You should know:**

1. Myasthenia gravis is a disease affecting skeletal muscles. It does not affect smooth muscle.

2. Graves disease patients have autoantibodies to the thyroid-stimulating hormone (TSH) receptor. Antibodies are not characteristic of other diseases causing hyperthyroidism.

3. Nearly all patients with Hashimoto's thyroiditis have antibodies to thyroglobulin and thyroid peroxidase.

4. 70% of patients who have pernicious anemia have anti–intrinsic factor antibodies. Less frequently, these patients have anti–parietal cell antibodies.

5. Anti–double-stranded DNA (anti-ds DNA) antibodies and anti-Smith (anti-SM) antibodies are considered to be rather highly specific for

systemic lupus erythematosus. However, they are clinically limited by their relative insensitivity.

GU, CV

E 132 A 62-year-old man has diabetic nephropathy with nephrotic syndrome. Which of the following is least likely to be noted in the patient?

A. Hyperlipidemia
B. Hypercoagulable state
C. Hypoalbuminemia
D. Oral fat bodies in the urine
E. Hypertension

Answer: E
E is correct because hypertension is *most unlikely* in nephrotic syndrome (NS) due to decreased circulating intravascular volume. This is caused by the low oncotic pressure related to hypoalbuminemia. Water moves out of the intravascular space into the interstitial area resulting in decreased circulating volume and low blood pressure. The hypoalbuminemia is due to the loss of this protein in the urine.

■ **You should know:**

1. Nephrotic syndrome (NS) is characterized by proteinuria (greater than 3.5 g/day), hypoalbuminemia, edema, and hyperlipidemia.

2. Nephrotic syndrome is a glomerular disease that may be due to primary glomerular disease or secondary to a systemic disease.

3. Primary glomerular diseases that may cause nephrotic syndrome include:
   • Minimal change disease
   • Focal segmented glomerulosclerosis
   • IgA nephropathy

4. Secondary glomerular diseases include:
   • Diabetes mellitus
   • Systemic lupus erythematosus
   • Amyloidosis
   • HIV nephropathy
   • Endocarditis

5. Treatment of nephrotic syndrome includes sodium and fat restriction in the diet, diuretics, ACEIs, HMG-CoA reductase inhibitors, and, if needed, heparin or warfarin for venous or arterial thrombosis.

6. Nephrotic syndrome is associated with a hypercoagulable state. There is an increased incidence of both arterial and venous thrombi, particularly deep vein thrombosis and renal vein thrombosis. The mechanism of hypercoagulability is complex, but is, in part, related to the loss of antithrombin in the urine.

7. Acute renal vein thrombosis should be suspected in the patient who has a hypercoagulable state and has flank pain, microscopic or gross hematuria, increased serum level of lactate dehydrogenase (LDH) without an increase in serum aminotransferases, and increased renal size on imaging.

8. The hyperlipidemia in nephrotic syndrome (NS) is related to hypercholesterolemia and hypertriglyceridemia that increase risk of cardiovascular disease.

Essentials is designed to promote critical thinking and enrich your knowledge base. Therefore, many questions will have more than one correct answer.

9. Lipid droplets in the urine may be free droplets or within hyaline casts (fatty casts).

HEME, CV

E 133   A 56-year-old man has a 2-week history of night sweats. Which of the following may be the underlying etiology?

A. Cushing's disease
B. Endocarditis
C. *Helicobacter pylori* gastric ulcer
D. Sarcoidosis
E. Lymphoma

Answer: B and E

B is correct because endocarditis is an infection that commonly causes night sweats. E is correct because 25% of Hodgkin's disease patients have night sweats. Less commonly, non-Hodgkin's lymphoma patients have nocturnal sweating.

■ **You should know:**

1. The infections most commonly associated with night sweats include tuberculosis, symptomatic HIV infection, and endocarditis.

2. Hodgkin's disease has a bimodal age distribution: 20 to 30 years and 50 to 60 years.

3. Medicines are a common cause of night sweats. All antidepressants, including tricyclics, selective serotonin reuptake inhibitors, venlafaxine, and bupropion, can cause night sweats.

4. In addition, medicine-induced hypoglycemia can cause night sweats.

5. Medicines may cause flushing (e.g., niacin, nitroglycerin, tamoxifen, sildenafil, and, in susceptible persons, alcohol).

6. The distinction between night sweats and menopausal hot flushes (flashes) may be difficult.

NEURO

E 134   Which of the following is the pathophysiologic abnormality in the brain that results in primary parkinsonism?

A. Dopamine depletion
B. Serotonin depletion
C. Increased activity of the reticulostriate system
D. Decreased parasympathetic tone
E. Increased neuronal uptake of norepinephrine

Answer: A

A is correct because primary (idiopathic) parkinsonism is due to a depletion in the brain of the neurotransmitter dopamine.

■ **You should know:**

1. Tremor, rigidity, postural instability, and bradykinesia are the primary features of parkinsonism.

2. Parkinsonism is characterized by resting tremor. Although typically bilateral, it may be unilateral for a protracted time. The tremor may involve the extremities, lips, and mouth. Gait has small, shuffling steps.

3. Weakness is not characteristic of parkinsonism. Deep tendon reflexes are normal.

4. Medical therapy of parkinsonism includes:
   • Amantadine
     (1) Best used in mild disease for rigidity and bradykinesia
     (2) Adverse effects include edema and livedo reticularis
   • Anticholinergic drugs
     (1) Reduce tremor and rigidity more than bradykinesia; are best in therapy of the younger patient when tremor is the dominant problem.
     (2) Adverse effects include dry mouth, blurred vision, confusion, and urinary outflow obstruction
   • Levodopa or levodopa/carbidopa combination
     (1) Particularly effective in bradykinesia
     (2) Adverse effects include nausea, vomiting, lethargy, orthostatic hypotension, confusion, and hallucinations
   • Dopamine agonists bromocriptine and pergolide
     (1) Are generally introduced in therapy before levodopa
     (2) Ineffective if patient does not respond to levodopa
   • Monoamine oxidase B inhibitor selegiline
     (1) May slow progression of disease
     (2) Adverse effects include headache and confusion
   • Catechol-*O*-methyltransferase inhibitors (COMT inhibitors) tolcapone and entacapone
     (1) Ineffective when given alone; potentiate the effect of levodopa
     (2) Adverse effects are the same as levodopa

5. Essential tremor, which may be familial, is characterized by an intention and postural tremor. (Postural tremor is evident when the patient is holding a weighted object [e.g., a glass of water when the arm is outstretched].) The hands, head, and voice are commonly affected. Otherwise, the neurologic examination is normal. Ingestion of alcohol temporarily suppresses the tremor. Propranolol is the preferred medicinal agent, but atenolol and primidone are also effective.

GI/N, ID

E 135   A 74-year-old man undergoes a partial gastrectomy for carcinoma of the stomach. Three hours after surgery, after the patient has been extubated, the patient's rectal temperature is 100.8°F. Other vital signs are normal. Lungs are clear to auscultation. A Foley catheter is anchored. Arterial blood gas values are normal. Which of the following is the most likely cause of the fever?

A. Atelectasis
B. Urinary tract infection
C. Surgical wound infection
D. Tissue release of cytokines
E. Aspiration pneumonia

Answer: D

D is correct because fever-associated cytokines, including interleukin, IL-6, and tissue necrosis factor, are produced in tissues and are released by the trauma of surgery. Therefore, fever (i.e., temperature greater than 100.4°F) is common in the first few days after surgery. Fever due to surgical trauma typically resolves in 2 to 3 days.

▪ **You should know:**

1. Postoperative fever may be due to infectious or noninfectious factors.

2. Causes of noninfectious fever beginning in the first few hours postoperatively include the following:
   - Medication or blood products—onset of fever is within hours of surgery
   - Inflammatory conditions (e.g., myocardial infarction or gout)
   - Group A streptococcus or *Clostridium perfringens* may cause a necrotizing skin infection and fever within a few hours after surgery
   - Malignant hyperthermia (MH) is related to inhalational anesthetics (e.g., halothane) or the depolarizing muscle relaxant succinylcholine. It may begin intraoperatively or within the first few hours postoperatively. Initially, the patient has masseter or generalized rigidity and hypotension, followed by fever and rhabdomyolysis.

3. Fever whose onset is within the first week of surgery may be related to:
   - Infection existing before surgery
   - Pneumonia, particularly in patients on mechanical ventilation
   - Urinary tract infection
   - Intravascular catheter infection
   - Pseudogout or gout
   - Occasionally, surgical site infection

4. Fever whose onset is 1 to 4 weeks after surgery may be related to:
   - Surgical site infection
   - Febrile reaction to medicines
   - Noninfectious inflammatory conditions (e.g., myocardial infarction, pulmonary embolism, deep vein thrombosis)

NEURO, CV

E 136   A 78-year-old man is diagnosed as having subclavian steal syndrome. Which of the following symptoms are consistent with this diagnosis?

   A. Monocular blurred vision
   B. Arm claudication
   C. Dizziness
   D. Diplopia
   E. Binocular blurred vision

Answer: B, C, D, and E

C, D, and E are correct because subclavian steal syndrome causes retrograde blood flow in the vertebral artery. The resultant vertebrobasilar artery insufficiency in the brain is associated with symptoms including dizziness, unstable gait, vertigo, diplopia, and bilateral blurred vision. B is correct because the subclavian artery stenosis may result in ischemia of the arm causing the patient to experience arm claudication or even arm numbness.

■ **You should know:**

1. Subclavian steal syndrome is most commonly due to atherosclerosis and is more common on the left side. In this condition, the subclavian artery is narrowed, resulting in retrograde flow in the ipsilateral vertebral artery.

2. Physical examination shows a significant difference in arm blood pressure (usually greater than 25 mm Hg lower systolic pressure on the affected side).

3. Diagnosis may be made using continuous wave Doppler, duplex ultrasonography, or angiography.

4. Treatment is surgical, either extrathoracic revascularization or percutaneous transluminal angioplasty.

5. Remember: *Transient monocular* visual loss is related to carotid artery disease; *transient binocular* visual loss suggests vertebrobasilar artery disease.

GU

E 137   A 26-year-old HIV-negative black man who suffers from heroin addiction acutely develops nephrotic syndrome. Which of the following is the most likely diagnosis?

A. Amyloidosis
B. Systemic lupus erythematosus
C. Multiple myeloma
D. Fibrillary glomerulonephritis
E. Focal glomerulosclerosis

Answer: E
E is correct because focal glomerulosclerosis is related to heroin nephropathy, and heroin nephropathy has a predilection for black patients.

■ **You should know:**

1. Focal glomerulosclerosis is an important cause of nephrotic syndrome in children, adolescents, and adults.

2. Focal glomerulosclerosis may be primary (idiopathic), which typically presents with acute onset of nephrotic syndrome. Secondary focal glomerulosclerosis is related to heroin nephropathy or HIV-associated nephropathy.

REPRO

E 138   Which of the following is a risk factor for sudden infant death syndrome (SIDS)?

A. Maternal smoking during pregnancy
B. Low-birth-weight infant
C. Prone sleeping position
D. Maternal history of diabetes mellitus
E. Patent foramen ovale in the infant

Answer: A, B, and C
A is correct because maternal smoking during pregnancy increases sudden infant death syndrome risk twofold to fourfold. It may be the most important preventable risk factor. B is correct because low birth weight infants are at a considerably increased risk compared with term infants. C is correct because the incidence of SIDS has dropped significantly since the recommendation that infants be placed in the supine position for sleeping.

Essentials is designed to promote critical thinking and enrich your knowledge base. Therefore, many questions will have more than one correct answer.

■ **You should know:**

1. In addition to the risk factors noted above, other risk factors for SIDS include maternal drug abuse, maternal age under 20 years, and use of a soft mattress for the infant.

2. SIDS (crib death) is the leading cause of death between 1 month and 1 year of age. SIDS usually occurs between the 2nd and 4th month of age.

3. The cause of SIDS cannot be identified in most cases. Long QT interval has been identified as one cause of SIDS.

4. Use of a pacifier by the infant appears to reduce the risk of SIDS.

REPRO, GU

E 139   Which of the following is an absolute contraindication to the use of combination oral contraceptives in a 36-year-old woman who smokes?

A. Diabetes mellitus
B. Benign tumor of the liver
C. History of spontaneous abortion
D. Chronic glomerulonephritis
E. Migraine with aura

Answer: B and E
B is correct because benign tumors of the liver (adenomas) are more likely to increase in number and size and more likely to bleed in women who take oral contraceptives (OCs). E is correct because the risk of ischemic stroke is increased in patients who have migraine with aura. OCs should not be taken by migraineurs who are over the age of 35, who smoke, or whose migraine is associated with aura.

■ **You should know:**

1. Oral contraceptives may be a combination of estrogen and progestin or a progestin minipill.

2. Absolute contraindications to use of a progestin/estrogen oral contraceptive include the following:
   • Pregnancy
   • Active hepatitis
   • Thrombogenic mutation (e.g., factor V Leiden, protein C, protein S, and antithrombin deficiency)
   • Coronary heart disease
   • History of stroke
   • Valvular heart disease with pulmonary hypertension, history of endocarditis, or atrial fibrillation
   • History of deep vein thrombosis or pulmonary embolism
   • Systolic blood pressure greater than 160 mm Hg
   • Benign tumor of the liver
   • Known or suspected cancer of the breast
   • Age over 35 years and smoking more than 15 cigarettes daily
   • Any condition requiring prolonged immobilization

3. The World Health Organization has specific recommendations for women who have migraine *without aura*:
   - Migraineurs under the age of 35 years may safely take an oral contraceptive whose estrogen content is less than 35 mcg.
   - The *risk of OCs in women over the age of 35 years* outweighs the benefits.

4. Barbiturates, phenytoin, primidone, carbamazepine, rifampin, and tetracycline decrease the efficacy of oral contraceptives (OCs).

5. Benefits of oral contraceptives (OCs) include decreased risk of ovarian and endometrial cancer.

ENDO, CV

E 140   A 62-year-old woman takes glyburide for type 2 diabetes mellitus. Additional therapy with which of the following medicines is most likely to facilitate the onset of hypoglycemia?

A. Propranolol
B. Indomethacin
C. Diltiazem
D. Chlorpromazine
E. Levodopa

Answer: A

A is correct because beta-adrenergic blockers inhibit both gluconeogenesis and glycogenolysis, thus facilitating hypoglycemia in the patient who takes an antidiabetic medication. In addition, beta blockers may mask the adrenergic manifestations of the low plasma glucose (e.g., sweating, anxiety, and palpitations).

■ **You should know:**

1. Epinephrine increases glucose production by promoting both glycogenolysis and gluconeogenesis, thus offering protection against the development of hypoglycemia.

2. In a brief summary, other medicines that cause hypoglycemia include the following:
   - In the type 2 diabetic, insulin secretagogues, sulfonylureas, and meglitinides (e.g., repaglinide and nateglinide)
   - Pentamidine, used in prophylaxis against *Pneumocystis jiroveci* pneumonia
   - Fluoroquinolones, particularly in diabetics (may also cause hyperglycemia)
   - Insulin-like growth factor (IGF-1), a mediator of growth hormone effects
   - Alcohol, particularly following a few days of binge-drinking with poor food intake

3. A brief summary of the treatment of hypoglycemia:
   - Mild symptoms: Intake of *glucose* tablets or fruit juice
   - Severe hypoglycemia: Intravenous glucose, if available, or glucagon (SC or IM)
   - For a patient who has *intentionally taken an overdose of a sulfonylurea*, intravenous glucose, if available, and parenteral octreotide, whose mechanism of action is to inhibit insulin release from beta-islet cells in the pancreas. (Route of administration of octreotide is dependent upon formulation.)

Essentials is designed to promote critical thinking and enrich your knowledge base. Therefore, many questions will have more than one correct answer.

4. Beta-adrenergic blockers slow the resting heart rate and are contraindicated in the patient with sick sinus syndrome unless the patient has an artificial pacemaker.

5. Beta blockers may increase airway resistance in patients with bronchospastic disease (e.g., asthma). Those blockers with beta-1 selectivity tend to cause a lesser degree of airway impairment.

6. Beta blockers increase symptoms of claudication in those with moderate to severe arterial occlusive disease. Further, this class of medicine is likely to worsen Raynaud's phenomenon.

ENDO, REPRO

E 141   A 24-year-old healthy primigravida of Native American ancestry should have plasma glucose determination after a 50-g oral glucose load at which of the following times during the pregnancy?

A. Between 16 and 20 weeks
B. Between 30 and 36 weeks
C. As soon as pregnancy is determined
D. Between 24 and 28 weeks
E. Only if ketonuria is present

Answer: D
D is correct because gestational diabetes screening should be performed between 24 and 28 weeks in women of Native American, African, Hispanic, Pacific Island, and South or East Asian ancestry.

■ You should know:

1. In both diabetic and nondiabetic women fasting glucose levels during pregnancy are lower than during the nonpregnant state.

2. Gestational screening should also be performed between 24 and 28 weeks in women who are overweight before the pregnancy and in women who have a history of diabetes mellitus in a 1st-degree relative.

3. In screening the pregnant woman for diabetes, the fasting patient is given an oral 50-g glucose load. Venous plasma glucose concentration is determined 1 hour later. A value of 130 mg/dL or higher indicates a need for a 100-g 3-hour oral glucose tolerance test.

4. In the United States, only insulin is used to treat gestational diabetes. (The U.S. Food and Drug Administration has not approved an oral hypoglycemic agent for treatment of diabetes mellitus in a pregnant woman.) A woman with diabetes who was taking an oral hypoglycemic agent before pregnancy should be converted to insulin therapy during the pregnancy.

5. A brief summary on exercise and insulin:
   • Exercise lowers plasma glucose concentration by increasing tissue sensitivity to glucose.
   • Insulin requirements are decreased during vigorous exercise.
   • In an effort to define the effect of exercise on the blood sugar level of an individual patient, it is advisable to measure glucose before, during, and after an exercise period.

- Generally, insulin requirements decrease by approximately 30% in that part of the day during which vigorous exercise occurs.

E 142   In the 23rd week of gestation, a previously normotensive 27-year-old primigravida has serial blood pressure determinations averaging 142/94 mm Hg. There is no proteinuria. In addition to restricted activity, which of the following is preferred management?

A. Initiate therapy with oral methyldopa
B. No medicinal therapy at this time
C. Initiate therapy with oral hydralazine
D. Initiate therapy with oral labetalol
E. Initiate therapy with sublingual nifedipine

Answer: B
B is correct because in the *nonpreeclampsia* patient, mild hypertension with systolic blood pressure in the 140 to 150 mm Hg range and diastolic pressure in the 90 to 100 mm Hg range is not treated.

■ **You should know:**

1. Although there are no strict criteria, it is prudent to initiate *antihypertensive therapy in a patient having preeclampsia* when systolic blood pressure is 160 mm Hg or higher and diastolic pressure is 105 mm Hg or higher.

2. Labetalol, methyldopa, and long-acting nifedipine are considered effective and safe medications in the pregnant woman. Thiazides appear to play little role overall in the management of hypertension in pregnancy because of the concern over hypovolemia.

3. Angiotensin-converting enzyme inhibitors (ACEI) and angiotensin-receptor blockers are contraindicated in all stages of pregnancy because they are teratogenic. Nitroprusside should be used only as an agent of last resort for intractable, severe hypertension.

4. Propranolol, labetalol, and metoprolol have *very little* medicine transfer into breast milk. However, breastfeeding should be avoided in the woman taking acebutolol or atenolol.

E 143   Which of the following is a cause of iron deficiency?

A. Intravascular hemolysis
B. Celiac disease
C. *Helicobacter pylori* gastritis
D. Carcinoma of the cecum
E. Graves disease

Answer: A, B, C, and D
A is correct because intravascular hemolysis results in urinary loss of iron in the form of hemosiderinuria and hemoglobinuria. B and C are correct because celiac disease and *Helicobacter pylori* gastritis are associated with decreased gastrointestinal absorption of iron. D is correct because carcinoma of the cecum commonly causes iron deficiency through fecal blood loss.

Essentials is designed to promote critical thinking and enrich your knowledge base.
Therefore, many questions will have more than one correct answer.

■ **You should know:**

1. Causes of iron deficiency include:
   - Blood loss: Gastrointestinal bleeding, blood-drawing in medical care, menometrorrhagia
   - Decreased iron ingestion
   - Decreased iron absorption: In addition to those previously noted, gastric achlorhydria also is associated with decreased absorption
   - Intravascular hemolysis

2. *Intravascular* hemolysis occurs in march hemoglobinuria, defective prosthetic heart valves, and paroxysmal cold hemoglobinuria.

3. *Extravascular* hemolysis occurs in the liver, spleen, and bone marrow. This type of hemolysis is noted in those conditions characterized by immune reactions in which complement coats the red blood cells, e.g., autoimmune hemolytic anemia.

4. A brief summary:
   - In both intravascular and extravascular hemolysis there is an *increase* in serum indirect bilirubin and lactate dehydrogenase values, an increase in reticulocyte percentage, and a *decrease* in serum haptoglobin concentration.

5. *An important clinical point: Iron stores can be totally depleted while the patient still has a hemoglobin level in the normal range.* These patients have a decreased serum ferritin, the storage iron protein. These patients will have fatigue and a sense of weakness from the depleted iron stores while the hemoglobin is still normal. Only a further depletion of iron stores will lead to clinically apparent iron deficiency anemia.

6. Iron deficiency is a recognized cause of restless legs syndrome (RLS). Patients have uncomfortable sensations (e.g., creeping, crawling, itching), which occur only at rest and are relieved immediately by movement. This discomfort is usually bilateral, and symptoms characteristically are noted below the knees.

7. The etiology of restless legs syndrome includes:
   - Primary, of unknown etiology
   - Secondary, associated with iron deficiency, pregnancy, end-stage renal disease, diabetes mellitus, and parkinsonism

8. The initial recommended medicinal treatment of RLS is pramipexole or ropinirole.

NEURO, GU

E 144   Serum alpha-fetoprotein levels are used to screen for which of the following conditions?

A. Neural tube defects
B. Tetralogy of Fallot
C. Wilms tumor of the kidney
D. Hepatic vein thrombosis
E. Germ cell tumor of the testis

Answer: A and E

A is correct because alpha-fetoprotein is a maternal serum marker for neural tube defects (NTDs). E is correct because serum alpha-fetoprotein is elevated in 90% of patients who have testicular germ cell tumors.

You should know:

1. Neural tube defects are secondary only to cardiac malformations in frequency of congenital anomalies.

2. Two neural tube defects are spina bifida and anencephaly.

3. NTDs risk factors (placing the mother at higher risk) include:
   • Folic acid deficiency in the mother
   • Medicines (folate antagonists, valproic acid, and carbamazepine)
   • Type 1 diabetes mellitus
   • Previous child with a NTD
   • Genetic factors

4. Alpha-fetoprotein is absent in the serum of nonpregnant normal adults.

5. All pregnant women should be offered screening for neural tube defects. Alpha-fetoprotein is a maternal serum marker. Maternal screening should be performed at 15 to 20 weeks of gestation.

6. Elevated level of maternal serum alpha-fetoprotein raises suspicion of neural tube defects. Ultrasonography and amniocentesis should then be done to assess whether a neural tube defect is present.

7. Folic acid supplements reduce the incidence of neural tube defects. All pregnant women should ingest daily folic acid supplements. The optimum dosage is not clearly identified. Those women considered to be at higher risk (see above) should ingest 4 mg/day during the preconception period and during the pregnancy.

8. Nonpregnant women of reproductive potential should ingest folic acid in a dose of 0.4 to 0.8 mg/day.

9. An increasing serum alpha-fetoprotein level in patients with cirrhosis should raise suspicion of hepatocellular carcinoma.

10. Serum alpha-fetoprotein is commonly elevated in the male with a germ cell tumor of the testis. It is occasionally elevated in a non–germ cell tumor of the testis. Further, in some testicular tumors there is elevation of the serum concentration of human chorionic gonadotropin hormone (hCG).

GU, HEME

E 145   A dipstick urinalysis in a 44-year-old man is positive for blood. Microscopic examination of the urine reveals no red blood cells. Presence of which of the following in the urine is most likely?

   A. Myoglobin
   B. Hemosiderin
   C. Phenazopyridine (Pyridium)
   D. Waxy casts
   E. Immunoglobulins

Essentials is designed to promote critical thinking and enrich your knowledge base. Therefore, many questions will have more than one correct answer.

Answer: A
A is correct because presence of myoglobin or hemoglobin in the urine will cause the dipstick to be positive for blood.

■ **You should know:**

1. A positive dipstick for blood may indicate three different conditions:
   • Red blood cells in the urine: This will be noted on microscopic urine sediment examination
   • Hemoglobinuria: No red blood cells will be seen on microscopic examination
   • Myoglobinuria: As occurs in skeletal muscle breakdown (rhabdomyolysis)

2. A *false-negative* dipstick for blood may occur in the presence of a high urinary concentration of ascorbic acid (vitamin C).

3. A *false-positive* dipstick for blood occurs in the presence of an alkaline urine with pH greater than 9.

4. Hemoglobinuria occurs in patients who have intravascular hemolysis, as may occur in patients with defective heart valves, march hemoglobinuria, and paroxysmal cold hemoglobinuria.

5. Oral intake of phenazopyridine in treatment of dysuria will cause red/orange discoloration of the urine. The urinary dipstick will not, however, become positive.

ID, DERM, EENT

E 146   A 12-year-old boy has a 5-day history of fever, headache, and rhinorrhea after which a rash appears. Examination shows a bilateral erythematous malar rash with circumoral pallor. Which of the following organisms is the most likely cause of the illness?

A. Adenovirus
B. *Streptococcus pyogenes*
C. Coxsackievirus
D. Parvovirus
E. Herpes simplex virus 1

Answer: D
D is correct because parvovirus is the etiologic agent causing fifth disease (erythema infectiosum) that is characterized by a mild febrile illness followed by development of a bilateral malar rash ("slapped cheeks").

■ **You should know:**

1. Children with erythema infectiosum are less likely to have joint manifestations, which, in contrast, are common in adults who have parvovirus infection.

2. The clinical manifestation of parvovirus infection depends upon the underlying host. Immunocompetent adults may have no symptoms or may experience a flulike illness followed 1 week later by arthralgia or arthritis.

3. The arthritis or arthralgia is typically symmetrical and involves small joints (e.g., hands, wrists, feet, and knees). Joint symptoms generally resolve in 3 to 4 weeks.

4. Patients with hematologic disease (e.g., sickle cell anemia, iron deficiency anemia) are at increased risk of developing an aplastic crisis with parvovirus infection.

5. Maternal infection with parvovirus during pregnancy can lead to fetal death.

6. In healthy persons the illness is usually self-limited, and there is no specific treatment that is necessary.

7. There is no vaccine to prevent erythema infectiosum.

ID

E 147   Which of the following is the pathophysiologic abnormality that is primarily responsible for opportunistic infection in the AIDS patient?

A. Hypercatabolism of immunoglobulin proteins
B. Decreased serum complement (C3) concentration
C. Impaired opsonization
D. Impaired cellular immunity
E. Immunoglobulin loss in urine

Answer: D
D is correct because HIV infection typically leads to CD4 T-cell depletion and impaired cellular immunity.

▓ **You should know:**

1. HIV type 1 is a human retrovirus that infects lymphocytes and other cells that bear the CD4 surface protein. Ultimately, the immune dysfunction caused by the virus produces clinical AIDS in which opportunistic infections and malignancies arise.

2. The time from initial HIV infection to appearance of clinical AIDS varies from months to years.

3. The virus is transmitted sexually and parenterally.

4. The Centers for Disease Control and Prevention (CDC) defines a patient as having AIDS if he or she has one of the following illnesses (called AIDS-defining illness) *with or without evidence of HIV infection*:
   • *Pneumocystis jiroveci* pneumonia
   • Esophageal candidiasis
   • Kaposi sarcoma
   • Extrapulmonary cryptococcosis
   • Disseminated *M. avium* infection

5. The Centers for Disease Control and Prevention (CDC) defines a patient as having AIDS if he or she has one of the following *illnesses with evidence of HIV infection*:
   • HIV encephalopathy
   • Disseminated coccidioidomycosis
   • Lymphoma of the brain
   • Pulmonary tuberculosis
   • Invasive cervical cancer

Essentials is designed to promote critical thinking and enrich your knowledge base.
Therefore, many questions will have more than one correct answer.

6. HIV therapy includes:
   - Antiretroviral therapy
   - Prophylaxis of opportunistic infection
   - Treatment of opportunistic infection
   - Immunomodulation

7. Antiretroviral medicines are grouped into five categories:
   - Nucleoside and nucleotide analog reverse transcriptase inhibitors (NRTIs); examples include tenofovir and emtricitabine
   - Protease inhibitors; examples include atazanavir and darunavir
   - Nonnucleoside reverse transcriptase inhibitors; an example is efavirenz
   - Integrase strand transfer inhibitors (INSTIs); an example is raltegravir
   - CCR5 antagonists; an example is maraviroc

8. Effective HIV therapy necessitates administration of three or more drugs from at least two classes. The goal of therapy is viral suppression to less than 50 cells/microL.

9. Treatment for asymptomatic HIV-infected persons should be initiated when the CD4 cell count is less than 500 cells/microL.

10. Zidovudine as part of combination therapy should be initiated in the HIV-infected pregnant patient, preferably by the 2nd trimester. However, this medicine may be given during labor or delivery and should be given to the newborn for 6 weeks.

11. All persons between the ages of 16 and 75 years should be offered HIV screening with appropriate confidentiality and informed consent.

12. In addition, HIV serology should be checked in the following persons:
    - High-risk persons (e.g., intravenous drug abusers, homosexual and bisexual men, hemophiliacs, sexual partner of known HIV-infected person, prostitutes and their partners, those with sexually transmitted diseases, those who received blood transfusions between 1977 and 1985, and those with multiple sex partners
    - Pregnant women
    - Patients with active tuberculosis
    - Hospitalized patients in communities in which HIV infection is considered to be significant
    - Donors of blood, semen, and organs
    - Selected health-care workers and those with occupational exposures

13. Screening for HIV infection is performed with an enzyme-labeled immunosorbent assay (ELISA) for HIV 1 and HIV 2.

14. In the patient with a positive enzyme-labeled immunosorbent assay, a repeat ELISA is performed in addition to a Western blot. An isolated positive ELISA must be confirmed by a positive Western blot before a definitive diagnosis of HIV infection is made.

15. A person with a positive serology and CD4 lymphocyte count less than 200 cells/microL or CD lymphocyte percentage less than 14% is considered to have AIDS. The CD4 count indicates the amount of HIV immune damage that is already experienced.

16. An HIV-positive patient should have the following tests:
    - CD4 cell count (normal is 600 to 1,500 cells/microL)
    - Virologic markers including RNA viral load (via polymerase chain reaction); this indicates the magnitude of HIV replication and its associated rate of CD4 cell destruction
    - Tuberculin skin test
    - Venereal Disease Research Laboratory (VDRL) test
    - Toxoplasma and cytomegalovirus titers
    - Hepatitis A, B (HBsAg, HBsAb, HBcAb), and C serologies
    - *Chlamydia* and gonococcus urine probe

17. HIV-positive persons should receive the following immunizations:
    - Pneumococcal
    - Hepatitis A and B
    - Influenza

ID

E 148 A 36-year-old man with AIDS has a CD4 cell count of less than 50 cells/microL. Tuberculin skin test shows 6 mm induration. He should not receive prophylaxis against which of the following infections?

A. *Mycobacterium avium* complex
B. Toxoplasmosis
C. *Pneumocystis*
D. *Candida*
E. Tuberculosis

Answer: D

D is correct because primary prophylaxis against *Candida* infection appears to promote resistance in *Candida* species.

■ You should know:

1. The use of prophylactic antibiotics has reduced the incidence of opportunistic infection (OI). Prophylaxis for OI includes:
   - *Pneumocystis* pneumonia for the patient with a CD4 cell count less than 200 cells/microL, or CD4 lymphocyte percentage less than 14%, or unexplained fever lasting longer than 2 weeks, or presence of oral candidiasis. Trimethoprim-sulfamethoxazole (TMP-SMX) is preferred therapy.
   - Tuberculosis (TBC) prophylaxis in the patient whose tuberculin test shows greater than 5 mm induration or who has had recent contact with a patient known to have active tuberculosis. Isoniazid (INH) with pyridoxine is preferred therapy.
   - *Toxoplasma* prophylaxis when CD4 count is less than 100 cells/microL. Trimethoprim-sulfamethoxazole (TMP-SMX) or dapsone/pyrimethamine is prescribed. If dapsone therapy is considered, the patient should have glucose-6-phosphate dehydrogenase (G-6-PD) screening prior to initiation of therapy. Further, the sulfone antibiotic dapsone may cause methemoglobinemia.
   - *Mycobacterium avium* complex prophylaxis is given when the CD4 cell count is less than 50 cells/microL. Azithromycin or clarithromycin is prescribed.

Essentials is designed to promote critical thinking and enrich your knowledge base.
Therefore, many questions will have more than one correct answer.

2. A brief review: Therapeutic indications for dapsone therapy:
   - Prophylaxis against *Pneumocystis* infection
   - Prophylaxis against *Toxoplasma* infection
   - Treatment of leprosy
   - Treatment of dermatitis herpetiformis
   - Treatment of chronic urticaria

3. Varicella zoster immune globulin should be given to the patient who has not had chickenpox and who is exposed to a patient with chickenpox or herpes zoster infection (shingles). *Zoster vaccination should not be given to an immuno-compromised patient* (e.g., HIV/AIDS).

E 149   After 4 days of aching discomfort in the right eye, a 52-year-old diabetic man has diplopia. Examination shows ptosis of the right eyelid, and the right eye is in a position of abduction. The pupils are normal in size and equal. Which of the following is the most likely diagnosis?

A. Subarachnoid hemorrhage
B. Lyme disease
C. Cranial nerve V mononeuropathy
D. Cervical spondylosis
E. Cranial nerve III mononeuropathy

Answer: E

E is correct because diabetic cranial mononeuropathy most commonly affects cranial nerves III, IV, and VI (the cranial nerves that innervate the extraocular muscles). Further, in 80% of cases of cranial nerve III palsy in the diabetic patient, the pupil size is *normal on the affected side* (in contrast to the usual case of cranial nerve III palsy in which the pupil is enlarged on the affected side).

■ You should know:

1. Diabetic neuropathy includes primarily:
   - Symmetrical polyneuropathy
   - Cranial nerve mononeuropathy
   - Peripheral nerve mononeuropathy
   - Autonomic neuropathy
   - Diabetic amyotrophy

2. Facial nerve (cranial nerve VII) mononeuropathy causing Bell's palsy occurs more frequently in the diabetic patient than in the nondiabetic patient. Bell's palsy is most commonly related to herpes simplex or zoster infection. It also is associated with Lyme disease and sarcoidosis.

3. Symmetrical distal polyneuropathy is the most common type of diabetic neuropathy. This is characterized by progressive sensory loss followed by motor weakness. Patients commonly have burning, tingling, and "pins and needles" followed by numbness. Examination shows loss of vibratory sensation, abnormal proprioception, and diminished pain, light touch, and temperature sensation.

4. Peripheral mononeuropathy includes carpal tunnel syndrome, ulnar neuropathy, and peroneal neuropathy, the last causing footdrop.

5. Diabetic amyotrophy is characterized by unilateral thigh pain, weakness, and muscle wasting. Spontaneous recovery occurs in months to years, but amyotrophy may recur on the opposite side.

(Autonomic neuropathy is considered in more detail in E 150.)

NEURO, ENDO, GU, CV

E 150   Which of the following is a manifestation of diabetic autonomic neuropathy?

A. Gastroparesis
B. Orthostatic hypotension
C. Nocturnal diarrhea
D. Retrograde ejaculation
E. Brady-tachy syndrome

Answer: A, B, C, and D
A and C are correct because gastroparesis, characterized by delayed emptying of the stomach, and nocturnal diarrhea are frequent gastrointestinal manifestations of diabetic neuropathy. The etiology of the gastroparesis is multifactorial; nocturnal diarrhea is related to abnormal motility and bacterial overgrowth. B is correct because diabetic neuropathy frequently causes functional disturbance in the sympathetic reflex arc resulting in the patient having orthostatic hypotension. D is correct because retrograde ejaculation in the diabetic results from impaired sphincter muscle control that is responsible for normal ejaculation.

▉ You should know:

1. Poor glycemic control is associated with development of diabetic autonomic neuropathy (DAN). Obversely, vigorous control of plasma glucose slows onset and later slows progression of DAN.

2. Diabetic autonomic neuropathy involves both the sympathetic and parasympathetic divisions of the autonomic nervous system.

3. Diabetic autonomic neuropathy affects different organ systems:
   • Cardiovascular
   • Genitourinary
   • Gastrointestinal
   • Sudomotor (sweating)
   • Ophthalmic
   • Neuroendocrine
   • Peripheral

4. Cardiovascular manifestations of diabetic autonomic neuropathy include:
   • Orthostatic hypotension: Diabetic autonomic neuropathy (DAN)–induced orthostatic hypotension is *not characterized by a compensatory heart rate increase* as the blood pressure drops. This is in contrast to hypovolemia-induced orthostatic hypotension in which the heart rate increases as blood pressure falls upon assumption of the standing position.
   • Lack of variation in heart rate, which is considered to be a risk factor for sudden cardiac death. A fixed heart rate between 80 and 90 per minute is associated with painless myocardial infarction and sudden cardiac death.

5. Gastrointestinal autonomic neuropathy may cause gastroparesis manifest by anorexia, nausea, vomiting, and wide swings in plasma glucose concentration

Essentials is designed to promote critical thinking and enrich your knowledge base.
Therefore, many questions will have more than one correct answer.

despite vigorous patient efforts. Another autonomic manifestation is nocturnal diarrhea.

6. Genitourinary manifestations of diabetic autonomic neuropathy include:
   - Retrograde ejaculation, often manifest as cloudy urine after intercourse
   - Erectile dysfunction
   - Dyspareunia related to decreased vaginal lubrication
   - Overflow incontinence of urine due to the patient's inability to sense a full bladder

7. Peripheral autonomic neuropathy may cause the patient to have distal anhidrosis (lack of sweating) with central hyperhidrosis. Further, this neuropathy may cause aching and tightness in the skin and the relatively painless
   Charcot deformity in the foot or ankle.

8. A neuroendocrine manifestation of DAN is decreased glucagon and epinephrine secretion in response to hypoglycemia.

REPRO

E 151   At 31 weeks of gestation, a 32-year-old G4 P2 woman has the sudden onset of profuse, painless vaginal bleeding. Which of the following is the most likely diagnosis?

A. Abruptio placentae
B. Threatened abortion
C. Ectopic pregnancy
D. Placenta previa
E. Hydatidiform mole

Answer: D
D is correct because placenta previa typically is characterized by 3rd-trimester
bleeding that is painless because there are no associated uterine contractions.

■ **You should know:**

1. 1st trimester vaginal bleeding occurs in approximately 30% of pregnant
   women.

2. The three major causes of *1st trimester bleeding* are:
   - Ectopic pregnancy
   - Threatened or imminent abortion
   - Disease of the cervix, uterus, or vagina

3. In the patient having bleeding in the 1st trimester, passage of blood clots,
   passage of tissue, or pelvic cramping make ectopic pregnancy and miscar-
   riage more likely.

4. Two or more consecutive pregnancy losses after 10 weeks of gestation suggest antiphospholipid antibody (APA) syndrome. This may be primary or
   associated with systemic lupus erythematosus. APA syndrome causes venous and arterial thrombosis, fetal loss, and thrombocytopenia.

5. After physical examination, ultrasonography is the preferred diagnostic
   test for evaluation of bleeding during early pregnancy.

6. The most common causes of *3rd trimester bleeding* include:
   - Placenta previa
   - Abruptio placentae

7. *Digital examination should not be performed in the patient presenting with late bleeding until placenta previa has been excluded.*

8. Risk factors for placenta previa include multiple cesarean sections and multiparity.

9. Clinically, abruptio placentae presents with vaginal bleeding, uterine contractions, and abdominal tenderness.

10. Risk factors for abruptio placentae include hypertension, smoking, cocaine use, prior abruptio placentae, advanced maternal age, and uterine fibroids.

11. Ultrasonography rarely shows abruption but is important to exclude placenta previa.

HEME

E 152   A 34-year-old woman is to undergo elective splenectomy for hereditary spherocytosis. Administration of which of the following is recommended prior to the surgery?

A. Oral folinic acid
B. Intravenous immunoglobulin
C. Oral metronidazole
D. *Haemophilus influenzae* conjugate vaccine
E. Platelet transfusion

Answer: D

D is correct because the postsplenectomy patient is at risk for sepsis caused by encapsulated bacteria (e.g., *Haemophilus influenzae, Streptococcus pneumoniae,* and *Neisseria meningitidis*).

▓ **You should know:**

1. The spleen is the primary site for production of IgM antibodies that opsonize encapsulated bacteria.

2. At least 2 weeks before elective splenectomy the patient should receive vaccines for infection by encapsulated bacteria (e.g., *Streptococcus pneumoniae* [pneumococcus], *Haemophilus* B, and *Neisseria meningitidis*).

3. Children who have undergone splenectomy or those with impaired splenic function (e.g., sickle cell anemia) should take daily penicillin for at least 3 to 5 years or until adulthood.

4. Remember, a patient who has a chronic hemolytic anemia such as sickle cell disease (SCD) is at increased risk of developing bilirubin gallstones. Acute cholecystitis is common in children who have SCD.

GI/N

E 153   A 47-year-old man has alcoholic cirrhosis with ascites. Which of the following is a precipitating cause of hepatic encephalopathy?

A. Hypovolemia
B. Hypokalemia
C. Gastrointestinal bleeding
D. Spironolactone therapy
E. Administration of a lactulose enema

Essentials is designed to promote critical thinking and enrich your knowledge base.
Therefore, many questions will have more than one correct answer.

Answer: A, B, and C

A and C are correct because both hypovolemia and gastrointestinal (GI) bleeding reduce oxygen delivery to the liver. Further, degradation of blood protein products in gastrointestinal bleeding leads to increased ammonia delivery to the liver. The diseased liver is unable to convert the ammonia to urea for renal excretion. B is correct because hypokalemia leads to *intracellular acidosis,* which in turn results in increased production of ammonia.

You should know:

1. The diagnosis of hepatic encephalopathy (HE) is not based upon blood ammonia concentration. However, ammonia is the most readily identified toxin in HE.

2. The clinical manifestations of HE are variable, ranging from mild confusion to drowsiness to coma.

3. Hepatic encephalopathy typically occurs in patients who have advanced chronic liver disease with signs including jaundice, ascites, palmar erythema, spider telangiectasia, and muscle wasting. Because the patient with chronic liver disease and ascites is not in right heart failure, the jugular venous pressure (JVP) is normal. (However, in the unusual case when the ascites is very tense, the JVP may be elevated. In this case, paracentesis will cause the jugular venous pressure to quickly decrease to normal levels. In contrast, in the patient who has ascites caused by constrictive pericarditis paracentesis will not reduce the JVP to normal.)

4. Other precipitating causes of hepatic encephalopathy include:
   • Hypoxemia
   • Sedatives/tranquilizers

5. Treatment of hepatic encephalopathy includes oral or rectal lactulose, dietary protein restriction, and oral rifampin. The lactulose increases ammonium excretion in the stool and modifies colonic bacterial flora so that fewer ammonia-producing bacteria are present. Oral rifampin reduces the number of ammonia-producing bacteria and is preferred over traditional neomycin therapy. Alternatively, metronidazole may be given in place of rifampin.

6. Treatment of ascites associated with cirrhosis usually includes a combination of spironolactone and furosemide.

GU, ENDO, HEME

E 154   A 67-year-old man with type 1 diabetes mellitus has end-stage renal disease. Which of the following is an expected laboratory abnormality to be noted in this patient?

A. Hypokalemia
B. Hypercalcemia
C. Hyperphosphatemia
D. Macrocytic, nonmegaloblastic anemia
E. Normocytic normochromic anemia

Answer: C and E

C is correct because the decreased glomerular filtration rate in advanced renal disease results in hyperphosphatemia. E is correct because the decreased renal production of erythropoietin in advanced renal disease leads to a normochromic normocytic anemia.

You should know:

1. Chronic renal disease is characterized by hyperkalemia, hypocalcemia, hyperphosphatemia, and metabolic acidosis.

2. Complications of chronic renal disease include:
   - Cardiovascular:
     (1) Hypertension
     (2) Pericarditis
     (3) Heart failure
   - Neurologic:
     (1) Uremic *encephalopathy* is manifest by confusion, lethargy, and coma. Signs include hyperreflexia, asterixis, and nystagmus.
     (2) Asterixis is *not specific* for uremic encephalopathy. Other causes include the following:
        (a) Hepatic encephalopathy
        (b) Metabolic encephalopathy caused by hyponatremia, drug overdose, or infection
     (3) Uremic *neuropathy* is manifest by a stocking glove sensorimotor polyneuropathy with loss of deep tendon reflexes.
     (4) A brief review: Disorders that are associated with a stocking glove peripheral neuropathy include the following:
        (a) Uremic neuropathy
        (b) Diabetes mellitus
        (c) Chronic alcohol abuse
        (d) Vitamin B_{12} deficiency
        (e) HIV infection
        (f) Lyme disease
   - Mineral metabolism
     (1) Osteitis fibrosa cystica from secondary hyperparathyroidism
     (2) Osteomalacia
   - Skin
     (1) Pruritus

GU, CV

E 155 A 78-year-old man has chronic systolic heart failure with a left ventricular ejection fraction of 24%. Therapy includes a loop diuretic, beta-adrenergic blocker, and angiotensin-converting enzyme inhibitor. The heart failure is most likely to be associated with which of the following?

A. Metabolic acidosis
B. Hyperchloremia
C. Hyperkalemia
D. Elevated serum osmolality
E. Hyponatremia

Answer: E
E is correct because the low cardiac output and reduced arterial pressure associated with systolic heart failure lead to increased secretion of antidiuretic hormone (ADH). Increased antidiuretic hormone (ADH) secretion causes hyponatremia.

Essentials is designed to promote critical thinking and enrich your knowledge base.
Therefore, many questions will have more than one correct answer.

You should know:

1. The hyponatremia (serum sodium less than 135 mEq/L) patient may be asymptomatic in mild cases. In more severe cases, nausea, vomiting, weakness, confusion, stupor, seizure, and coma may be present.

2. Hyponatremia is categorized by:
   • Serum osmolality (normal: 280 to 285 mOsm/kg)
   • Extracellular fluid (ECF) volume

3. Serum osmolality determination enables hyponatremia to be categorized by:
   • Isotonic hyponatremia
   • Hypertonic hyponatremia
   • Hypotonic hyponatremia

4. *Isotonic* hyponatremia is usually caused by marked elevation in serum proteins or lipids (e.g., triglycerides or chylomicrons).

5. *Hypertonic* hyponatremia is most commonly due to marked hyperglycemia.

6. *Hypotonic* hyponatremia is divided by extracellular volume into three categories:
   • Volume depletion, with orthostatic hypotension and poor turgor
   • Volume expansion, with peripheral edema
   • Euvolemia (normal extracellular fluid [ECF] volume)

7. Volume depletion hyponatremia occurs in cases of excessive nonrenal losses of sodium and water, replaced by excess water alone or water with inadequate salt intake (as might occur in a long-distance runner) or by adrenal insufficiency.

8. Euvolemic hyponatremia occurs typically in syndrome of inappropriate antidiuretic hormone secretion (SIADH) that may occur in central nervous system tumor or infection, in malignancy (small cell carcinoma of lung, carcinoma of pancreas, lymphoma) or due to medicines (e.g., tricyclic antidepressants, cyclophosphamide, thiothixene, carbamazepine).

9. Increased extracellular volume (volume expansion) hyponatremia occurs in the following:
   • Heart failure
   • Cirrhosis with ascites
   • Nephrotic syndrome

CV, GU

E 156   Which of the following conditions may precipitate generalized seizures?

   A. Hyponatremia
   B. Hypocalcemia
   C. Transient ischemic attack
   D. Uremia
   E. Encephalitis

Answer: A, B, D, and E

A, B, and D are correct because hyponatremia (or hypernatremia), hypocalcemia, and uremia are brain *nonstructural* causes of seizures. E is correct because encephalitis is a *structural* (i.e., inflammatory) brain disorder that may be associated with seizures. Seizures of any etiology are caused by abnormal neuron firing in the brain that is related to a biochemical process affecting the action potentials of the neuron.

▓ **You should know:**

1. Other causes of nonstructural seizures include:
   - Acute withdrawal of drugs (e.g., benzodiazepines)
   - Drug intoxication (e.g., cocaine, methamphetamine)
   - Medicine effects (e.g., cyclosporine, imipenem)
   - Epilepsy

2. Other causes of structural seizures include:
   - Primary or metastatic brain tumor
   - Brain infections (e.g., meningitis, encephalitis)
   - Brain trauma or hemorrhage
   - Cerebrovascular accident

3. Transient ischemic attacks (TIAs) last minutes to hours. They generally are associated with "negative" manifestations (e.g., weakness, visual loss, or numbness).

4. In contrast, seizures are associated with "positive" neurologic symptoms and signs (e.g., jerking, stiffness, or visual hallucinations).

5. Encephalitis should be suspected in the patient who has fever and neurologic signs, especially personality change, motor or sensory deficits, seizures, but without meningeal signs. Herpes simplex virus is the most common cause of encephalitis.

6. In contrast to encephalitis, patients with acute meningitis initially have headache and nuchal rigidity.

GU

E 157   Over a period of 3 days, an 87-year-old man who is bedridden has worsening mental status and then becomes delirious. Serum sodium is 156 mEq/L. Which of the following is the most likely cause?

A. Hepatic encephalopathy
B. Hyperglycemia
C. Acute adrenal insufficiency
D. Hypertriglyceridemia
E. Dehydration

Answer: E

E is correct because dehydration occurs when there is a lack of replacement of usual or increased body water loss. The water loss leads to hypernatremia, an increase in plasma sodium concentration.

▓ **You should know:**

1. Hypernatremia is caused by:
   - Dehydration
   - Renal loss of water
     (1) Central diabetes insipidus (involvement of the pituitary or hypothalamus by tumor, trauma, infection, or stroke)
     (2) Nephrogenic diabetes insipidus (genetic or related to therapy with lithium or demeclocycline [Declomycin])
     (3) Osmotic diuresis (related to glycosuria or tube feedings)
   - Extrarenal loss of water (sweating, burns)
   - Increased sodium intake (hypertonic saline)

Essentials is designed to promote critical thinking and enrich your knowledge base.
Therefore, many questions will have more than one correct answer.

E 158   Which of the following may be a clinical manifestation of hypoglycemia?

A. Sweating
B. Confusion
C. Seizures
D. Thirst
E. Polyuria

Answer: A, B, and C
A is correct because sweating is an *autonomic* (adrenergic) manifestation of hypoglycemia. B and C are correct because confusion and seizures are *neuroglycopenic* manifestations of hypoglycemia.

■ **You should know:**

1. Hypoglycemia most commonly occurs in the diabetic population due to inappropriate glycemic therapy, either insulin or oral preparations.

2. Hypoglycemic symptoms are either autonomic or neuroglycopenic.

3. Autonomic symptoms include:
   • Tremulousness
   • Sweating
   • Palpitations
   • Hunger
   • Tingling sensation

4. Neuroglycopenic manifestations include:
   • Impaired concentration
   • Confusion
   • Seizures
   • Coma

5. An important clinical point: Hypoglycemia may cause *localized neurologic signs* (e.g., hemiplegia).

6. Fasting hypoglycemia may be due to:
   • Insulinoma, an insulin-secreting tumor
   • Alcohol abuse
   • Advanced hepatic or renal disease
   • Glucocorticoid deficit (adrenal or pituitary insufficiency)

7. *Postprandial hypoglycemia* may be due to:
   • Gastrectomy or Roux-en-Y procedure that may be done in bariatric surgery. Hypoglycemia after either procedure may occur caused by hyperinsulinism related to rapid gastric emptying. This tends to occur approximately 2 to 3 hours after eating.
   • Functional (reactive) hypoglycemia, an imprecise term related to patients who have adrenergic symptoms 3 to 5 hours after meals. In these patients there is no clear correlation between symptoms and plasma glucose levels.

8. Hypoglycemia associated with alcohol intake may be related to decreased food intake, reduced hepatic glycogen storage, or deficiency of the enzyme

that metabolizes alcohol. Hypoglycemia, manifest by coma or seizures, may occur with binge alcohol drinking and can be mistaken for alcohol intoxication or withdrawal.

9. *Dumping syndrome* that may occur after gastrectomy or Roux-en-Y surgery should not be confused with hypoglycemia, although the symptoms are similar. Symptoms occur 15 minutes to 1 hour after eating and may be related to contraction of plasma volume due to fluid shifts into the bowel.

10. A brief review: Gastrectomy or Roux-en-Y procedure may provoke *both dumping syndrome and hypoglycemia.*

ID, GU

E 159   Infection with human papillomavirus may cause which of the following conditions?
   A. Carcinoma of the cervix
   B. Chancroid
   C. Granuloma inguinale
   D. Condylomata acuminata
   E. Plantar warts

Answer: A, D, and E
A is correct because virtually all cases of carcinoma of the cervix are related to chronic human papillomavirus (HPV) infection. D is correct because condylomata acuminata, caused by human papillomavirus infection, is an anogenital cutaneous lesion and is the most common viral, sexually transmitted disease in the United States. E is correct because another cutaneous manifestation of human papillomavirus infection is plantar warts.

▮ You should know:

1. HPV infection most commonly causes cutaneous and anogenital diseases.

2. Cutaneous manifestations of HPV infection include:
   • Common warts (verruca vulgaris)
   • Plantar warts
   • Flat (juvenile) warts

3. Anogenital manifestations of human papillomavirus (HPV) infection include:
   • Condylomata acuminata
   • Carcinoma of the cervix, anus, vulva, penis, and vagina

4. Laboratory diagnosis of human papillomavirus (HPV) infection includes:
   • Cytology (Papanicolaou smear)
   • Molecular-based methods, including human papillomavirus (HPV) DNA testing in selected patients

5. Immunization with human papillomavirus (HPV) vaccine is *recommended* in females 11 to 12 years of age, with "catch-up" immunization in females 13 to 26 years of age.

6. Immunization with human papillomavirus (HPV) vaccine is *suggested* in males 9 to 26 years of age.

NEURO, GI/N

E 160   Forty-eight hours after his last alcohol drink, a 67-year-old man with chronic alcohol abuse has hallucinations, disorientation, and agitation. Examination shows a confused patient with profuse diaphoresis, low-grade fever, and tachycardia. Which of the following is the most likely diagnosis?

A. Delirium tremens
B. Alcoholic hallucinosis
C. Pheochromocytoma
D. Malignant neuroleptic syndrome
E. Korsakoff's syndrome

Answer: A
A is correct because delirium tremens in the patient with a history of sustained alcohol intake characteristically starts with 48 to 96 hours of abstinence. Hallucinations, disorientation, low-grade fever, agitation, and diaphoresis are common manifestations.

■ **You should know:**

1. Alcohol withdrawal syndromes include:
   • Minor withdrawal
   • Withdrawal seizures
   • Alcoholic hallucinosis
   • Delirium tremens

2. Minor withdrawal usually occurs 5 to 30 hours after the last drink and is manifest by insomnia, tremulousness, headache, and sweating.

3. Withdrawal seizures are generalized tonic-clonic convulsions that usually occur 6 to 48 hours after the last drink. Benzodiazepines are used in seizure therapy; other anticonvulsants are not used unless the patient has a preexisting seizure disorder.

4. Alcoholic hallucinosis, occurring typically 12 to 48 hours after the last drink, is characterized most frequently by visual hallucinations, although auditory or tactile hallucinations may occur. The sensorium is not clouded.

5. Thiamine, either intramuscularly or intravenously, should promptly be given to all patients with alcohol withdrawal symptoms or signs.

6. Benzodiazepines are the first-line agents for all alcohol withdrawal clinical syndromes. Antipsychotic medications should *not* be given.

GI/N

E 161   A 3-week-old infant male has immediate postprandial, nonbilious vomiting. Examination shows a small rounded mass at the lateral edge of the rectus abdominis muscle in the right upper quadrant. Which of the following is the most likely diagnosis?

A. Hypertrophic pyloric stenosis
B. Intussusception
C. Hirschsprung's disease
D. Congenital diaphragmatic hernia
E. Umbilical hernia

Answer: A

A is correct because the typical presentation of infantile hypertrophic pyloric stenosis (IHPS) is a 3-to-6-week-old baby who has immediate postprandial, nonbilious vomiting.

■ You should know:

1. IHPS is four to six times more common in male infants.

2. IHPS is linked to hyperbilirubinemia, more commonly unconjugated hyperbilirubinemia, and is called "icteropyloric syndrome." The elevation in serum bilirubin resolves soon after operation.

3. Neonatal administration of a macrolide antibiotic appears to increase the incidence of IHPS. (Macrolide may be given to the newborn for treatment of chlamydial conjunctivitis or pneumonia or for prophylaxis against pertussis.)

4. Ultrasound or upper gastrointestinal contrast study can be used for diagnosis.

5. Definitive therapy is surgical.

6. A brief review: Causes of vomiting in infancy include the following conditions:
   • Pyloric stenosis
   • Gastroesophageal reflux
   • Milk protein–induced enteritis
   • Intestinal obstruction
   • Adrenal insufficiency

ENDO

E 162　A 66-year-old woman has type 2 diabetes mellitus. Metformin therapy has resulted in fasting plasma glucose levels in the 160 to 170 mg/dL range. Blood urea nitrogen, serum creatinine, and liver function values are normal. Which of the following is the preferred additional therapy?

A. NPH insulin
B. Acarbose
C. Glipizide
D. Nateglinide
E. Rosiglitazone

Answer: C

C is correct because the patient whose plasma glucose cannot be controlled with metformin requires therapy with a second medicine that has a different mechanism of action in lowering the glucose levels. It is common to use a sulfonylurea (e.g., glipizide) in addition to the metformin.

■ You should know:

1. Diagnosis of diabetes mellitus: Criteria include two fasting plasma glucose values greater than 126 mg/dL or a HbA_{1c} value 6.5% or higher. A random glucose level, the least acceptable test for diagnosis, greater than 200 mg/dL, in the presence of diabetic symptoms, indicates diabetes mellitus. A 2-hour glucose tolerance test value greater than 200 mg/dL is diagnostic.

2. Target values of HbA_{1c} should be individualized for the patient. However, an HbA_{1c} value less than 7% is considered optimum control in most patients.

Essentials is designed to promote critical thinking and enrich your knowledge base.
Therefore, many questions will have more than one correct answer.

3. Rigorous glycemic control in both type 1 and type 2 diabetes reduces the risk of *microvascular* diabetic complications. Microvascular complications refer to diabetic retinopathy, diabetic nephropathy, and diabetic neuropathy.

4. Biguanides (e.g., metformin) suppress hepatic glucose production, decrease intestinal absorption of glucose, and improve insulin sensitivity.

5. Sulfonylureas increase pancreatic secretion of insulin.

6. Thiazolidinediones (e.g., rosiglitazone and pioglitazone) increase sensitivity to insulin. This class of medicine is *contraindicated* in the patient who is in heart failure.

7. Alpha-glucosidase inhibitors (e.g., acarbose and miglitol) reduce gastrointestinal absorption of carbohydrates.

8. Meglitinides (e.g., repaglinide and nateglinide) increase pancreatic secretion of insulin.

9. Urine glucose testing is not recommended because it does not adequately assess glycemic status.

PSY/LE

E 163   During a commercial airline flight, the captain requests assistance from an onboard passenger who is a medical professional. Under which of the following conditions does the Samaritan lose legal protection under the Aviation Medical Assistance Act of 1998?

A. Fails to hold current professional licensure
B. Fails to obtain sick passenger's consent
C. Fails to produce written documentation of intervention
D. Fails to directly communicate with captain
E. Receives monetary compensation

Answer: E

E is correct because the Aviation Medical Assistance Act of 1998 states that legal immunity from malpractice litigation is, in part, based upon the Samaritan not receiving compensation for the medical intervention. Seat upgrades and travel vouchers do not count as compensation.

▨ **You should know:**

1. The Aviation Medical Assistance Act of 1998 offers legal protection against malpractice litigation if the following conditions are met:
   • Samaritan is medically qualified to perform service
   • Samaritan acts voluntarily
   • Samaritan acts in good faith
   • Samaritan does not engage in gross negligence
   • Samaritan receives no compensation

2. The aircraft cabin environment during flight is characterized by:
   • Reduced oxygen pressure
   • Pressurization to 5,000 to 8,000 feet above sea level
   • Low humidity (10% to 20%)

- Ventilation system maintains low bacteria and fungi counts
- Significant vibration

3. The low humidity can trigger medical problems, especially in patients with asthma and chronic obstructive lung disease, due to drying of mucus in the bronchial airways.

HEME, ID

E 164   Intravenous immune globulin may be administered to a patient who has which of the following conditions?

A. Multiple myeloma
B. Multiple sclerosis
C. Polyarteritis nodosa
D. Idiopathic thrombocytopenic purpura
E. Kawasaki disease

Answer: D and E
D is correct because intravenous immune globulin is highly effective in raising the platelet count in idiopathic thrombocytopenic purpura (ITP), but its effect lasts only 1 to 2 weeks. E is correct because immune globulin plus aspirin reduces the risk of coronary artery aneurysm in Kawasaki disease patients.

■ **You should know:**

1. Intravenous immune globulin administration in idiopathic thrombocytopenic purpura (ITP) is generally reserved for cases of bleeding emergencies and, at times, preparing a patient for surgery. However, it may be given in initial ITP therapy in combination with a glucocorticoid.

2. The primary therapy of ITP in children and adults is a glucocorticoid, typically prednisone, in a tapering course over 4 to 6 weeks after the platelet count has returned to normal. Patients who are resistant to the glucocorticoid may be treated with the monoclonal antibody rituximab or anti-Rho (D) immunoglobulin, although the latter is associated with intravascular hemolysis.

3. Kawasaki disease, a childhood vasculitis of immune etiology, is characterized by fever, conjunctivitis, erythema of lips and oral mucosa, "strawberry" tongue, and adenopathy. The major complication is coronary artery aneurysm formation, which may lead to acute myocardial infarction, arrhythmia, and sudden cardiac death.

4. A brief review of intravenous immune globulin (IVIG):
   - An immunoglobulin derived from thousands of donors
   - IVIG is used in the treatment of the following conditions:
     (1) Kawasaki disease (IVIG, administered in conjunction with aspirin)
     (2) Guillain-Barré syndrome (as effective as plasma exchange transfusion)
     (3) Idiopathic thrombocytopenic purpura (ITP)
     (4) Myasthenia gravis
     (5) Autoimmune hemolytic anemia
     (6) Pediatric HIV patients
     (7) Antibody deficiency disorders

Essentials is designed to promote critical thinking and enrich your knowledge base.
Therefore, many questions will have more than one correct answer.

GI/N

E 165   Presence of which of the following differentiates chronic liver failure from the previously healthy patient who now has acute, fulminant liver failure?

A. Jaundice
B. Spider angiomata
C. Ascites
D. Asterixis
E. Encephalopathy

Answer: B

B is correct because spider angiomata result from alterations in sex hormone metabolism that occur in chronic liver disease. The increase in estradiol/free testosterone ratio is thought to be related to the development of these vascular lesions that have a central arteriole surrounded by smaller vessels.

▓ **You should know:**

1. Stigmata of (chronic) hepatic cirrhosis include:
   • Palmar erythema
   • Abdominal wall collateral veins (caput medusae)
   • Gynecomastia
   • Ascites
   • Dupuytren's contracture
   • Jaundice
   • Testicular atrophy
   • Peripheral neuropathy (sensory or sensorimotor—not autonomic)
   • Esophageal and gastric varices due to portal hypertension

2. The cardinal manifestations of acute liver failure include the following:
   • Encephalopathy caused by cerebral edema
   • Bleeding (gastrointestinal, mucosal, puncture sites) caused by decreased hepatic production of coagulation factors

3. There are many causes of acute liver failure including the following:
   • Viral infection, particularly hepatitis B but including hepatitis C and hepatitis D
   • Medicines (e.g., acetaminophen and amiodarone)
   • Vascular disease (e.g., ischemic hepatic injury)
   • Wilson's disease

4. A brief review: A comparison of the manifestations of acute and chronic liver failure:

	Encephalopathy	Jaundice	Bleeding	Ascites	Edema	Portal Hypertension	Spider Angiomata
Acute	Yes	Yes	Yes	Yes	Yes	No	No
Chronic	Yes	Yes	Yes	Yes	Yes	Yes	Yes

E 166   Which of the following is an absolute contraindication to oral contraceptive therapy?

A. Hypertriglyceridemia
B. Chronic active hepatitis
C. History of deep vein thrombosis
D. 1st-degree relative with ovarian cancer
E. Atrial fibrillation

Answer: B and C
B is correct because oral contraceptives (OCs) can worsen liver function in patients who have active liver disease. C is correct because OCs increase risk of thrombosis in women who have a history of thrombosis (e.g., stroke or deep vein thrombosis).

■ **You should know:**

1. Oral contraceptives increase the risk of thrombosis in women older than 35 years of age who smoke 15 or more cigarettes per day.

2. Before initiating OC therapy, determine whether concomitant medicinal intake by the patient could influence the efficacy of the oral contraceptives. Phenytoin, rifampin, and St. John's wort decrease OC effectiveness.

3. Oral contraceptives reduce the risk of ovarian cancer.

4. Oral contraceptives increase the risk of stroke in women who have a history of migraine with aura. Therefore, migraine with aura is an absolute contraindication to OC therapy.

5. Hypertriglyceridemia (HTG) is the third most common cause of acute pancreatitis, after biliary stones and alcohol ingestion. HTG-induced pancreatitis occurs when the serum TG level is 1,000 mg/dL or greater.

6. The clinical manifestations of HTG-induced pancreatitis are the same as pancreatitis of other etiology.

7. Although OCs do increase serum TG levels, they are not contraindicated in the patient who has mild to moderate hypertriglyceridemia.

E 167   Which of the following is associated with hyperglycemia?

A. Polycystic ovary syndrome
B. Hypercortisolism
C. Acromegaly
D. Pheochromocytoma
E. Medullary carcinoma of the thyroid

Answer: A, B, C, and D
A is correct because polycystic ovary syndrome is associated with increased insulin resistance. Therefore, diabetes mellitus is common. B is correct because hypercortisolism increases insulin resistance that induces hyperglycemia. C is correct because growth hormone antagonizes the action of insulin causing hyperglycemia. D is correct because the increased catecholamine secretion in pheochromocytoma promotes gluconeogenesis and glycogenolysis and induces tissue resistance to insulin.

Essentials is designed to promote critical thinking and enrich your knowledge base. Therefore, many questions will have more than one correct answer.

■ **You should know:**

1. Polycystic ovary syndrome is characterized by infertility, obesity, hirsutism, and oligomenorrhea (or amenorrhea). Abnormal laboratory values include high testosterone, estrogen, and luteinizing hormone levels in the serum. Insulin resistance and diabetes mellitus are common.

2. Hypercortisolism due to pituitary adenoma (Cushing's disease), adrenal hyperplasia or carcinoma, or exogenous glucocorticoid therapy is associated with hyperglycemia secondary to insulin resistance. These patients often have hypertension, truncal obesity, ecchymoses, rounded face (moon facies), and psychological manifestations that may include euphoria, depression, and even psychosis.

3. Acromegaly results from excess growth hormone secretion by a pituitary adenoma. It is characterized by enlargement of the hands, feet, and jaw, coarsening of facial features, hypertension (50%), and diabetes mellitus (30%). The adenoma secretes both growth hormone and prolactin.

4. Pheochromocytomas are tumors that secrete excessive quantities of norepinephrine and epinephrine. Most patients have sustained hypertension (a smaller percentage having paroxysmal hypertension). Episodic sweats, headache, and palpitation lasting minutes to hours are characteristic. Diagnosis is established in most cases by assay of urinary catecholamines and metanephrines. Only pheochromocytoma is associated with hypertension and orthostatic hypotension.

5. A brief review: In the patient who has *hypertension and hyperglycemia*, think of the following disorders:
   • Pheochromocytoma
   • Hypercortisolism
   • Acromegaly
   • The diabetic patient who develops hypertension secondary to progressive renal involvement

6. A brief review: In the patient who has *hypertension and hypokalemia*, think of the following disorders:
   • Primary hyperaldosteronism
   • Renovascular disease (e.g., unilateral renal artery stenosis—hypersecretion of renin causes a sequential increase in angiotensin II and aldosterone levels)
   • Cushing's syndrome (most commonly when associated with ectopic ACTH production)
   • Excessive licorice ingestion
   • Diuretic therapy that is surreptitious

7. Medullary carcinoma of the thyroid may produce one or more chemicals, including calcitonin, serotonin, prostaglandin, and adrenocorticotropic hormone. Flushing and diarrhea may be presenting symptoms.

E 168   Which of the following medicines may cause hypertension?

A. Lithium

B. Doxazosin

C. Fluoxetine

D. Naproxen

E. Sildenafil

Answer: D

D is correct because nonaspirin, nonselective, nonsteroidal anti-inflammatory drugs (NSAIDs) *inhibit renal vasodilator prostaglandins.* As a result, blood pressure increases.

■ **You should know:**

1. NSAIDs increase salt and water reabsorption in the kidney. Thus, a normal person will gain 0.5 to 1 kg in weight. Those with cirrhosis or heart failure may gain much more weight due to exaggerated salt and water retention.

2. Adverse effects of NSAIDs include:
   - Skin rashes of varying nature, including the serious condition toxic epidermal necrolysis
   - Edema
   - Peptic ulcer
   - Prerenal failure, especially in the hypovolemic patient
   - Hyperkalemia, most commonly in the patient who takes the NSAID in conjunction with an angiotensin-converting enzyme inhibitor or the chronic renal disease patient who takes an NSAID
   - Colitis associated with gross rectal bleeding
   - Postsurgical oozing due to the antiplatelet effect of NSAIDs that is similar to that of aspirin
   - Drug-induced lichen planus (other medicines that can cause lichen planus include ACEIs, beta-adrenergic blockers, lithium, sulfonylureas, and quinine)

3. Phosphodiesterase-5 inhibitors (e.g., sildenafil, vardenafil, and tadalafil) can cause profound hypotension when taken in conjunction with a nitrate. Additionally, this class of medicine must be used with caution in men who take alpha-adrenergic blockers.

E 169   Which of the following diseases is associated with eosinophilia?

A. Trichinellosis

B. Ascariasis

C. Systemic lupus erythematosus

D. Multiple sclerosis

E. Meningococcemia

Answer: A and B

A and B are correct because trichinellosis and ascariasis are parasitic diseases that invade tissue. The tissue invasion elicits an immune response resulting in eosinophilia. Eosinophils attack parasites but not bacteria.

Essentials is designed to promote critical thinking and enrich your knowledge base.
Therefore, many questions will have more than one correct answer.

▥ **You should know:**

1. Trichinellosis is caused by the parasite *Trichinella* and is often related to ingestion of uncooked meat. Initial symptoms may be nausea, vomiting, and diarrhea, or the patient may be asymptomatic until skeletal muscles are invaded.

2. In trichinellosis, skeletal muscle pain is typical, often associated with fever. Splinter hemorrhages, periorbital edema, and conjunctival hemorrhages occur at this time

3. *Ascaris lumbricoides,* a roundworm, causes varied clinical manifestations, including:
   • Pulmonary involvement, with pneumonia.
   • Intestinal involvement, with nausea, vomiting, and diarrhea. In children between ages 1 and 5 years, intestinal obstruction is common.

4. Systemic lupus erythematosus (SLE) is typically associated with leukopenia, thrombocytopenia, and occasionally hemolytic anemia. Some systemic lupus erythematosus (SLE) patients have antiphospholipid antibodies that increase the risk of venous and arterial thrombosis.

5. A brief review: Causes of splinter hemorrhages include the following conditions:
   • Trichinellosis
   • Infective endocarditis
   • Antiphospholipid antibody syndrome
   • Psoriasis
   • Medication (e.g., sorafenib, a tyrosine kinase inhibitor)
   • Atherosclerotic emboli to fingers or toes, as in subclavian steal syndrome

CV

E 170   Which of the following is a risk factor for dissection of the aorta?

A. Hypertension
B. Muscular dystrophy
C. Use of crack cocaine
D. Tetralogy of Fallot
E. Marfan syndrome

Answer: A, C, and E
A is correct because hypertension is the most important predisposing cause of dissection. C is correct because the abrupt, transient increase in blood pressure associated with crack cocaine use results in an intimal tear in the aorta with attendant dissection. E is correct because Marfan syndrome, an inherited disorder of connective tissue, causes weakening of the aorta media predisposing to dissection.

▥ **You should know:**

1. Aortic dissection begins with an intimal tear followed by development of a dissecting hematoma in the media of the aorta wall.

2. In a patient who has acute chest pain, clinical clues suggesting dissection of the ascending aorta include the following:
   • A new murmur of aortic valve regurgitation, occurring in one half to two thirds of cases
   • Unequal blood pressure in the arms, occurring in approximately 15% to 20% of cases

3. Adult patients most commonly have the dissection in the 5th through 7th decades. In this group, hypertension is the most common predisposing factor.

4. Younger patients with dissection generally have a congenital anomaly or inherited defect in connective tissue.

5. Congenital anomalies associated with dissection include:
   - Coarctation of aorta
   - Bicuspid aortic valve, particularly in the pregnant woman

6. Connective tissue disorders associated with dissection include:
   - Marfan syndrome
   - Ehlers-Danlos syndrome

7. Diagnostic modalities employed in the diagnosis of acute dissection of the aorta include the following:
   - CT imaging with contrast
   - MRI imaging with gadolinium
   - Transesophageal echocardiography (TEE)

NEURO, EENT

E 171 Presence of which of the following differentiates vertigo related to brainstem disease ("central" vertigo) from vertigo related to inner ear disease ("peripheral" vertigo)?

A. Dysmetria
B. Nystagmus
C. Head extension exacerbates vertigo
D. Association with herpes zoster
E. Tinnitus

Answer: A

A is correct because central vertigo is associated with other neurologic symptoms and signs including diplopia, ataxia, visual loss, slurred speech, weakness, and numbness. Physical examination may show dysmetria and abnormal reflexes.

■ **You should know:**

1. Dizziness is nonspecific and may refer to vertigo, presyncope, and disequilibrium.

2. Vertigo is a sensation of movement. It can be related to peripheral or central vestibular dysfunction.

3. The peripheral system refers to the inner ear; the central, to the brainstem and cerebellum.

4. Benign positional vertigo and Ménière's disease are peripheral causes of vertigo. Vertebrobasilar artery insufficiency, brainstem infarction, and cerebellar infarction are central causes.

5. Peripheral vertigo is typically not associated with other neurologic symptoms.

6. Nausea and vomiting can occur with *both* central and peripheral vertigo.

7. Nystagmus may be noted in patients having *both* central and peripheral vertigo.

Essentials is designed to promote critical thinking and enrich your knowledge base. Therefore, many questions will have more than one correct answer.

8. A patient with vertigo who also has tinnitus suggests a peripheral origin of the vertigo.

9. Presyncope refers to "almost blacking out" from cerebral hypoperfusion. This may occur with orthostatic hypotension or cardiac arrhythmia.

10. Disequilibrium is imbalance in walking. Peripheral neuropathy, cervical spondylosis, and muscular diseases may cause gait instability.

11. A brief review: A comparison of the clinical manifestations of peripheral and central vertigo:

	Vertigo	Nausea/Vomiting	Nystagmus	Tinnitus	Dysmetria
Peripheral	Yes	Yes	Yes	Yes	No
Central	Yes	Yes	Yes	No	Yes

NEURO, HEME

E 172 A 22-year-old man who lives in a residence with a poorly functioning heating system has a severe headache and mild confusion. Which of the following is the preferred diagnostic test for carbon monoxide poisoning?
A. Pulse oximetry
B. Systemic arterial Po_2 (Pao_2) level
C. Venous cyanohemoglobin level
D. Systemic arterial methemoglobin level
E. Systemic arterial carboxyhemoglobin level

Answer: E
E is correct because carbon monoxide binds with the iron in hemoglobin resulting in formation of carboxyhemoglobin. *Pulse oximetry cannot screen for carbon monoxide poisoning* because oximetry cannot differentiate between normal oxyhemoglobin and abnormal carboxyhemoglobin.

▊ **You should know:**

1. Carbon monoxide (CO) is colorless, odorless, and tasteless.

2. Smoke inhalation is the most common cause of CO poisoning (e.g., exposure to a poorly ventilated, fuel-burning heater or a poorly functioning heating system).

3. Headache is the most common presenting system. Nausea and dizziness followed by change in mental status (confusion to coma) may follow.

4. Systemic arterial Po_2 (Pao_2) is usually *normal* in carbon monoxide poisoning because Po_2 (Po_2) reflects oxygen that is dissolved in blood.

5. The "cherry red" skin sign in carbon monoxide (CO) poisoning is very insensitive.

6. Carbon monoxide poisoning is treated with high-flow, face mask oxygen inhalation.

7. *Methemoglobin* is an abnormal state of hemoglobin in which iron in heme is in the *ferric* state (Fe^{3+}). Methemoglobinemia may be congenital or acquired,

the latter caused by medicines, including the local anesthetic benzocaine, dapsone, and phenazopyridine (Pyridium). Methemoglobin cannot carry oxygen; patients are cyanotic, but systemic arterial Pao_2 is normal. The preferred treatment is administration of intravenous methylene blue that reduces ionic iron back to the normal ferrous (Fe^{2+}) state.

8. A comparison of oxyhemoglobin, methemoglobin, and carboxyhemoglobin follows:

	Oxyhemoglobin	Methemoglobin	Carboxyhemoglobin
Ionic iron state	Ferrous (Fe^{2+})	Ferric (Fe^{3+})	Ferrous (Fe^{2+})
Precipitating factor	Normal	Acquired or congenital	Carbon monoxide
Arterial Pao_2	Normal	Normal	Normal
Pulse oximetry	Accurate	Inaccurate	Inaccurate
Treatment		Methylene blue	Inhaled oxygen

GU

E 173   Presence of which of the following clinical signs differentiates torsion of the appendix testis from testicular torsion?

A. Fever and chills
B. Urethral discharge
C. Long axis of testis is oriented horizontally
D. Abdominal wall reflexes
E. Cremasteric reflex

Answer: E

E is correct because the cremasteric reflex is typically present in the patient who has torsion of the appendix testis but is absent in the patient who has testicular torsion.

■ **You should know:**

1. The differential diagnosis of acute scrotal pain in children and adolescents includes:
   • Testicular torsion
   • Torsion of appendix testis
   • Epididymitis
   • Orchitis
   • Henoch-Schönlein purpura
   • Inguinal hernia

2. Color Doppler ultrasonography is the preferred diagnostic test used to differentiate among these conditions.

3. Testicular torsion is occasionally seen in neonates but most commonly occurs in postpubertal boys (although it can occur at any age). Pain is sudden in onset and often occurs several hours after strenuous physical activity. Physical examination shows an exquisitely tender, high-riding testis on the affected side, with the long axis of the testis oriented transversely ("bell-clapper deformity"). The cremasteric reflex is usually absent. Immediate surgical intervention is necessary.

Essentials is designed to promote critical thinking and enrich your knowledge base. Therefore, many questions will have more than one correct answer.

4. The onset of pain is usually more gradual in torsion of the appendix testis. This is the most common cause of acute scrotal pain. Eighty percent of cases occur between the ages of 7 and 14 years. Inspection of the scrotal wall may show a "blue dot" sign representing infarction of the appendix testis. Treatment may be conservative (e.g., a nonsteroidal anti-inflammatory drug [NSAID]) or surgical.

5. Epididymitis may be acute but also occurs in a subacute form. *Acute* epididymitis is characterized by severe pain and swelling, usually associated with fever, chills, and voiding symptoms. Physical examination shows induration, swelling, and exquisite tenderness of the involved epididymis. In the sexually active male, *Chlamydia trachomatis* is the most common infecting organism, although gonococcus and other gram-negative organisms may be causative.

6. Orchitis may be caused by multiple viruses (e.g., mumps, coxsackie, and others). It is characterized by scrotal swelling and shininess of the skin and tenderness of the testis.

7. *Subacute* epididymitis usually occurs in healthy men related to sexual activity, heavy physical exertion, or bicycle/motorcycle riding.

NEURO

E 174   A 52-year-old man has a 3-hour history of diffuse headache. Presence of which of the following historical factors is suggestive of a life-threatening headache?

A. Sudden onset
B. Association with nasal congestion
C. Association with tearing
D. Pulsating quality
E. Onset with physical exertion

Answer: A and E
A is correct because a headache that starts suddenly and reaches maximum intensity within seconds is suggestive of subarachnoid hemorrhage (SAH). E is correct because a headache that starts with exertion (e.g., walking or Valsalva strain) suggests intracranial hemorrhage, carotid artery dissection, or pheochromocytoma.

▌ **You should know:**

1. The clinician must differentiate life-threatening headache (e.g., meningitis, subarachnoid hemorrhage [SAH], or brain tumor) from benign headache (e.g., cluster, migraine, and tension).

2. Patients who have subarachnoid hemorrhage typically have sudden onset of the headache with nausea and vomiting. This is followed very quickly, in many cases, by seizures and loss of consciousness. SAHs are due to rupture of cerebral aneurysm, cocaine/amphetamine abuse, and arteriovenous malformations.

3. Cluster headache is always unilateral. It is deep and excruciating in the area of the eye or temple. The headache is accompanied by autonomic signs (e.g., tearing, nasal congestion, and Horner's syndrome). Alcohol is a common precipitating factor. *Acute* cluster headache can be treated with administration of subcutaneous sumatriptan or octreotide and inhalation of 100% oxygen via

nonrebreathing mask. Medications given to *prevent* recurrent cluster headache include verapamil, prednisone, and lithium.

E 175   A 27-year-old healthy, nonpregnant woman has a 2-day history of dysuria and urinary frequency without fever or vaginal discharge. Microscopic analysis of a clean-catch urine specimen shows pyuria and bacteriuria. Which of the following is the most appropriate management?

A. 1 day of nitrofurantoin therapy
B. 3 days of fluoroquinolone therapy
C. 1 day of trimethoprim-sulfamethoxazole therapy
D. 7 days of ampicillin therapy
E. 7 days of tetracycline therapy

Answer: B
B is correct because uncomplicated cystitis in the healthy, nonpregnant woman is preferentially treated with either 3 days of a fluoroquinolone or 5 days of nitrofurantoin. Trimethoprim-sulfamethoxazole (TMP-SMX) is now less often used in empiric therapy of cystitis because of significant bacterial resistance.

■ **You should know:**

1. Dysuria in women, manifest by pain or burning upon urination, is caused by inflammation of the urethra, bladder, or vagina. The inflammation may or may not be related to infection.

2. Common infectious causes of dysuria include bacterial cystitis, chlamydial urethritis, acute pyelonephritis, gonococcal urethritis, *Trichomonas* urethritis, and vaginitis. Vaginal itching or discharge significantly reduces the likelihood of cystitis.

3. Pyuria is almost always noted in the patient who has bacterial cystitis, pyelonephritis, and chlamydial or gonococcal urethritis. Pyuria is not typically present in the woman with vaginitis. The presence of hematuria effectively rules out vaginitis.

4. The urinalysis is the most important diagnostic test in the healthy, young, nonpregnant woman with dysuria. Pyuria with bacteriuria is found in bacterial cystitis, most commonly due to *Escherichia coli, Staphylococcus saprophyticus,* and enterococci. Urine culture and sensitivity should be reserved for those suspected of having a complicated urinary tract infection.

5. Complicated urinary infections occur in those who have the following conditions:
   • Diabetes mellitus
   • History of childhood urinary tract infections
   • Three urinary tract infections in the past year
   • Indwelling urethral catheter
   • Hospital-acquired urinary infection

6. The examination of the urine in the patient with chlamydial urethritis shows pyuria but no bacteria. No blood is noted. Of the available diagnostic tests, nucleic acid amplification techniques (NAAT) appear to be most sensitive and specific. NAAT may be performed on urethral specimen or

urine. Other diagnostic modalities include culture, direct immunofluorescence, and ELISA. The nonpregnant patient is treated with azithromycin or
doxycycline.

7. In addition to dysuria, the woman with a gonococcal infection may have a
   purulent urethral discharge. Urinalysis shows pyuria without bacteriuria,
   but Gram stain of the urethral discharge shows gram-negative diplococci.
   Ceftriaxone or cefpodoxime is the preferred therapy. Sex partners should
   be treated. Patients should be empirically treated for *Chlamydia*.

8. Bacterial vaginosis (BV) is the most common cause of vaginitis in women
   of childbearing age. It is due to an increase in the number of many organisms, most notably *Gardnerella*. The patient frequently has a "fishy
   smelling," thin vaginal discharge. Diagnosis is based upon a positive whiff-
   amine test, defined as a fishy odor when 10% potassium hydroxide is
   added to vaginal discharge specimens. Clue cells, vaginal epithelial cells
   with adherent coccobacilli, are the most reliable predictor of bacterial vaginosis (BV). Oral metronidazole or intravaginal clindamycin is an effective
   therapy.

9. *Trichomonas vaginalis* may be an asymptomatic condition but classically
   causes vaginal burning and pruritus, dysuria, and a malodorous, thin vaginal discharge. Examination shows a "strawberry" cervix (i.e., punctate
   hemorrhages on the cervix) and a green-yellow frothy discharge. Wet
   mount preparations show motile trichomonads. Therapy of the nonpregnant patient is metronidazole. Sexual partners should be treated.

10. Patients with chlamydial or gonococcal urethritis should be tested for HIV
    infection and syphilis.

ID, GU

E 176   A 32-year-old man has a 2-day history of fever, dysuria, urinary frequency, and
perineal discomfort. Examination shows a tender, swollen prostate. Which of the
following are likely infecting organisms?

A. *Enterobacter* species
B. *Acinetobacter* species
C. *Moraxella catarrhalis*
D. *Proteus vulgaris*
E. *Escherichia coli*

Answer: D and E
E is correct because *Escherichia coli* and *Proteus* are the two most common organisms
causing acute bacterial prostatitis. Gram-positive enterococci are less frequent infecting organisms.

■ **You should know:**

1. *Acute bacterial prostatitis* is characterized by fever, chills, dysuria, and discomfort, often in the low back and perineum. The patient may require hospitalization if hypotension or mental changes are evident, for this patient is susceptible to gram-negative septicemia. Gram-negative rods are treated with
   quinolones or trimethoprim-sulfamethoxazole (TMX-SMX). Gram-positive
   enterococci are treated with ampicillin or amoxicillin. After completion of

antibiotic therapy, urine culture and sensitivity and prostatic secretion examination should be performed. *If urinary retention occurs, urethral catheterization is contraindicated in the patient who has acute bacterial prostatitis.* Suprapubic drainage of the urinary bladder should be performed.

2. *Chronic bacterial prostatitis* may be related to both gram-negative and gram-positive organisms. Patients commonly have dysuria and frequency. Analysis of the urine is frequently normal. Prostatic secretion analysis shows increased number of leukocytes (greater than 10/high-power field). Diagnosis is based upon culture of prostatic secretions or postmassage urine specimen. The preferred therapy is a fluoroquinolone for 4 to 12 weeks. Alternatively, trimethoprim-sulfamethoxazole may be given.

3. Nonbacterial prostatitis is common and is of unknown etiology. Patients have dysuria and discomfort in the perineal and suprapubic areas. Prostatic secretions show an increased number of leukocytes, but all cultures are sterile. A combination of an alpha-adrenergic blocking agent and a fluoroquinolone for 4 weeks is helpful in many patients.

NEURO

E 177 Which of the following is most likely to be considered a normal variant upon examination of a vigorous 81-year-old man?

A. Loss of proprioception in the toes
B. Unilateral facial anhidrosis
C. Stocking glove sensory loss in the lower legs
D. Unilateral extensor Babinski response
E. Absence of bilateral ankle deep tendon reflexes

Answer: E
E is correct because absence of ankle deep tendon reflexes is noted in 50% of persons between the ages of 81 and 90 years who have no recognized nervous system disease.

You should know:

1. Horner's syndrome is characterized by miosis, ptosis, and facial anhidrosis. It may arise from lesions in the brainstem and cervical/thoracic spinal cord in which sympathetic fibers are disrupted. Causes of Horner's syndrome include the following:
   - Bronchogenic carcinoma with tumor spread into the inferior sympathetic ganglion
   - Cluster headache
   - Cerebellar infarction due to thrombosis of inferior cerebellar artery
   - Dissection of carotid artery

2. An extensor plantar reflex (extensor Babinski sign) occurs when there is damage to central (upper) nervous system motor pathways. The abnormal response is characterized by great toe extension (dorsiflexion) with the other toes fanning out.

3. Stocking glove sensory loss occurs in polyneuropathy related to:
   - Diabetes mellitus
   - Alcohol abuse

Essentials is designed to promote critical thinking and enrich your knowledge base. Therefore, many questions will have more than one correct answer.

- Vitamin B$_{12}$ deficiency
- HIV infection
- Syphilis

4. Proprioceptive loss occurs in neuropathy due to diabetes mellitus and vitamin B$_{12}$ deficiency. Loss of proprioception may be caused by disease affecting the posterior spinal column or peripheral nerve or nerve root.

DERM

E 178   A 46-year-old woman has a 1-week history of a rash involving her chest, scalp, and inguinal areas. The rash is depicted in the photograph. Which of the following is the most likely diagnosis?

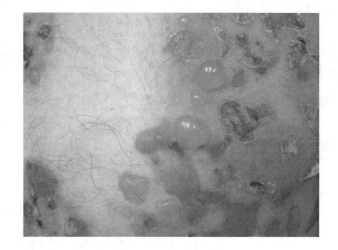

A. Lichen simplex chronicus
B. Miliaria
C. Pemphigus
D. Contact dermatitis
E. Atopic dermatitis

Answer: C
C is correct because pemphigus is an autoimmune disease that causes formation of bullae (blisters).

■ **You should know:**

1. Blistering diseases include pemphigus, bullous pemphigoid, dermatitis herpetiformis, erythema multiforme, porphyria cutanea tarda, and toxic epidermal necrolysis.

2. Nikolsky's sign is a mechanical sign that is often found in a patient with pemphigus. Application of pressure to the skin causes the superficial skin to separate from the deeper layers. The sign may be elicited on normal skin or at the margin of a blister.

3. Miliaria is a rash characterized by vesicles, papules, or pustules typically on the trunk and in intertriginous areas. It is most frequently noted in patients who live in hot, humid environments. It is due to plugging of eccrine sweat glands. Differential diagnosis includes drug rash and folliculitis.

E 179   A 52-year-old obese man has a 1-week history of burning in the groin area. The area is shown in the photograph. Which of the following is the preferred initial diagnostic test?

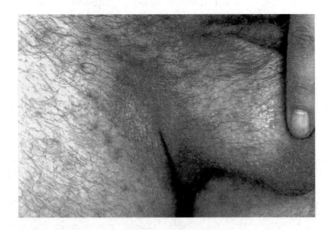

A. Potassium hydroxide preparation of rash debris
B. Bacterial culture and sensitivity of rash debris
C. Polymerase chain reaction
D. Anti–streptolysin O titer
E. Examination under Wood's lamp

Answer: A

A is correct because the diagnosis of candidiasis is made by potassium hydroxide (KOH) preparation on rash scrapings. Examination of the preparation shows budding yeasts with or without pseudohyphae.

▓ **You should know:**

1. *Candida* are normal flora in the gastrointestinal and genitourinary tracts of humans.

2. Cutaneous candidiasis is particularly likely to occur in patients with diabetes mellitus or in obese persons who perspire freely.

3. Oral candidiasis (thrush) is seen in infants, those who wear dentures, patients on antibiotic therapy, chemotherapy, or radiation therapy to the head and neck, and those patients with AIDS.

4. Esophageal candidiasis is an AIDS-defining illness. The patient may or may not have coexisting thrush.

5. Vulvovaginal candidiasis most often occurs in patients who have increased estrogen levels (e.g., pregnancy, oral contraceptive intake, or estrogen therapy). Other risk factors include diabetes mellitus, corticosteroid therapy, intrauterine devices, and diaphragm use.

6. A brief review: Microscopic examination of skin scrapings using *KOH preparation* is used in the diagnosis of the following fungal and yeast disorders:
   • Tinea corporis
   • Tinea pedis

Essentials is designed to promote critical thinking and enrich your knowledge base.
Therefore, many questions will have more than one correct answer.

- Tinea capitis
- Tinea cruris
- Tinea versicolor
- Candidiasis

7. *Wood's lamp* examination is used in the diagnosis of tinea capitis due to *Microsporum canis* or *Microsporum audouinii* (approximately 15% of cases of tinea capitis), erythrasma, and porphyria cutanea tarda.

CV

E 180   Upon routine examination, an asymptomatic 14-year-old boy is noted to have a heart murmur. His electrocardiogram is shown. Which of the following is the most likely diagnosis?

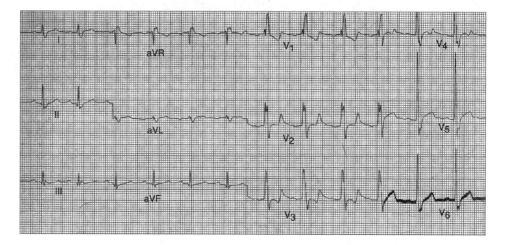

A. Atrial septal defect
B. Ventricular septal defect
C. Aortic valve stenosis
D. Tetralogy of Fallot
E. Mitral valve prolapse

Answer: A
A is correct because complete right bundle branch block (CRBBB) or incomplete right bundle branch block is present on electrocardiographic study in nearly all patients who have an atrial septal defect.

■ **You should know:**

1. The electrocardiogram (ECG) in ventricular septal defect may be normal or may demonstrate left ventricular hypertrophy or biventricular hypertrophy depending upon the size of the shunt.

2. Electrocardiography in the patient with tetralogy of Fallot typically demonstrates right ventricular hypertrophy and right axis deviation.

3. In the typical case of mitral valve prolapse the ECG is normal.

4. Electrocardiographic study in the patient with aortic valve stenosis commonly demonstrates left ventricular hypertrophy that may lead to diastolic heart failure. (Remember that left ventricular hypertrophy causes the

ventricle to become stiff [noncompliant], and a stiff left ventricle is the underlying factor leading to onset of diastolic heart failure.)

5. Complete RBBB is infrequently considered to be a normal variant.

6. Pathologic causes of right bundle branch block include:
   • Myocardial ischemia/infarction
   • Myocarditis
   • Cor pulmonale (conditions associated with chronically increased right ventricular pressure)
   • Cardiomyopathy (e.g., sarcoid granulomas affecting the cardiac conduction system)
   • Congenital heart disease (e.g., atrial septal defect)
   • Degenerative disease of the conduction system in an otherwise healthy patient

7. Cardiac auscultation in the patient with CRBBB will show a persistently split second heart sound (S2) that splits further during inspiration.

8. Complete left bundle branch block (CLBBB) is rarely considered to be a normal variant.

9. Pathologic causes of CLBBB include the following:
   • Hypertension
   • Myocardial ischemia/infarction
   • Degenerative disease of the conduction system in an otherwise healthy patient
   • Valvular disease
   • Dilated cardiomyopathy

10. Cardiac auscultation in the patient with CLBBB will show a paradoxically split second heart sound (S2).

CV

E 181   A 26-year-old woman has the sudden onset of palpitations described as very fast and regular. Blood pressure is 110/60 mm Hg and respiratory rate is 24/min. The patient is alert and pink. No heart murmur or gallop is heard. Chest radiography is normal. The patient's electrocardiogram is shown. Which of the following is the preferred initial medicinal therapy?

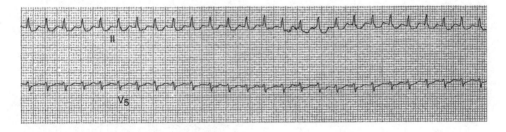

   A. Intravenous lidocaine
   B. Oral verapamil
   C. Sublingual nifedipine
   D. Intravenous adenosine
   E. Emergent cardioversion

Essentials is designed to promote critical thinking and enrich your knowledge base.
Therefore, many questions will have more than one correct answer.

Answer: **D**

D is correct because intravenous adenosine is effective (90%) in terminating paroxysmal supraventricular tachycardia (PSVT). Further, it has a very short half-life (approximately 6 seconds). (The electrocardiogram in this patient demonstrates a regular, normal QRS tachycardia at a rate of 220/min.)

You should know:

1. The initial treatment of paroxysmal supraventricular tachycardia is vagal stimulation including carotid sinus massage, Valsalva strain maneuver, or splashing cold water on the face.

2. *Never exert bilateral carotid sinus pressure at the same time.*

3. Do *not* employ carotid sinus pressure if the patient has a carotid artery bruit on either side.

4. If PSVT is refractory to vagal stimulation, intravenous administration of adenosine is preferred. If the arrhythmia is refractory to adenosine, then the arrhythmia is often terminated by the intravenous administration of a calcium channel blocker (verapamil or diltiazem), beta-adrenergic blocker, or digoxin.

5. The primary mechanism of action of adenosine is to slow atrioventricular (AV) conduction. Therefore, transient atrioventricular block, even advanced block, may occur.

6. Adenosine may provoke bronchospasm in patients with reactive airways disease (e.g., asthma).

7. Tachycardias are generally categorized by normal QRS (less than 120 msec) or widened QRS (equal to or greater than 120 msec).

8. A *narrow QRS* suggests that the depolarization of the ventricles originates in or above the atrioventricular (AV) node.

9. A *wide QRS* suggests that the arrhythmia originates in the ventricle—that is, ventricular tachycardia *or* the arrhythmia is supraventricular with a preexisting conduction defect or a rate-related aberrant conduction.

E 182   During a very hot and humid summer, a 34-year-old man has a 1-week history of a rash on his trunk. The rash does not involve the palms and soles. The rash is shown in the photograph. Which of the following is the most likely diagnosis?

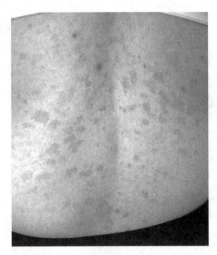

A. Secondary syphilis
B. Erythema multiforme
C. Bullous pemphigoid
D. Rocky Mountain spotted fever
E. Tinea versicolor

Answer: E

E is correct because tinea versicolor (TV) is a rash characterized by oval-to-round macules of various colors (white, orange-brown, and dark-brown) with overlying fine scales.

■ **You should know:**

1. Tinea versicolor (TV) is a superficial infection caused by *Malassezia furfur*, saprophytic yeast. Adolescents and young adults are most commonly affected.

2. Hot and humid weather, hyperhidrosis, skin oils, and immunosuppression appear to cause the clinical disease.

3. The diagnosis is confirmed by microscopic examination of skin scales using a 10% potassium hydroxide preparation.

4. Many topical preparations may be used in treatment of tinea versicolor, including clotrimazole, econazole, ketoconazole, and selenium sulfide. Alternatively, an oral medication (e.g., ketoconazole) may be used for therapy of extensive disease or resistant infection.

5. The rash of secondary syphilis is a symmetrical macular or papular eruption involving the entire trunk, including the palms and soles.

Essentials is designed to promote critical thinking and enrich your knowledge base. Therefore, many questions will have more than one correct answer.

DERM, REPRO

E 183   A 27-year-old woman has a 1-month history of an asymptomatic rash on both cheeks. The rash is shown in the photograph. Which of the following is the most likely associated condition?

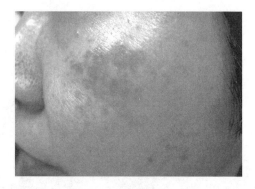

   A. Cushing's disease
   B. Oral intake of diltiazem
   C. Oral intake of omeprazole
   D. Pregnancy
   E. Rheumatoid arthritis

Answer: D
D is correct because approximately 75% of pregnant women have melasma, a hyperpigmentation that affects the cheeks, forehead, chin, and nose.

■ **You should know:**

   1. The cause of melasma is unknown.

   2. Other factors that favor development of melasma include intake of oral contraceptives, exposure to the sun, and certain antiepileptic medications.

   3. Melasma associated with pregnancy usually recedes within 1 year after delivery.

   4. In the differential diagnosis, other splotchy hyperpigmentation disorders, including acne, eczema, and contact dermatitis, should be considered.

   5. Therapy of melasma includes sunscreen, bleaching agents (hydroquinone, azelaic acid, tretinoin), and chemical peels.

DERM, ID

E 184 A 41-year-old man has a 2-day history of a rash that is shown in the photographs. The skin disorder is most likely to be associated with which of the following?

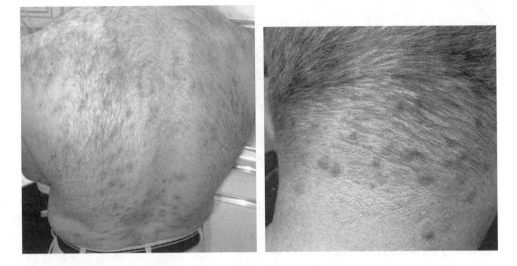

- A. Bathing in a hot tub
- B. Exposure to ultraviolet radiation
- C. Ingestion of sulfites
- D. Vitamin A poisoning
- E. Adverse reaction to verapamil

Answer: A
A is correct because folliculitis due to *Pseudomonas aeruginosa* may occur from bathing in hot tubs that are inadequately chlorinated. Hot tub folliculitis usually resolves without treatment if the patient is not exposed to the contaminated water.

■ **You should know:**

1. Folliculitis is a pustular eruption of the skin follicles. When not related to infection from a contaminated hot tub, it is most commonly due to infection with *Staphylococcus aureus*.

2. Staphylococcal folliculitis is most commonly treated with topical agents including mupirocin or ethyl alcohol containing aluminum chloride.

3. Nasal carriage of *Staphylococcus* may cause recurrent folliculitis. Mupirocin ointment applied to the anterior nares is effective in eradicating *Staphylococcus aureus* colonization.

4. Less often, folliculitis is caused by infection by *Candida*, especially in patients taking broad-spectrum antibiotics.

5. Impetigo is a superficial vesiculopustular eruption that typically arises at sites of insect bites or abrasions. The pustules rupture causing a crusting with a golden appearance. *Staphylococcus aureus* and group A streptococci are the most common infecting organisms. Streptococcal impetigo may be associated with poststreptococcal glomerulonephritis in children.

Essentials is designed to promote critical thinking and enrich your knowledge base. Therefore, many questions will have more than one correct answer.

6. A brief review: Streptococcal *pharyngitis* may be complicated by acute rheumatic fever or glomerulonephritis. Streptococcal *impetigo* may be complicated by glomerulonephritis but not rheumatic fever.

ID, PUL

E 185   A healthy 34-year-old man who lives in Arizona has a 3-day history of fever, minimally productive cough, and right pleuritic chest pain. He now has erythema nodosum on the anterior surface of both lower legs. Which of the following is the preferred initial diagnostic test to confirm the diagnosis of coccidioidomycosis?

   A. Sputum culture and sensitivity
   B. Skin test to coccidioidomycosis antigens
   C. Immunodiffusion assay for IgG and IgM
   D. Latex test
   E. Biopsy of erythema nodosum lesion

Answer: C
C is correct because serologic tests are most commonly used for the diagnosis of coccidioidomycosis. Immunodiffusion assay is considered to be the most specific serologic assay for this disease.

   ■ **You should know:**

   1. Coccidioidomycosis is endemic in arid areas of the southwestern United States, Mexico, and Central and South Americas.

   2. Coccidioidomycosis organisms grow a few inches under desert soil. Inhalation of conidia causes clinical infection.

   3. The illness has a wide clinical spectrum, varying from insignificant illness to community-acquired pneumonia (CAP) to disseminated disease with meningitis, pulmonary cavitation or abscess formation, and bone lesions.

   4. Increased risk for disseminated disease occurs in the following:
      • HIV-infected patients
      • Diabetes mellitus patients
      • Those on immunosuppressive or chemotherapy
      • Pregnant women

   5. Sputum culture is not routinely obtained for diagnosis. Dermal hypersensitivity to the coccidioidomycosis antigen remains for life. A positive skin test may reflect distant infection rather than current illness.

   6. Healthy persons whose illness is limited to the chest do not need antifungal therapy. Antimicrobial therapy is for those who manifest progressive disease.

NEURO, ENDO

E 186   A 57-year-old woman has recurrent numbness and tingling in her fingers, toes, and the perioral area around her lips. Which of the following conditions is associated with the patient having paresthesias?

   A. Vertebrobasilar artery insufficiency
   B. Primary hypoparathyroidism
   C. Hypoglycemia
   D. Diabetic polyneuropathy
   E. Organic mercury poisoning

Answer: A, B, C, D, and E
There are several underlying disorders that can cause the patient to experience paresthesias. These include metabolic disturbances (e.g., hypocalcemia and hypoglycemia), poisoning, brain ischemia, and peripheral neuropathy.

▨ **You should know:**

1. Paresthesias are subjective sensations often described as pins-and-needles, tingling, or even numbness, without external sensory stimulation.

2. Paresthesias may arise from a neurologic disorder that anatomically may range from the peripheral nerve to the sensory cortex of the brain. Consequently, the subjective sensations may be noted by the patient who has sensory seizures, ulnar or median nerve compression syndromes, or peripheral neuropathy (e.g., diabetic, uremic, or alcohol-related).

3. The distal symmetrical polyneuropathy of diabetes, uremia, and chronic alcohol abuse is functionally similar. Paresthesias are the early symptoms with examination showing a loss of sensation (e.g., vibratory, proprioceptive, light touch, and temperature). Later, motor symptoms (e.g., weakness) and signs may be present.

4. Parathyroid hormone and vitamin D affect the serum calcium level via their effects on the gastrointestinal tract, kidney, and bone. A decreased serum level of ionized calcium that may occur in hypoparathyroidism or vitamin D deficiency increases the excitability of nerves causing the patient to have paresthesias in the extremities and in the perioral area of the face.

5. Adrenergic manifestations of hypoglycemia include sweating, palpitations, tremulousness, and paresthesias. The paresthesias involve the extremities and the perioral area of the face. Note that both hypocalcemia and hypoglycemia may be associated with perioral paresthesias; however, only hypoglycemia has the adrenergic symptoms of sweating and palpitations.

6. Vertebrobasilar artery insufficiency may be associated with paresthesias of the trunk, extremities, or face (perioral area), *binocular* blurred vision or diplopia, ataxia, vertigo, and weakness. (In contrast, amaurosis fugax, most commonly caused by atherosclerosis in the carotid artery, is characterized by *monocular* blurred vision.)

7. Organic mercury poisoning, as may occur with exposure to contaminated fish, may cause paresthesias, notably perioral, ataxia, tremors, and convulsions.

8. A brief review: Perioral paresthesias may occur in the patient who has hypocalcemia, hypoglycemia, vertebrobasilar artery insufficiency, or organic mercury poisoning.

9. In contrast, *chronic lead poisoning* typically causes a motor neuropathy (e.g., wrist drop) without an associated sensory neuropathy.

Essentials is designed to promote critical thinking and enrich your knowledge base. Therefore, many questions will have more than one correct answer.

E 187   Presence of which of the following differentiates respiratory distress syndrome (hyaline membrane disease) from transient tachypnea of the newborn?

A. Occurs in premature infants
B. "Sunburst" hilar pattern on chest radiography
C. Deficiency of pulmonary surfactant
D. Occurs in infants of diabetic mothers
E. Is considered a benign disorder

Answer: C

Although respiratory distress syndrome and transient tachypnea of the newborn have certain features in common (e.g., both occurring more frequently in premature infants and occurring in infants of diabetic mothers), the pathophysiology, prognosis, and radiographic features must be differentiated.

▓ **You should know:**

1. Transient tachypnea of the newborn (TTN) is a benign disorder; respiratory distress syndrome (RDS) is serious.

2. *Both* TTN and RDS occur more frequently in premature infants.

3. *Both* TTN and RDS are associated with mothers who have diabetes mellitus.

4. *Only* TTN appears to be associated with mothers who have asthma.

5. *Only* TTN appears to be associated with cesarean section at term.

6. The following table compares and contrasts other clinical differences between TTN and RDS:

	Pathophysiology	**Chest Radiography**	**Treatment**
TTN	Delayed resorption of fetal alveolar fluid	"Sunburst" pulmonary edema pattern	Supplemental oxygen
RDS	Deficiency of surfactant	Ground-glass pattern with air bronchogram	Oxygen; inhaled surfactant; CPAP

(CPAP = continuous positive airway pressure)

E 188   Which of the following conditions is characterized by an elevated serum gastrin level (hypergastrinemia)?

A. Pernicious anemia
B. Barrett's esophagus
C. Celiac disease
D. Zollinger-Ellison syndrome
E. Acromegaly

Answer: A and D

Pernicious anemia (PA) is characterized by achlorhydria that causes a secondary increase in serum gastrin levels. Gastrin-producing tumors cause atypical peptic ulcer disease known as Zollinger-Ellison syndrome.

■ **You should know:**

1. Gastrin is produced primarily in the antrum of the stomach. It is secreted in response to a meal or to a high pH in the stomach.

2. The fundamental pathologic lesion in PA is chronic atrophic gastritis with achlorhydria and failure to secrete intrinsic factor. Further, the deficiency in intrinsic factor is related to autoimmune anti–intrinsic factor antibodies. Thus, there is both deficient production of intrinsic factor and presence of antibodies to intrinsic factor that lead to vitamin B_{12} deficiency in the body.

3. The upper limit of normal of serum gastrin is 100 pg/mL. In the patient who has PA, the serum gastrin level may be as high as 1,000 pg/mL.

4. In contrast, high serum gastrin levels, typically greater than 1,000 pg/mL, may be a *primary disorder* in which gastrin-producing tumors lead to excessive gastric acid secretion and development of intractable peptic ulcer disease, ulcers with diarrhea, and ulcers in atypical locations (e.g., the second and third portions of the duodenum). This is Zollinger-Ellison syndrome.

5. In the patient who has a very high serum gastrin level the clinician must differentiate between PA and Zollinger-Ellison syndrome. Measurement of gastric pH will enable the clinician to quickly make the distinction.

CV, GI/N, ENDO

E 189   Family screening should be performed in 1st-degree relatives of patients who have which of the following conditions?

A. Atherosclerotic heart disease
B. Hemochromatosis
C. Ovarian cancer
D. Hypertrophic obstructive cardiomyopathy
E. Melanoma

Answer: A, B, C, D, and E
The clinician must determine when family screening of a patient should be performed in an effort to prevent clinical disease in the relative and potentially to prevent premature death in that family member.

■ **You should know:**

1. There are genetic and environmental factors that contribute to development of premature coronary heart disease. First-degree relatives of a patient who has premature coronary disease (i.e., under the age of 45 years) should be screened. Relatives should be evaluated for serum levels of cholesterol (and lipid fractions), glucose, and insulin. (Many family members may not have overt hyperglycemia but will exhibit a hyperinsulinemic response to an oral glucose load.)

2. First-degree relatives of a patient who has hemochromatosis should have measured serum levels of transferrin and ferritin. If elevated, genetic testing should be considered. The appropriate age for family screening is between 18 and 30 years.

3. The strongest risk factor for ovarian cancer is family history. Family screening should be performed when there is a patient who has familial ovarian cancer

syndrome—that is, ovarian cancer occurring under the age of 50 years and in at least two generations in the family. Screening should include serial measurement of CA 125, testing for *BRCA1* and *BRCA2* genetic mutations, and transvaginal ultrasonography.

4. Hypertrophic obstructive cardiomyopathy (HOCM) is an autosomal dominant disorder. First-degree relatives should undergo history and physical examination, electrocardiography, and echocardiography. Screening of children should begin at age 12 years *unless the child has clinical manifestations of HOCM or is going to participate in vigorous sports.* Screening should be performed annually from age 12 to 18 years, for the hypertrophy may not begin until adolescence. After age 18 years, evaluation should be performed approximately every 5 years.

5. There is a familial melanoma syndrome. There should be family screening in the melanoma patient who has a family history of more than one 1st-degree relative with the skin disease.

6. Those individuals who have a 1st-degree relative younger than age 60 years with *colorectal cancer* or who have two 1st-degree relatives diagnosed at any age should have a screening colonoscopy at age 40 years or 10 years younger than the earliest diagnosis in the family.

7. *Scabies is not an inherited disorder.* It is transmitted by skin-to-skin contact. Therefore, it is suggested that *all family members and close contacts* of a patient with scabies be treated in an effort to prevent reinfection.

DERM

E 190 Which of the following skin diseases is characterized by target-like lesions on the skin and erosions on the lips and oral mucosa?

A. Stevens-Johnson syndrome
B. Erythema multiforme
C. Pemphigus
D. Pityriasis rosea
E. Rocky Mountain spotted fever

Answer: A and B
A is correct because Stevens-Johnson syndrome (SJS) is characterized by target-like skin lesions, vesicles, bullae, and oral and buccal mucosa erosions. SJS is an idiosyncratic reaction that is commonly related to medicines, including allopurinol, sulfonamides, penicillins, carbamazepine, diphenylhydantoin, phenobarbital, and piroxicam. B is correct because erythema multiforme (EM) is also characterized by target skin lesions and oral erosions. EM is an immune-mediated skin disorder that is most commonly associated with herpes simplex virus infection.

▓ **You should know:**

1. *Pemphigus* is a chronic autoimmune skin disorder that is characterized by flaccid bullae in the oropharynx followed by scalp, chest, axillae, and groin involvement. These bullae spontaneously rupture. Target skin lesions are not found in pemphigus.

2. *Stevens-Johnson syndrome* is characterized by fever and influenza-like symptoms followed by skin and oral mucosal lesions that may become necrotic and slough.

3. In SJS, medicine exposure commonly precedes the onset of symptoms and rash by 1 to 3 weeks.

4. Toxic epidermal necrolysis and SJS are overlapping conditions. There is a lack of consensus whether they are variants of the same condition or, alternatively, are separate disorders.

5. *Erythema multiforme* is usually self-limited, resolving within a few weeks. Although herpes simplex virus is considered to be the most important cause of EM, other infectious organisms (viral, bacterial, and fungal) are implicated. Other noninfectious conditions that have been implicated include sarcoidosis, radiation therapy, and medications.

6. The following table compares and contrasts EM and SJS:

	EM	SJS
Target lesions	Yes	Yes, atypical
Etiology	Infection (90%)	Medicines (50%)
Pathophysiology	Immune-mediated	Idiosyncratic
Mucous membranes	Occasionally involved	Always involved
Skin necrosis	No	Yes

7. A brief review of the *"erythemas"*:
   • Erythema multiforme: See above.
   • Erythema migrans: A skin lesion in early Lyme disease that appears 3 to 32 days after a tick bite.
   • Erythema marginatum: The ring- or crescent-shaped skin lesion that is a major criterion in the diagnosis of acute rheumatic fever. Other "major" criteria include carditis, arthritis, chorea, and subcutaneous nodules.
   • Erythema nodosum: An inflammatory lesion in the subcutaneous fat typically in the anterior portion of the lower leg. It is associated with many infections (e.g., bacterial, fungal, or spirochetal) in addition to medicines, pregnancy, sarcoidosis, and inflammatory bowel disease.
   • Erythema toxicum neonatorum: A rash of unknown etiology that appears 24 to 48 hours after birth. It is characterized by erythematous macules and papules 1 to 3 mm in diameter on the trunk and proximal extremities (sparing the palms and soles) that progress to pustular lesions. The rash typically resolves spontaneously without treatment.

ID, GI/N

E 191   A 6-year-old child has a 5-day history of bloody diarrhea and abdominal pain. Enterohemorrhagic *E. coli* (EHEC) diarrhea is diagnosed. Which of the following is the least likely clinical finding to be noted?

A. White blood count 14,000/microL
B. Oral temperature 102°F
C. Blood urea nitrogen 46 mg/L
D. Schistocytes on peripheral blood smear
E. Presence of fecal leukocytes

Essentials is designed to promote critical thinking and enrich your knowledge base. Therefore, many questions will have more than one correct answer.

Answer: B

B is correct because *fever is not a clinical presentation* of EHEC-related hemorrhagic colitis. However, leukocytosis (white blood count greater than 10,000/microL), abdominal pain and tenderness, and presence of fecal leukocytes are characteristic. Approximately 10% of EHEC colitis is complicated by hemolytic-uremic syndrome (HUS).

■ You should know:

1. EHEC produce Shiga toxin that causes a hemorrhagic colitis (bloody diarrhea).

2. *An important clinical point*: Fever is *not* a characteristic presentation of EHEC bloody diarrhea. In contrast, other bacterial causes of bloody diarrhea include *Campylobacter, Shigella* species, and *Salmonella*; in these patients fever is prominent. Amebiasis, caused by the protozoan *Entamoeba histolytica*, also produces bloody diarrhea; fever is noted in approximately 25% of amebiasis cases.

3. *The clinician should not exclude an infectious cause of bloody diarrhea if the patient is afebrile.* Noninfectious causes of (afebrile) bloody diarrhea include intussusception, ischemic bowel, and inflammatory bowel disease.

4. Outbreaks of EHEC-related colitis have been related to consumption of lettuce, spinach, sprouts, and undercooked beef.

5. HUS occurs in approximately 10% of EHEC colitis. HUS is characterized by acute renal failure, microangiopathic hemolytic anemia, and thrombocytopenia.

6. Microangiopathic hemolytic anemia is caused by nonautoimmune destruction of red blood cells in the microvasculature. Schistocytes are noted on examination of a peripheral blood smear. Other features of a hemolytic anemia are noted (e.g., increased serum indirect bilirubin, low serum haptoglobin, and reticulocytosis).

7. Thrombocytopenia in HUS is caused by platelet clumping in the microvasculature.

8. HUS is treated with plasma exchange; antibiotics do not appear to be beneficial.

HEME/ONC, CV

E 192   Which of the following is the primary mechanism of action of dabigatran?
   A. Direct thrombin inhibitor
   B. Blocks adenosine diphosphate (ADP) receptor on platelets
   C. Cyclooxygenase (COX) inhibition
   D. Inhibits glycoprotein IIb/IIIa receptors
   E. Inhibits vitamin K coagulation factors

Answer: A

Dabigatran directly inhibits thrombin, the last enzyme in the coagulation cascade that catalyzes fibrinogen into fibrin.

■ You should know:

1. Thrombin is the enzyme that links the extrinsic pathway and the intrinsic pathway of the coagulation cascade in the production of fibrin.

2. Dabigatran is an oral medication that is approved for stroke prevention in patients who have *nonvalvular* atrial fibrillation.

3. Its half-life is 12 to 14 hours in patients who have normal renal function. Eighty percent is excreted unchanged in the urine. Therefore, patients who have renal insufficiency require lower dosage.

4. Advantages of dabigatran include the following:
   • No interaction with food
   • No anticoagulant monitoring (except in certain patients with azotemia)

5. In order to ensure stability and loss of potency from moisture, dabigatran should be stored in its original bottle or blister package. It should not be put in a pill box or pill organizer.

6. There is no specific antidote to dabigatran. In order to reverse its anticoagulant effect, the medication must be discontinued and the following measures may be employed:
   • Hemodialysis
   • Charcoal ingestion to remove nonabsorbed drug from the gastrointestinal tract
   • Administration of three-factor prothrombin complex concentrate

7. The following list indicates drug interactions with dabigatran:
   • *Decreased* dabigatran concentration (*administer dabigatran at least 2 hours before these medications*): Acid suppressive medications, including antacids, H2 antagonists, and proton pump inhibitors
   • *Decreased* dabigatran concentration (*avoid concurrent use, if possible*): Carbamazepine, dexamethasone, St. John's wort, doxorubicin
   • *Increased* dabigatran concentration (*these medicines inhibit P-glycoproteins that act to eliminate drugs into the urine, bile, and stool*): Amiodarone, cyclosporine, verapamil, and protease inhibitors

8. Clinical studies have demonstrated the efficacy of dabigatran in *prevention* of venous thromboembolism after knee or hip replacement. Further, this medication is equivalent to warfarin (after parenteral anticoagulation) in *treatment* of venous thromboembolism. However, as of July 1, 2012, the Food and Drug Administration has not approved dabigatran in either prevention or treatment of venous thromboembolism.

HEME/ONC

E 193   In which of the following diseases is thrombocytopenia caused by autoimmune antibody destruction of platelets?

   A. Rocky Mountain spotted fever
   B. Idiopathic thrombocytopenic purpura
   C. Heparin-related thrombocytopenia
   D. Parvovirus infection
   E. Splenomegaly caused by portal hypertension

Answer: B and C
Idiopathic thrombocytopenic purpura (ITP) and heparin-related thrombocytopenia are caused by immune destruction of platelets by antibodies.

■ **You should know:**

1. Major causes of thrombocytopenia include increased platelet destruction, decreased platelet production by the bone marrow, and redistribution of platelets in the circulation.

2. Increased platelet destruction may be on an immune or nonimmune basis. *Immune* (antibody) destruction occurs in ITP, heparin therapy, abciximab administration, and systemic lupus erythematosus.

3. Approximately 2.5% of patients receiving unfractionated heparin for more than 4 days will develop thrombocytopenia. Low molecular weight heparin can also cause thrombocytopenia but less frequently than unfractionated. Abciximab is an intravenous glycoprotein IIa/IIIb inhibitor of platelet aggregation. It can cause a marked reduction in platelet count within 24 hours of initial administration, often within several hours.

4. A *nonimmune* cause of increased platelet destruction is Rocky Mountain spotted fever. The decreased platelet count is related to the generalized endothelial damage from the infectious vasculitis. Another is disseminated intravascular coagulation (DIC) in which platelets are consumed in the uncontrolled triggering of coagulation. In addition to thrombocytopenia, DIC is characterized by depletion of fibrinogen and coagulation factors.

5. Decreased platelet production may occur on a nonimmune basis in viral infections (notably, parvovirus, varicella, mumps, hepatitis C), chemotherapy administration, extensive radiotherapy, and vitamin B_{12} or folate deficiency.

6. Splenomegaly, particularly related to portal hypertension, will cause the spleen to sequester increased number of platelets resulting in thrombocytopenia.

GI/N

E 194 Roux-en-Y gastric bypass surgery is performed in a 46-year-old markedly obese man in an effort to cause weight loss. The patient is likely to develop a deficiency of which of the following nutrients?

A. Iron
B. Vitamin D
C. Vitamin K
D. Vitamin B_{12}
E. Folate

Answer: A, B, C, D, and E
Micronutrient deficiency is common after Roux-en-Y surgery caused by alterations in digestive anatomy related to the surgical procedure.

■ **You should know:**

1. The following nutrients should be given as supplements to the patient who has undergone Roux-en-Y surgery:
   • Vitamins A, B_1, D, E, K, B_{12}
   • Iron
   • Folate
   • Biotin, selenium, zinc
   • Calcium

2. Another important complication of this operation is the development of cholelithiasis, thought to be related to rapid weight loss. A 6-month

prophylactic course of ursodeoxycholic acid given after surgery reduces gallstone formation.

3. In addition to the Roux-en-Y procedure, the clinician should remember other factors that are associated with increased risk of cholelithiasis:

Cholesterol stones:
- Obesity
- Diabetes mellitus
- Native American ethnicity
- Medicines
  (1) Clofibrate
  (2) Estrogen
  (3) Octreotide

Bilirubin stones:
- Crohn's inflammatory disease of the bowel
- Chronic hemolytic anemia (e.g., sickle cell disease or congenital spherocytosis)

HEENT

E 195　Presence of which of the following differentiates perennial allergic rhinitis from vasomotor rhinitis?

A. Elevated serum level of IgG
B. Eosinophils on nasal cytology
C. Association with sarcoidosis
D. Association with asthma
E. Positive immediate hypersensitivity skin testing

Answer: B, D, and E

Perennial allergic rhinitis is triggered by responses to allergens that are present throughout the year, including animal dander, mold spores, or dust containing mites. Manifestations of allergy include eosinophils on nasal cytology, association with asthma, and positive skin testing.

▓ **You should know:**

1. Vasomotor rhinitis is of unknown etiology and is characterized by perennial clear nasal discharge that is related to food intake, especially spicy foods or alcohol (gustatory rhinitis), changes in temperature or humidity, or chemical odors.

2. The following table differentiates perennial allergic rhinitis (PAR) from vaso-motor rhinitis (VR):

	PAR	VR
Chronology	Perennial	Perennial
Associated symptoms	Nasal and ocular itching	None
Nasal cytology	Eosinophils	No eosinophils
Association with asthma	Yes	No
Treatment	Oral or topical antihistamines; intranasal glucocorticoids	Intranasal anticholinergic (ipratropium)

Essentials is designed to promote critical thinking and enrich your knowledge base. Therefore, many questions will have more than one correct answer.

3. Medications that can cause rhinorrhea include the following:
   - Beta-adrenergic blockers
   - Estrogen and progesterone
   - Angiotensin-converting enzyme inhibitors (ACEIs)
   - Nonsteroidal anti-inflammatory drugs (NSAIDs)
   - Phosphodiesterase-5 inhibitors (PDE-5 inhibitors)

HEME/ONC, MS

E 196   A 72-year-old man is to undergo elective right total hip replacement. Which of the following is an advantage of low molecular weight heparin over unfractionated heparin?

A. Greater bioavailability
B. Decreased risk of thrombocytopenia
C. Twice-daily dosing
D. Decreased risk of chemical hepatitis
E. Decreased risk of fetal congenital defects

Answer: A, B, and C
Low molecular weight heparin (LMWH) has *greater bioavailability* meaning that more of the injected medication has the desired anticoagulant effect, rather than a fraction of the medicine binding to tissue and plasma proteins and not having its pharmacologic action. In contrast to LMWH, some unfractionated heparin (UFH) does bind to proteins and thereby loses anticoagulant action. LMWH can be administered in twice-daily dosing for it has a longer half-life than UFH. LMWH has a lesser risk of inducing antibodies to platelets with development of thrombocytopenia.

▓ **You should know:**

1. The anticoagulant effect of LMWH is directly related to body weight. Therefore, patients receiving LMWH do not require serial laboratory monitoring of anticoagulant effect. (In contrast, patients who are receiving unfractionated heparin require serial measurement of activated partial thromboplastin time [aPTT].)

2. LMWH induces less bone loss than does UFH. UFH decreases bone formation and may increase bone resorption.

3. Comparing LMWH and UFH in anticoagulation of the pregnant woman:
   - UFH has a high molecular weight and does not cross the placenta. There is no teratogenic risk to the fetus.
   - The LMWH heparin, enoxaparin, is considered by the Food and Drug Administration as Category B. (Animal studies have failed to demonstrate risk to the fetus and there are no well-controlled studies in pregnant women.)

4. In *reversing* the anticoagulant effect, LMWH has a lesser response to protamine.

E 197   All 50 U.S. states, the District of Columbia, Puerto Rico, U.S. Virgin Islands, and Guam provide universal screening of newborns for which of the following disorders?

A. Sickle cell disease
B. Congenital hypothyroidism
C. Phenylketonuria
D. Congenital adrenal hyperplasia
E. Biotinidase

Answer: B and C
There is universal screening for congenital hypothyroidism and phenylketonuria in the above legal jurisdictions.

■ **You should know:**

1. *Nearly all* states screen for galactosemia and hemoglobinopathies. The American College of Medical Genetics recommends a panel of 26 genetic and metabolic disorders for screening. Approximately half of the states have implemented this panel.

2. Congenital hypothyroidism is manifest by hypothermia, hoarse cry, large fontanels, lethargy, slow movement, and macroglossia.

3. Phenylketonuria will cause mental retardation.

E 198   A 73-year-old woman who takes levothyroxine in therapy of hypothyroidism purposefully doubles her medication dosage in an effort to lose weight. Which of the following is a potential cardiovascular complication?

A. Angina pectoris caused by coronary artery spasm
B. Atrial fibrillation
C. Orthostatic hypotension
D. Leg claudication
E. High cardiac output heart failure

Answer: B and E
Cardiovascular effects of hyperthyroidism include increased cardiac output (CO) and tachycardia. The increase in CO is caused by increased peripheral oxygen requirements and increased ventricular contractility. High cardiac output heart failure may develop. Atrial fibrillation occurs in 10% to 20% of hyperthyroid patients and is more common in the patient over the age of 45 years.

■ **You should know:**

1. In the patient who has *coexisting coronary artery atherosclerosis,* the tachycardia and increased ventricular contractility in hyperthyroidism may cause development of angina pectoris.

2. Patients who have *subclinical hyperthyroidism,* characterized by a low serum TSH value with normal serum free T_4 and T_3 levels, also have an increased likelihood of developing atrial fibrillation.

Essentials is designed to promote critical thinking and enrich your knowledge base. Therefore, many questions will have more than one correct answer.

3. In the treatment of *hypothyroidism,* the clinician should recognize the following:
   - If the onset of hypothyroidism is insidious, levothyroxine (T_4) should be administered rather than the short-acting T_3. The initial dosage should be very small (e.g., 25 mcg daily) with small incremental increases in dosage at 3- to 6-week intervals.

4. Levothyroxine should be taken on an empty stomach, preferably 1 hour before breakfast. Absorption of the medication is reduced when food is taken at a shorter interval.

5. Physical signs of *hyperthyroidism* include the following:
   - Stare and lid lag
   - Tachycardia, widened pulse pressure, systolic hypertension
   - Warm, smooth skin
   - Palpation of the thyroid
     (1) Diffusely enlarged thyroid in Graves disease
     (2) Single or multiple thyroid nodules in nonautoimmune hyperthyroidism
   - *Only in Graves disease are exophthalmos and pretibial myxedema noted.* Pretibial myxedema is characterized by a thickening and induration of the skin, often with an orange peel texture.

Please refer to Essentials questions E 192 and E 199 for additional information on atrial fibrillation and its treatment.

CV

E 199   An 82-year-old man has a 1-week history of worsening fatigue. Blood pressure is 106/72 mm Hg; pulse, 122/min irregularly irregular; and respirations, 22/min. Examination shows normal jugular venous pressure and lung fields clear to auscultation. The apical impulse is in the sixth intercostal space in the anterior axillary line. A 2/6 holosystolic murmur and S3 gallop are heard at the apex. Electrocardiography shows new atrial fibrillation. Which of the following is the preferred initial therapy?

A. Aspirin
B. Clopidogrel (Plavix)
C. Abciximab (ReoPro)
D. Unfractionated heparin
E. Dabigatran

Answer: **D**
D is correct because a patient who has valvular heart disease and atrial fibrillation is at high risk of systemic thromboembolism. The patient should receive unfractionated heparin while waiting to achieve target levels for oral warfarin anticoagulation. Alternatively, low molecular weight heparin may be administered.

▨ **You should know:**

1. Common causes of atrial fibrillation (AF) include hypertension, coronary heart disease, valvular heart disease, cardiomyopathy, and hyperthyroidism.

2. AF is considered:
   - *Paroxysmal:* Episodes of AF terminate spontaneously in fewer than 7 days (often within 24 hours).
   - *Persistent:* Episodes of AF last more than 7 days or require an intervention to restore sinus rhythm.

- *Permanent*: AF is continuous and efforts to restore sinus rhythm have been unsuccessful or have not been attempted.

3. *Lone* AF refers to AF in the absence of structural heart disease. These patients are typically men 40 to 50 years of age, and symptoms of AF occur at night, at rest, following vigorous exercise, or with alcohol ingestion.

4. The three reasons to treat AF include:
   - Reduce symptoms
   - Prevent thromboembolism
   - Prevent cardiomyopathy (a ventricular rate persistently greater than 100/min may cause development of a dilated cardiomyopathy and systolic heart failure)

5. In the AF patient who does *not have structural heart disease, rhythm control*—namely, reversion to sinus rhythm—is generally indicated. Patients should receive medication to control the heart rate and adequate anticoagulation of AF lasting more than 48 hours before pharmacologic cardioversion or elective direct current electrical cardioversion. In these patients who do not have structural heart disease, medications for cardioversion include flecainide, propafenone, and amiodarone. (Flecainide and propafenone should not be administered to patients who have structural heart disease.)

6. In most patients with AF, particularly those with structural heart disease, the preferred strategy is *rate control*—namely, allowing the patient to remain in AF with therapy directed toward control of heart rate and anticoagulation.

7. Clinical studies have compared rhythm control and rate control in management of AF:
   - Rhythm control *does not improve mortality, hospitalization, stroke, or quality of life* compared with rate control.

8. Medications that slow the ventricular rate in AF include the following:
   - Beta-adrenergic blockers
   - Nondihydropyridine calcium channel blockers (verapamil and diltiazem)
   - Digoxin (not useful for rate control with exercise)

9. Patients with paroxysmal, persistent, and permanent AF *have the same indications for anticoagulation*. Those with *valvular heart disease* are considered to be at high risk for thromboembolism and should receive indefinite anticoagulation. Those who have *nonvalvular AF* are considered for anticoagulation based upon CHADS guidelines.

10. CHADS
    - C = Cardiac failure
    - H = Hypertension
    - A = Age greater than 75 years
    - D = Diabetes mellitus
    - S = Stroke

11. Dabigatran is presently FDA approved *only for treatment of nonvalvular AF*.

12. Clopidogrel is a thienopyridine that blocks the ADP receptor P2Y12 on the platelet, thus retarding platelet aggregation. Clopidogrel must be metabolized to an active form in the body. It is used in conjunction with

Essentials is designed to promote critical thinking and enrich your knowledge base.
Therefore, many questions will have more than one correct answer.

aspirin in patients who have acute coronary syndrome, either managed conservatively or with early percutaneous coronary intervention and stent placement.

13. Abciximab is a glycoprotein IIb/IIIa inhibitor that reduces platelet aggregation. This class of medication is used in treatment of the following:
    - ST elevation acute myocardial infarction (STEMI) in conjunction with fibrinolytic agents
    - Percutaneous coronary intervention in patients with acute coronary artery syndromes. The Glycoprotein IIb/IIIa agent is used in conjunction with aspirin and clopidogrel.

Please see Essential questions E 192 and E 196 for discussion of dabigatran and low molecular weight heparin.

ENDO

E 200 A 23-year-old woman with type 1 diabetes mellitus wishes to become pregnant. She should be counseled that which of the following is a recognized complication in the infant of a diabetic mother?

A. Macrosomia
B. Transposition of the great arteries
C. Spina bifida
D. Strabismus
E. Anomalous origin of a coronary artery

Answer: A, B, and C
Congenital anomalies occur in infants of mothers who have either pregestational or gestational diabetes, although they are more common in mothers with pregestational hyperglycemia. Nearly two thirds of the congenital anomalies involve the cardiovascular or the central nervous system. Macrosomia is related to fetal hyperinsulinemia that stimulates growth of fetal tissues.

■ **You should know:**

1. Diabetes mellitus is the most common complication of pregnancy. The diabetes may be *gestational*, meaning that the diabetes appeared during the pregnancy. Alternatively, the diabetes may be *pregestational*, meaning that the woman was known to be diabetic at the onset of pregnancy.

2. Cardiovascular anomalies in the infants of diabetic mothers include notably transposition of the great arteries, but coarctation of the aorta, atrial and ventricular septal defects, coarctation of the aorta, and others may be found.

3. Congenital neurologic anomalies in the infants of diabetic mothers include neural tube defects, anencephaly, and microcephaly.

4. Maternal hyperglycemia causes fetal hyperglycemia. Macrosomia is caused by fetal hyperglycemia producing pancreatic hyperinsulinemia in the fetus. The increased insulin in the fetus stimulates growth of subcutaneous fat, skeletal and cardiac muscle, and liver, producing a large newborn.

5. Transient tachypnea of the newborn and respiratory distress syndrome are both more common in the infant of a diabetic mother.

6. Strabismus is an ocular anomaly that may be congenital or acquired and is characterized by malalignment of the eyes. One eye is deviated in (esodeviation) or out (exodeviation).

Please see Essentials question E 187 related to transient tachypnea of the newborn and respiratory distress syndrome.

DERM, RESP, GI/N

E 201   A 12-month-old girl has egg allergy manifest by urticaria. She may receive which of the following immunizations?

A. Typhoid vaccine
B. Yellow fever
C. Measles-mumps-rubella
D. Herpes zoster
E. Pneumococcal

Answer: C
Egg protein is found in negligible amounts in measles-mumps-rubella (MMR) vaccine, and therefore MMR may be administered to a child with known egg allergy.

■ **You should know:**

1. Egg protein is found in influenza vaccine, yellow fever vaccine, and in negligible amounts in MMR and purified chick embryo rabies vaccine. Therefore, MMR and rabies vaccine may be given to the child with known egg allergy.

2. Pneumococcal vaccine is not to be given to a child under the age of 24 months.

3. Herpes zoster vaccine is indicated only in immunocompetent persons who are over the age of 60 years.

4. Both *inactivated and intranasal live-attenuated influenza vaccines* contain egg protein. The content of the egg protein, ovalbumin, in the vaccine varies among vaccines made by different manufacturers. Safe administration of *low* ovalbumin influenza vaccine to infants with egg allergy has been reported. The clinician must weigh the risk and benefits of vaccine administration in each patient.

5. The primary series of *Haemophilus influenzae* type b conjugate vaccine (Hib) is administered before the age of 7 months. It may be given to the child with egg allergy, for there are no known contraindications to this vaccine.

ID, GU, CV

E 202   An adult patient who has a history of which of the following should receive antimicrobial prophylaxis?

A. Rheumatic fever
B. Recurrent urinary tract infection in a nonpregnant woman
C. Spontaneous bacterial peritonitis in a cirrhotic patient
D. Influenza
E. Pneumococcal pneumonia

Answer: A, B, C, and D
Continuous antibiotic prophylaxis prevents recurrent episodes of acute rheumatic fever (RF) and is indicated in all patients with a history of RF. Nonpregnant women

with three or more uncomplicated urinary tract infections within 12 months should receive either continuous low-dose antibiotic prophylaxis or patient-initiated treatment after onset of symptoms. Prolonged (i.e., indefinite duration) secondary prophylaxis is indicated in those patients with a history of spontaneous bacterial peritonitis. Chemoprophylaxis of influenza A and B infection with inhaled zanamivir or oral oseltamivir is effective in prophylaxis after exposure in unvaccinated high-risk patients and unvaccinated health-care professionals in an outbreak setting.

■ **You should know:**

1. Antimicrobial prophylaxis may be considered:
   - *Primary*: Prevention of an initial infection
   - *Secondary*: Prevention of recurrence or reactivation of infection
   - *Other*: Elimination of a colonizing organism

2. Primary prevention of acute rheumatic fever requires appropriate treatment of streptococcal pharyngitis. Secondary prevention of RF is indicated in all patients with a history of RF whether or not the initial attack was associated with carditis. (Carditis in acute rheumatic fever may be manifest as valvulitis [mitral or aortic regurgitation], myocarditis with left ventricular dilation or atrioventricular block, or pericarditis.) The duration of RF prophylaxis is dependent upon whether the patient has residual rheumatic heart disease and personal factors (e.g., exposure to children having streptococcal pharyngitis).

3. The woman who has recurrent urinary tract infections should be evaluated for the presence of underlying structural abnormality of the urinary tract. Several antibiotics may be used in prophylaxis. The duration of continuous prophylaxis is commonly 6 months. Monthly urine cultures should be obtained to monitor for bacteriuria and the development of antibiotic resistance. The woman should be counseled to avoid spermicide-containing products taken in an effort to prevent pregnancy.

4. Aerobic gram-negative bacteria and streptococci are the most frequent infectious causes of spontaneous bacterial peritonitis (SBP). Although *secondary* prophylaxis is indicated in those patients with a history of SBP, there is presently no consensus whether patients with cirrhosis and ascites should take primary prophylaxis in order to prevent an *initial* episode of SBP.

5. Chemoprophylaxis for influenza should not be administered 48 hours before or 2 weeks after administration of the intranasal live-attenuated FluMist influenza vaccine. Chemoprophylaxis has no effect on the inactivated vaccine.

6. Antimicrobial prophylaxis is also indicated in the prevention of the following:
   - Infective endocarditis. (Please see Essentials question E 079.)
   - Meningococcal meningitis: "Close contacts" of the patient with meningococcal meningitis should receive chemoprophylaxis. "Close contact" generally includes persons with more than 8 hours of contact within 3 feet of the patient or those exposed to oral secretions of the meningitis patient starting 1 week before onset of the patient's symptoms until 24 hours after initiation of antibiotic therapy.
   - Travelers' diarrhea: (Please see Essentials question E 113.)
   - Bite wound infection: Dog bites, cat bites, and human bites commonly become secondarily infected and may lead to septic arthritis, tenosynovitis,

severe soft tissue infection, or sepsis. Chemoprophylaxis should be administered when the bites are through the dermis, are in areas of venous or lymphatic compromise, occur close to bone or a joint, occur in an immunocompromised person, or when the bite requires surgical intervention. Those who have sustained *human bites* should be evaluated for HIV and hepatitis B infection. Tetanus immune globulin and tetanus toxoid should be administered to those who have not been immunized or toxoid alone to the person who has not received a tetanus booster within the past 5 years.

- Children with sickle cell disease are at increased risk of infection and bacteremia from encapsulated bacteria (*S. pneumoniae, H. influenzae,* and *N. meningitidis*). They should receive daily oral penicillin for at least 3 to 5 years but may continue into adulthood. (Please see Essentials E 152.)

CV

E 203   Late for school, an active 8-year-old girl suddenly collapses and dies while anxiously running into her school building. Autopsy shows no evidence of structural heart disease. Which of the following cardiac conditions may be the cause of death?

A. Long QT syndrome
B. Preexcitation syndrome
C. Anomalous origin of a coronary artery
D. Hypertrophic cardiomyopathy
E. Brugada syndrome

Answer: A, B, and E
Nonstructural causes of sudden cardiac death may or may not be inherited. Long QT syndrome and Brugada syndrome are *inherited* disorders that predispose to sudden cardiac death. Preexcitation syndrome is a cause of sudden death that *rarely has a genetic pattern.*

You should know:

1. A primary electrical disturbance—that is, abnormality in depolarization or repolarization of myocardial cells—may cause sudden cardiac death in persons who have no structural heart disease. These include long QT syndrome, preexcitation syndrome, Brugada syndrome, and commotio cordis.

2. The primary electrical disturbance may be related to *inherited genetic mutations.* Long QT syndrome and Brugada syndrome are examples of inherited, nonstructural disorders causing sudden death. Long QT syndrome may have autosomal dominant or autosomal recessive inheritance. Brugada syndrome has an autosomal dominant pattern.

3. In the patient who has inherited long QT syndrome, the QT interval may fluctuate during the day. Therefore, a single electrocardiogram demonstrating a normal QT interval *does not preclude the diagnosis.* Serial electrocardiograms should be taken with measurement of QT interval.

4. Long QT syndrome often causes syncope or death during periods of heightened sympathetic nervous system activity. In these cases, the heart rhythm catapults into polymorphous ventricular tachycardia called torsades de

Essentials is designed to promote critical thinking and enrich your knowledge base.
Therefore, many questions will have more than one correct answer.

pointes. (In the above question scenario, the child had exaggerated sympathetic tone related to her physical exertion and anxiety.)

5. Long QT syndrome may also be *acquired*. Causes of long QT interval include drugs, hypokalemia, and hypomagnesemia. A list of the many drugs that prolong the QT interval may be found at www.torsades.org.

6. Intravenous magnesium is commonly the initial medication used to treat torsades de pointes, even in patients who have a normal serum magnesium concentration (in addition to correction of any electrolyte deficiency, if present).

7. Although Brugada syndrome is most commonly diagnosed in adults (average age at diagnosis is 41 years), it does occur in children. Patients who have Brugada syndrome typically demonstrate a *fluctuating electrocardiographic abnormality* manifest by right bundle branch block with elevation of the ST segment.

8. Patients who have preexcitation syndrome are born with accessory conduction pathways that connect atria to ventricles bypassing the atrioventricular node. These patients are prone to develop atrial fibrillation with very high ventricular rates (e.g., 300 per minute) that may degenerate into ventricular fibrillation and sudden death. Because genetic inheritance is rare, it is not recommended to screen children of parents who have preexcitation.

9. Commotio cordis is ventricular fibrillation (VF) caused by a sudden chest wall impact. In order to catapult the normal heart into VF, the blow must be over the heart and occur during the early portion of the T wave in the cardiac cycle.

10. In contrast, *structural heart defects* that increase the risk of sudden death in children include anomalous origin of a coronary artery, hypertrophic cardiomyopathy, and arrhythmogenic right ventricular dysplasia (ARVD).

11. ARVD is an inherited disorder in which fat replaces the myocardium of the right ventricle. Presentation is most common between the ages of 10 and 50 years. Ventricular tachycardia related to the fatty infiltration causes syncope, dyspnea, palpitations, and sudden cardiac death.

12. The following table summarizes disorders that increase the risk of sudden cardiac death in children:

	Inherited	**Structural Heart Disease**
Long QT syndrome	Yes, autosomal dominant or recessive; may be acquired	No
Brugada syndrome	Yes, autosomal dominant	No
Preexcitation	Rarely	No
Commotio cordis	No	No
Anomalous origin coronary artery	No	Yes
Hypertrophic cardiomyopathy	Yes, autosomal dominant; sporadic cases occur	Yes
Arrhythmogenic RV dysplasia	Yes, autosomal dominant or recessive	Yes

13. *Sudden cardiac death in the adult is generally related to structural heart disease.* Major causes of sudden death in the adult include the following:
    • Coronary heart disease with myocardial infarction or angina pectoris
    • Dilated cardiomyopathy of any etiology
    • Hypertrophic cardiomyopathy
    • Myocarditis

MS, NEURO, GU

E 204   Generalized muscle weakness and muscle cramps are common manifestations of which of the following disorders?

A. Hypokalemia
B. Hypomagnesemia
C. Hypocalcemia
D. Metabolic acidosis
E. Myasthenia gravis

Answer: A, B, and C
Hypokalemia and hypomagnesemia affect action potentials of skeletal and cardiac muscle and may cause skeletal muscle weakness and cramps in addition to cardiac ectopic arrhythmias. Hypocalcemia increases the irritability of the nervous system, specifically causing spontaneous discharge of nerve fibers causing muscle spasms. Further, low serum calcium concentration interferes with muscle contraction causing weakness.

You should know:

1. Common causes of hypokalemia include loop and thiazide diuretics, vomiting or diarrhea, and alkalosis, both metabolic and respiratory. (In alkalosis, hydrogen ions come out of cells into the serum; potassium moves from the serum into cells.)

2. The etiology of hypomagnesemia includes loop and thiazide diuretics and gastrointestinal electrolyte loss via vomiting or diarrhea. Further, hypomagnesemia is common in those who suffer from chronic alcohol abuse, for alcohol intake causes loss of magnesium in the urine.

3. Because the causes of hypokalemia and hypomagnesemia are the same, it is common for both electrolyte deficiencies to occur together in a patient.

4. The electrocardiographic manifestations of hypokalemia and hypomagnesemia are the same—namely, ST segment depression, flattening of the T wave, and increased amplitude of the U wave. (Many consider this prolongation of the QT interval.)

5. Calcium is found in the blood in three fractions: bound to anions (e.g., phosphate), bound to albumin, and in an ionized state. Hypoalbuminemia (as will occur in nephrotic syndrome or liver cirrhosis) will cause the total albumin level in the blood to be low, but the ionized fraction will be normal. A low serum ionized calcium concentration will cause muscle weakness and cramps.

6. Low ionized calcium concentration may be found in hypoparathyroidism, vitamin D deficiency, and magnesium depletion. Magnesium deficiency directly causes hypocalcemia. Hypocalcemia causes prolongation of the QT interval on electrocardiography.

Essentials is designed to promote critical thinking and enrich your knowledge base. Therefore, many questions will have more than one correct answer.

7. Myasthenia gravis, an autoimmune disease characterized by the presence of antibodies to acetylcholine receptors, will cause weakness but not muscle cramps.

8. A brief review: Hypokalemia, hypomagnesemia, and hypocalcemia can cause weakness and muscle cramps.

	Hypokalemia	Hypomagnesemia	Hypocalcemia
Causes	Loop and thiazides; vomiting or diarrhea	Loop and thiazides; vomiting or diarrhea	Hypoparathyroidism; vitamin D deficiency; magnesium deficiency
ECG	ST depression; flattening of T wave; increased amplitude of U wave	ST depression; flattening of T wave; increased amplitude of U wave	Prolongation of QT interval

HEME/ONC, ID

E 205   An elevation of serum immunoglobulin E (IgE) level and peripheral eosinophilia would be expected to be present in which of the following conditions?

A. Asthma
B. Atopic dermatitis
C. Allergic bronchopulmonary aspergillosis
D. Interstitial nephritis
E. Ascariasis

Answer: A, B, C, and E
Elevation of serum IgE level and peripheral eosinophilia are present in two very different clinical settings—namely, *noninfectious* allergic disorders and *infectious* diseases caused by helminth (worm) parasites. Less commonly, eosinophilia is associated with neoplasms, connective tissue disorders, drugs, and endocrine disease.

■ You should know:

1. The normal eosinophil count in peripheral blood is 40 to 500/microL. Greater than 500/microL is considered eosinophilia.

2. The normal serum immunoglobulin E level is 0 to 0.002 mg/mL.

3. IgE binds to receptors on eosinophils, mast cells, and basophils. In allergic disorders, the allergen (antigen) interacts with IgE that is bound to these cells. Chemical pharmacologic mediators including histamine and cytokines are released from the cells resulting in bronchospasm and allergic inflammation.

4. Elevated serum IgE and eosinophilia are found in allergy patients who have asthma, allergic rhinitis, and atopic dermatitis.

5. The body's primary defense against worm infestation, particularly round worm (nematode) infestation, is the eosinophil with bound IgE that kills the worm.

6. When eosinophilia and elevated serum IgE level are unexplained, the clinician should initiate a prompt search for occult roundworm infection.

7. Allergic bronchopulmonary aspergillosis occurs in patients who have asthma or cystic fibrosis. The illness is related to an allergic response to the

Aspergillus fungus. Clinical manifestations include productive cough, and bronchial obstruction with radiographic findings including atelectasis, bronchiectasis, and pulmonary infiltrates.

8. Hodgkin's disease, chronic adrenal insufficiency, sarcoidosis, and drugs (penicillins, nonaspirin nonsteroidal anti-inflammatory drugs [NSAIDs], allopurinol, and phenytoin) may be associated with eosinophilia.

ID, GI/N, GU

E 206   Gram-negative septicemia is a recognized complication in which of the following diseases?

A. Diverticulitis
B. Ascending cholangitis
C. Pyelonephritis
D. Lyme disease
E. *Klebsiella* pneumonia

Answer: A, B, C, and E
The most common infections that predispose to gram-negative bacteremia are those in the urinary tract (pyelonephritis), hepatobiliary tree (ascending cholangitis), gastrointestinal tract (perforated diverticulitis), and lungs (*Klebsiella* pneumonia).

■ **You should know:**

1. With rare exception, gram-negative bacteremia (GNB) occurs in association with infection at another site in the body (i.e., a primary source of infection). Commonly, abscess formation secondary to perforated bowel, ascending biliary infection related to a common bile duct stone, and hematogenous spread from pyelonephritis are the underlying infections.

2. Whether community-acquired or hospital-acquired, the most common gram-negative bacteria that are associated with GNB include the following:
   • *E. coli*
   • *Pseudomonas aeruginosa*
   • *Klebsiella* pneumonia
   • *Enterobacter* species

3. Other clinical factors that increase the risk of GNB include the following:
   • Intravascular catheters or surgical drainage tubes
   • Stem cell transplant
   • Hematogenous malignancy
   • Diabetes mellitus
   • Liver failure

4. GNB is arbitrarily classified as sepsis, severe sepsis, and septic shock, based upon physical examination, hemodynamics, and need for intravenous volume expansion and vasopressors.

5. The most serious expression of GNB is septic shock that is characterized by fever and chills (a minority will have hypothermia), disorientation, oliguria, and hypotension. Multiple organ failure and disseminated intravascular coagulation (DIC) may follow.

6. The pathophysiology of *septic shock* relates to a release of cytokines (endotoxin) that excites a diffuse inflammatory reaction and vasodilation. The

Essentials is designed to promote critical thinking and enrich your knowledge base.
Therefore, many questions will have more than one correct answer.

initial hemodynamic manifestation of septic shock is vasodilatory with the patient appearing warm, dry, and flushed. Later, intense vasoconstriction may occur.

7. The treatment of septic shock from GNB includes removal of indwelling catheters, antibiotic administration, intravenous fluid (normal saline or albumin), vasopressors, and drainage of a localized abscess. Antibiotic therapy should be promptly initiated when GNB is suspected but after blood cultures have been obtained. The recommended initial empiric antibiotic therapy should include the following:
   - Cephalosporin: Ceftazidime or cefepime *or*
   - Beta-lactam/beta-lactamase inhibitor: Piperacillin-tazobactam *or*
   - Carbapenem (imipenem, meropenem, or ertapenem)

8. Ringer's lactate solution should not be administered to a patient who has metabolic acidosis.

9. The value of the administration of intravenous glucocorticoid and mineralocorticoid in treatment of septic shock is still undecided.

10. "Cotton fever" may occur in heroin users who filter the heroin through cotton that is colonizing *Enterobacter* species. The patient has the acute onset of fever approximately 10 minutes after injection. While considered benign, the patient requires antibiotic therapy.

11. Combat-injured military personnel in Iraq and Afghanistan have an increased risk of GNB caused by *Acinetobacter* infection found at field hospitals.

12. *Cardiogenic shock* is most commonly related to acute myocardial infarction but may be related to acute mitral regurgitation or rupture of the ventricular septum or free wall. The pathophysiology is a dramatic reduction in stroke volume and cardiac output resulting in tissue hypoxia and lactic acidosis. Cardiogenic shock is characterized by hypotension, oliguria, confusion or disorientation, and moist, cold skin caused by intense vasoconstriction. Most patients in cardiogenic shock have pulmonary congestion.

13. The following table compares septic shock related to gram-negative bacteremia and cardiogenic shock:

	Septic Shock	Cardiogenic Shock
Pathophysiology	Infection; release of cytokines (endotoxin)	Dramatic reduction in stroke volume
Blood pressure	Low	Low
Urine volume	Low	Low
Disorientation	Yes	Yes
Skin	Warm and flushed (vasodilation); later, vasoconstriction may occur	Cold and clammy (vasoconstriction)
Disseminated intravascular coagulation	May occur	No
Acid-base status	Respiratory alkalosis, early; metabolic (lactic) acidosis, later	Metabolic (lactic) acidosis

ID

E 207   Fluoroquinolones should not be prescribed for which of the following patients?

A. 32-year-old pregnant woman
B. 12-year-old girl
C. 28-year-old with gonococcal urethritis
D. 22-year-old woman with uncomplicated urinary tract infection
E. 23-year-old with skin infection caused by methicillin-resistant *S. aureus*

Answer: A, B, C, and E
Contraindications to fluoroquinolone therapy relate to pregnancy, age, and resistant microbial organisms.

■ **You should know:**

1. Fluoroquinolones are highly effective against gram-negative aerobic bacteria. Newer medications in this class have significant activity against gram-positive and anaerobic organisms.

2. *However,* resistant organisms are appearing. Therefore, fluoroquinolones should *not* be used in the treatment of urethritis caused by *Neisseria gonorrhoeae* or in therapy of skin and soft tissue infections caused by methicillin-resistant *S. aureus* (MRSA).

3. Fluoroquinolones are not recommended for patients under the age of 18 years because of the risk of erosion in joint cartilage.

4. Tendinopathy and tendon rupture have been reported in *adults*. The Food and Drug Administration (FDA) recommends that patients taking this class of medicine discontinue treatment at the first indication of tendon pain or swelling, avoid exercise, and promptly report to their caregiver.

5. The FDA product information for levofloxacin, gemifloxacin, and norfloxacin states that prolongation of the QT interval on electrocardiography may occur. Fluoroquinolones should not be given to the patient who is taking another medicine known to cause prolongation of the QT interval or in the patient who has hypokalemia, hypomagnesemia, or hypocalcemia, all of which can cause QT prolongation.

6. The safety of fluoroquinolones in pregnancy is not established. Further, these medications are excreted in breast milk. Therefore, intake should be avoided in nursing mothers.

7. The presence of renal insufficiency, elderly age, and an underlying brain disorder increase the patient's risk of having neurotoxicity from fluoroquinolones. Patients may experience hallucinations, seizures, and psychosis.

8. The patient who takes a fluoroquinolone may develop phototoxicity related to ultraviolet (UV-A) irradiation. The skin rash appears to be exaggerated sunburn; bullae may appear.

Please see Essentials question E 208 for discussion of methicillin-resistant *Staphylococcus aureus* (MRSA) infection.

E 208   One week after scraping his leg on a sports locker door, a 14-year-old boy has a furuncle on his lower leg. Which of the following is the most likely infecting bacteria?

A. *Streptococcus pyogenes*
 B. *Staphylococcus aureus*
C. *Pseudomonas aeruginosa*
D. *Corynebacterium diphtheriae*
 E. *Bacteroides fragilis*

Answer: B

B is correct because methicillin-resistant *S. aureus* (MRSA) is a common infecting organism in locker rooms of sports teams that may cause community-acquired skin and soft tissue infections.

▪ **You should know:**

1. MRSA transmission requires contact with a contaminated surface or with a person who colonizes the bacteria.

2. The U.S. Centers for Disease Control and Prevention has subdivided MRSA infection into two categories:
   • Health care–associated (HCA), meaning that the infection started more than 48 hours after hospitalization
   • Community-associated

3. *Health care–associated* MRSA
   • Characterized by severe, invasive disease, often complicated by bacteremia or pneumonia
   • Risk factors for HCA
     (1) Prolonged hospitalization
     (2) Hemodialysis
     (3) Intensive care
     (4) Contact with a person who colonizes the bacteria
   • MRSA is often found contaminating the following in the hospital:
     (1) Endotracheal tubes, intravenous and urinary catheters
     (2) Environmental surfaces (e.g., beds, blood pressure cuffs, and stethoscopes)

4. *Community-acquired MRSA*
   • Associated with skin and soft tissue infection in young, healthy persons
   • Commonly occurs in child care centers, sport teams, military personnel, prison inmates and guards, and men who have sex with men
   • Risk factors include the following:
     (1) Skin abrasions or lacerations
     (2) Tattoos
     (3) Shared shaving equipment without proper cleansing
     (4) Close contact with a person who colonizes the bacteria

5. Treatment of MRSA skin and soft tissue infection
   • Fluctuant infections should be treated with incision and drainage (I&D), with appropriate culture and sensitivity testing.
   • Larger abscesses with or without systemic signs of infection should be treated with I&D and antibiotic administration.

- Oral antibiotics include clindamycin, trimethoprim-sulfamethoxazole, minocycline, and linezolid.
- Parenteral antibiotics should be administered to those patients who are in the following categories:
  (1) Diabetes mellitus
  (2) Immunocompromised state
  (3) Have extensive soft tissue infection
- Vancomycin is the preferred initial antibiotic for parenteral administration.

6. *Colonization* of MRSA is a reservoir for infection. Colonization occurs in healthy persons in the general population, health-care workers, and hospitalized patients. Colonization of the bacteria occurs most commonly in the anterior nares but may also occur in the throat, axillae, perineum, and on the hands.

7. *The role of antibiotic decolonization in control of MRSA is uncertain. At this time, general decolonization is not recommended.* However, in the setting of a MRSA outbreak where there is evidence that points to a specific health-care worker as the source of infection, decolonization is indicated. The colonizing person should receive topical mupirocin in the nose in addition to bathing in chlorhexidine.

8. Hand hygiene, either washing with soap and water or use of alcohol-based gel or foam, before and after each patient contact is the single most important measure to reduce transmission of microorganisms from one person to another.

GI/N

E 209　A 34-year-old woman has a 3-month history of intestinal gas and diarrhea without associated weight loss. Which of the following conditions could cause this symptom complex?

A. Celiac disease
B. Ingestion of sorbitol
C. Ingestion of fructose
D. Intake of lisinopril
E. Lactase deficiency

Answer: A, B, C, and E
A is correct because bacterial digestion of malabsorbed nutrients causes intestinal bloating and diarrhea in the patient who has celiac disease. B and C are correct because both ingested sorbitol and fructose cause an osmotic diarrhea. E is correct because the malabsorbed lactose is fermented by intestinal bacteria producing gas and osmotic diarrhea.

■ You should know:

1. Although the autoimmune celiac disease causing gluten enteropathy classically presents during infancy or early childhood, it is common for the disease to be associated with onset of symptoms during adulthood. Gastrointestinal symptoms in the adult are often *less severe than in the child*; therefore, the adult may have only mild intestinal bloating and diarrhea. A minority of adult celiac patients have the full manifestations of malabsorption syndrome characterized by weight loss, steatorrhea, fat-soluble vitamin deficiency, and iron and folate deficiency.

2. Serologic tests for celiac disease include IgA endomysial antibodies and anti–tissue transglutaminase (IgA tTG) antibodies. Confirmation of the

Essentials is designed to promote critical thinking and enrich your knowledge base.
Therefore, many questions will have more than one correct answer.

diagnosis of celiac disease is made by endoscopic biopsy of the distal duo-denum or proximal jejunum.

3. Sorbitol is a sugar alcohol that is commercially used as a "sugar-free" candy or chewing gum. It is minimally absorbed in the gastrointestinal tract. The sorbitol increases the osmolality of the intestinal contents causing secretion of water into the bowel.

4. Fructose is a natural sugar that does not require insulin for metabolism. It is poorly absorbed in the small bowel resulting in osmotic diarrhea.

5. A deficiency of the enzyme lactase results in impaired breakdown of lactose to glucose. The malabsorbed lactose is fermented by intestinal bacteria pro-ducing gas and osmotic diarrhea.

6. In any patient who has intestinal bloating and diarrhea, the clinician should inquire about ingestion of low-calorie or "sugar-free" sweeteners.

7. A brief review: What do lactase deficiency, ingestion of fructose, and inges-tion of sorbitol have in common?
   - Lactose, fructose, and sorbitol are all poorly absorbed in the small intestine.
   - All have high osmolality that causes secretion of water into the bowel re-sulting in osmotic diarrhea.

ID, DERM, CV

E 210   Which of the following is a common denominator when comparing streptococcal toxic shock syndrome and staphylococcal toxic shock syndrome?

A. Both are mediated by exotoxins
B. Both are associated with bullous skin eruptions
C. Both are associated with acute glomerulonephritis
D. Both are associated with normal anion gap metabolic acidosis
E. Both are associated with elevated cardiac output

Answer: A
A is correct because exotoxins released from both streptococci and staphylococci ac-tivate T cells to release cytokines that provoke the inflammatory and hemodynamic effects in toxic shock syndromes (TSS).

You should know:

1. Both group A streptococcus (GAS) and *Staphylococcus aureus* produce exotox-ins. These exotoxins are called *superantigens* because they activate T cells into massive cytokine production. The cytokines provoke a massive inflamma-tory response producing the symptoms and signs of toxic shock syndrome.

Streptococcus:
2. The gram-positive **group A streptococcus** (e.g., *S. pyogenes*) can cause pharyngitis and skin diseases including cellulitis and erysipelas.

3. Less frequently, GAS can cause *invasive disease*. Invasive GAS infections are characterized by the following:
   - Pneumonia
   - Bacteremia
   - Necrotizing fasciitis and gangrenous myositis
   - Toxic shock syndrome and organ failure

4. Risk factors for invasive GAS infection include the following:
   - Trauma causing hematoma
   - Surgical procedures
   - Viral infection (e.g., influenza)

5. *The clinical presentation of* **streptococcal toxic shock syndrome** *includes the following*:
   - The abrupt onset of pain in soft tissue, usually an extremity. (The pain may be followed by loss of sensation in the affected area.)
   - Erythema and localized swelling in the soft tissue followed by ecchymosis and sloughing of skin that may lead to fasciitis or myositis.
   - Hemodynamic shock may follow, related to hypovolemia caused by capillary leakage and diffuse vasodilation.

6. Complications of streptococcal TSS include the following:
   - Adult respiratory distress syndrome (ARDS)
   - Disseminated intravascular coagulation (DIC)
   - Multiple organ failure, particularly renal failure

7. Treatment of streptococcal TSS includes the following:
   - Massive infusion of intravenous fluids
   - Aggressive debridement of infected tissue
   - Antibiotic therapy: Intravenous clindamycin and intravenous penicillin G are administered

Staphylococcus

8. The specific staphylococcal exotoxin that causes toxic shock syndrome is *toxic shock syndrome toxin-1 (TSST-1)*.

9. In addition to TSST-1, *S. aureus* may produce two other exotoxins:
   - *Exfoliative exotoxin*, which causes scalded skin syndrome
   - *Enterotoxin*, which causes food poisoning

10. **Staphylococcal toxic shock syndrome** occurs in two clinical settings:
    - Menstrual, with TSS developing during the menstrual period in the woman using a highly absorbent tampon
    - Nonmenstrual, occurring in association with surgical wound infection, osteomyelitis, sinusitis, or pulmonary infection following influenza

11. *The clinical presentation of* **staphylococcal toxic shock syndrome** includes the following:
    - Fever with chills, hypotension, vomiting, and diarrhea
    - Diffuse erythroderma ("sunburn") that involves the palms and soles

12. Complications of staphylococcal toxic shock syndrome include multiple organ failure:
    - Brain: Confusion, agitation, and hallucinations
    - Kidney: Acute renal failure
    - Lungs: Pulmonary edema and pleural effusion

13. Treatment of staphylococcal toxic shock syndrome includes the following:
    - Massive infusion of intravenous fluids
    - Antibiotic therapy: Intravenous clindamycin and another antibiotic are administered. (The second antibiotic is dependent upon whether the organism is or is not methicillin-sensitive.)

Essentials is designed to promote critical thinking and enrich your knowledge base.
Therefore, many questions will have more than one correct answer.

14. Intravenous immunoglobulin (IVIG) has been administered in both strep-tococcal and staphylococcal toxic shock syndromes. The efficacy of the IVIG is not clear.

RESP

E 211 Which of the following is a clinical manifestation of obstructive sleep apnea?

A. Snoring
B. Daytime sleepiness
C. Increased risk of motor vehicle accidents
D. Increased all-cause mortality
E. Is caused by a primary brainstem disorder

Answer: A, B, C, and D
A is correct because snoring occurs in almost all patients who have obstructive sleep apnea (OSA) that is caused by narrowing of the nasopharyngeal airways. B and C are correct because the disturbed sleep in OSA results in daytime sleepiness and loss of concentration. E is correct because patients who have OSA have a three- to six-fold increase in all-cause mortality thought to be related to increased risk of coronary heart disease and stroke.

You should know:

1. OSA is *obstructive* apnea or hypopnea (continued breathing but with decreased ventilation) at night caused by repetitive *collapse of the upper airways during sleep*. The disturbed breathing leads to intermittent hypoxemia and hypercapnia.

2. OSA is characterized by the following:
   • Snoring (in almost all cases) with restless sleep
   • Daytime sleepiness and loss of concentration
   • Cognitive defects and mood swings

3. Important clinical points:
   • *All patients who snore should be asked about daytime sleepiness*. The presence of significant daytime sleepiness should indicate evaluation for OSA. Virtually all patients with OSA snore; not all patients who snore have OSA.
   • *OSA occurs in children* and is an important cause of behavioral problems in children. The American Academy of Pediatrics recommends that the caregivers of children be routinely asked about snoring. Any child who snores on most or all nights should undergo evaluation for OSA.

4. Risk factors for the development of OSA include the following:
   • Increased neck size: greater than 17 inches in men; greater than 16 inches in women (neck circumference appears to be more important than obesity)
   • Craniofacial structural abnormalities
   • Enlargement of tonsils and adenoids

5. OSA causes systemic hypertension and, to a lesser degree, pulmonary hypertension. It is also associated with nocturnal arrhythmias, including supraventricular tachycardias, ventricular tachycardia, and bradycardia (sinus bradycardia, asystole, and atrioventricular block).

6. Polysomnography is the preferred diagnostic modality to confirm OSA.

7. The treatment of OSA includes the following:
   • Weight loss
   • Avoidance of alcohol and hypnotic medications
   • Nasal continuous positive airway pressure
   • Surgical resection of soft tissue in selected cases

8. Cheyne-Stokes respiration is characterized by cyclic apnea and hyperpnea caused by impaired brainstem respiratory center responsiveness to systemic arterial P_{CO_2}. It most frequently occurs in patients who have severe systolic heart failure or who are in coma caused by stroke.

9. The following table differentiates OSA and Cheyne-Stokes respiration:

	OSA	**Cheyne-Stokes**
Underlying cause	Narrowed upper airways	Systolic heart failure; stroke
Pathophysiology	Obstructed breathing	Decreased brainstem reflexes
Breathing pattern	Intermittent; noncyclic apneic periods	Cyclic periods of apnea and hyperpnea
Snoring	Almost always	No

HEME/ONC, REPRO

E 212   Genetic testing in a 45-year-old woman shows the presence of mutations in the tumor suppressor genes breast cancer type 1 and type 2 susceptibility genes (*BRCA1* and *BRCA2*). The patient should be counseled that she is at increased risk for which of the following malignancies?

A. Non-Hodgkin's lymphoma
B. Kaposi sarcoma
C. Cancer of the breast
D. Cancer of the pancreas
E. Cancer of the ovary

Answer: C, D, and E
C, D, and E are correct because *BRCA1* and *BRCA2* mutations increase the risk of cancer of the ovary in women and cancer of the breast and pancreas in both sexes.

■ **You should know:**

1. The most common cause of hereditary breast and ovarian cancers is mutations in tumor suppressor genes breast cancer type 1 and type 2 susceptibility genes (*BRCA1* and *BRCA2*).

2. The presence of *BRCA1* and *BRCA2* mutations is increased in certain ethnic groups, notably Ashkenazi Jews, from central and eastern Europe. However, populations in other areas (e.g., Ireland and French Canada) also have an increased incidence of the mutations.

3. The following clinical features suggest hereditary breast and ovarian cancer (HBOC) syndrome:
   • Young age at diagnosis
   • Men or women with two *primary* breast cancers
   • Woman with breast and ovarian (including fallopian tube) cancer

Essentials is designed to promote critical thinking and enrich your knowledge base.
Therefore, many questions will have more than one correct answer.

- Multiple blood relatives with early-onset breast or ovarian cancer or male breast cancer

4. Mutations in *BRCA* genes are inherited in an autosomal dominant fashion.

5. *Women* with *BRCA1* and *BRCA2* mutations have an increased risk of developing the following cancers:
   - Breast cancer (lifetime risk 50% to 85%)
   - Ovarian cancer (lifetime risk 15% to 40%)

6. For *women* with *BRCA1* and *BRCA2* mutations, the recommendation of expert groups has two tracks:
   - Bilateral salpingo-oophorectomy at the end of childbearing and prophylactic bilateral mastectomy *or*
   - Frequent personal breast examinations
   - Annual mammography
   - Annual MRI of the breasts
   - Annual transvaginal ultrasonography
   - Annual serum CA-125 levels

7. *Men* with *BRCA1* and *BRCA2* mutations have an increased risk of developing the following cancers:
   - Breast
   - Prostate

8. For *men* with *BRCA1* and *BRCA2* mutations, the recommendations are as follows:
   - Frequent personal breast examinations
   - Prostate cancer screening via digital rectal examinations and serum prostate specific antigen (PSA) levels
   - Annual mammography in selected cases

9. Because of increased risk for cancer of the pancreas, *men* and *women* with *BRCA1* and *BRCA2* mutations should undergo serial endoscopic retrograde cholangiopancreatography (ERCP) and serum CEA and CA 19-9 concentrations.

10. The U.S. Preventive Services Task Force has recommendations on who should be offered genetic testing for *BRCA* mutations, and the National Comprehensive Cancer Network has criteria for consideration of *BRCA1/BRCA2* genetic testing. The criteria are based upon the following:
    - Age of individual at time of cancer diagnosis
    - Frequency and age of relatives who have had female or male breast cancer and ovarian or fallopian tube cancer

HEME/ONC

E 213 Which of the following medications must be metabolized in order to have an anticoagulant effect?

   A. Enoxaparin (Lovenox)
   B. Abciximab (ReoPro)
   C. Warfarin
   D. Aspirin
   E. Clopidogrel (Plavix)

Answer: E

E is correct because clopidogrel must be metabolized by hepatic action by the CYP 450 family of enzymes to an active form. The active metabolite is uncharacterized and is labile and highly reactive.

■ **You should know:**

1. Clopidogrel is a thienopyridine that antagonizes platelet agglutination by blocking the adenosine diphosphate (ADP) receptor P2Y12 on platelets. The antiplatelet effect of clopidogrel is additive to the effect of aspirin.

2. A hepatic cytochrome P-450 system enzyme called CYP2C19 is necessary for metabolism of clopidogrel to an active form. Some persons have a genetic allele (a version of a gene) that impairs enzymatic conversion of the medicine to an active form. Those with the genetic variant are called "poor metabolizers." The impaired conversion has two effects—namely, reduced antiplatelet activity and increased blood levels of the medication.

3. Indications for clopidogrel therapy include the following:
   • All patients with acute coronary syndrome whether managed conservatively or with early invasive therapy
   • After percutaneous intervention (PCI)
   • After coronary artery bypass surgery

4. Clopidogrel is most commonly taken together with aspirin but may be taken alone.

5. As of July 1, 2012, major medical societies do not recommend *routine testing* of patients for clopidogrel resistance whether by in vitro tests or by genetic testing for CYP2C19 poor metabolizers.

6. Patients who take clopidogrel should not take the protein pump inhibitor (PPI) omeprazole, for there is competition of omeprazole and clopidogrel with the same hepatic enzyme system. The concomitant intake of clopidogrel and omeprazole causes a decreased concentration of the active metabolite of clopidogrel and decreased anticoagulant effect. Whether this is a class effect of PPIs is not known.

NEURO, GU, ENDO

E 214 A 56-year-old man has the sudden onset of a generalized tonic-clonic seizure. Which of the following may be the cause of the seizure?

A. Hypoglycemia
B. Normal pressure hydrocephalus
C. Epilepsy
D. Hyponatremia
E. Theophylline poisoning

Answer: A, C, D, and E

Hypoglycemia can cause generalized seizures; infrequently, hypoglycemia may present with *focal* neurologic signs. Approximately 10% of patients with inherited epilepsy have generalized seizures. Hyponatremia and theophylline toxicity are examples of metabolic and medication-related generalized seizures.

Essentials is designed to promote critical thinking and enrich your knowledge base.
Therefore, many questions will have more than one correct answer.

■ **You should know:**

1. Hypoglycemic symptoms are of two types, *autonomic* and *neuroglycopenic*.
   - Autonomic symptoms and signs include the following:
     (1) Sweating
     (2) Palpitations
     (3) Tremulousness
     (4) Hunger
     (5) Paresthesias
   - Neuroglycopenic symptoms and signs include the following:
     (1) Confusion
     (2) Fatigue
     (3) Seizures

2. In addition to hypoglycemia, other causes of *toxic metabolic encephalopathy* and generalized seizures include the following:
   - Medications (a wide range of medicines, including antibiotics, antidepressants, analgesics, antineoplastic agents, and bronchodilators [e.g., theophylline])
   - Hyponatremia, hypernatremia, hypocalcemia
   - Uremia
   - Poisoning (a wide range of agents, including tabun and sarin [organophosphates], strychnine, cyanide, mercury, methanol, and petroleum solvents)

3. Hyponatremia is clinically divided by *serum osmolality* into three categories: *normal (isotonic), low (hypotonic),* and *high (hypertonic)*.
   - Isotonic hyponatremia is typically associated with hyperproteinemia or hyperlipidemia.
   - Hypertonic hyponatremia is commonly associated with hyperglycemia or intake of mannitol, glycerol, sorbitol, or maltose.
   - Hypotonic hyponatremia must be further categorized into *hypovolemic, euvolemic,* and *hypervolemic states.*
     (1) Hypovolemic hypotonic hyponatremia includes dehydration, diuretic therapy, and mineralocorticoid deficiency
     (2) Euvolemic hypotonic hyponatremia includes syndrome of inappropriate ADH secretion, psychogenic polydipsia, and endurance exercise.
     (3) Hypervolemic hypotonic hyponatremia includes heart failure, advanced liver disease, and nephrotic syndrome.

4. Theophylline toxicity may be precipitated by overdose or, more commonly, by drug interaction. Theophylline is metabolized by the hepatic cytochrome oxidase CYP enzymes. Medicines that inhibit this enzyme will cause elevated levels of theophylline and onset of toxic manifestations. Generalized seizures are frequently the first sign of toxicity. Medications that increase theophylline levels include the following:
   - Macrolide antibiotics
   - Ciprofloxacin
   - Amiodarone

5. Seizures may occur in acute cerebrovascular accidents. Seizures may occur at the *onset of a subarachnoid hemorrhage, intracranial hemorrhage,* or *embolic infarction* but are rare at the *onset of a thrombotic stroke.* Seizures associated with thrombotic stroke typically start weeks, even years, after clinical presentation of the stroke.

6. Normal pressure hydrocephalus presents as dementia, gait disturbance (typically, short steps with a widened base), and urinary symptoms (usually starting with urgency and then progressing to incontinence).

E 215   A 53-year-old man who suffers from chronic alcohol abuse has a 3-month history of progressive weight loss and foul-smelling bulky stools. Chronic pancreatitis is diagnosed. Malabsorption of which of the following nutrients would be expected?

A. Vitamin D
B. Vitamin B_{12}
C. Vitamin K
D. Iron
E. Fat

Answer: A, B, C, and E
A, B, C, and E are correct because a deficiency in exocrine pancreas secretion of lipase causes malabsorption of fats and the fat-soluble vitamins A, D, E, and K. Although not a fat-soluble vitamin, pancreatic insufficiency causes a malabsorption of vitamin B_{12}.

■ **You should know:**

1. The *endocrine pancreas* secretes the following:
   • Beta cells producing insulin
     (1) Insulin stimulates glucose uptake by muscle and fat and drives potassium into cells
   • Alpha cells producing glucagon
     (1) Glucagon acts in the liver to raise blood glucose by stimulation of both glycogenolysis and gluconeogenesis

2. The *exocrine pancreas* secretes the following:
   • Lipase for fat digestion
   • Amylase for carbohydrate digestion
   • Protease for protein digestion

3. *In the patient who has chronic pancreatitis (CP):*
   • Endocrine dysfunction may lead to diabetes mellitus requiring insulin therapy. A clinical point: In contrast to type 1 diabetes mellitus in which autoimmune destruction of beta cells occurs, in CP there is nonautoimmune destruction of both beta cells that produce insulin and alpha cells that produce glucagon.
   • Exocrine dysfunction leads to fat malabsorption, malabsorption of vitamin B_{12}, and impaired absorption of the fat-soluble vitamins. Tests for protein malabsorption are difficult to perform.

4. Chronic pancreatitis (CP):
   • Eighty percent of cases of CP are caused by chronic alcohol abuse.
   • Malabsorption leads to weight loss, bulky foul-smelling stools, and chemical evidence of fat-soluble vitamin deficiency (e.g., low levels of vitamin D, vitamin B_{12}, calcium, and prolonged prothrombin time).
   • Mechanical complications include pseudocyst formation, bile duct or duodenal obstruction, and pancreatic ascitic or pleural effusions (a very

high amylase concentration, typically greater than 1,000 IU/L, is found the fluid)

- Treatment of CP includes the following:
  - (1) Low-fat diet
  - (2) Pancreatic enzyme supplements
  - (3) Insulin
  - (4) Surgery in selected cases

5. Celiac disease (CD) is another disease that causes malabsorption. It is characterized by an immune response to gluten that causes T cell–mediated mucosal damage in the proximal small bowel. Endoscopy in the patient who has CD shows atrophy or scalloping of duodenal folds. Biopsy of the proximal small bowel reveals blunting of villi with cellular infiltration.

6. Celiac disease (CD) has *different clinical manifestations in the infant or child compared to the adult.*
   - In the infant or child, diarrhea and abdominal distention with pain are common symptoms. Steatorrhea and nutritional deficiencies are evident, including iron, vitamin B_{12}, vitamin D, calcium, magnesium, and carotene. Dermatitis herpetiformis (DH) is a papulovesicular rash that is associated with CD but is *uncommon before puberty.*
   - In the adult, gastrointestinal symptoms are mild (mimicking irritable bowel syndrome) or not present. Osteoporosis and iron deficiency are common. Less commonly, dental enamel defects and peripheral neuropathy are noted. Dermatitis herpetiformis is common in the adult patient who has CD. The skin lesions respond to a gluten-free diet.
   - *In all patients who have celiac disease,* the diagnosis is suggested by the presence of IgA endomysial or IgA transglutaminase (tTG) antibodies. Small bowel biopsy confirms the diagnosis.

7. The D-xylose test measures the ability of the small intestine to absorb and therefore whether a defect in the intestinal mucosal epithelium is responsible for malabsorption. The D-xylose test is abnormal in the patient who has CD but is normal in the patient who has pancreatic disease, for pancreatic enzymes are not required for xylose absorption.

8. The following table compares chronic pancreatitis and celiac disease in the adult patient:

	Chronic Pancreatitis	**Celiac Disease in Adult**
Pathophysiology	Deficiency in pancreatic lipase, protease, and amylase	Antibodies to gluten causing changes in intestinal mucosal epithelium
Steatorrhea	Yes	Very infrequently
Iron deficiency	No	Yes
Osteoporosis	Yes	Yes
D-xylose test	Normal	Abnormal
Diagnostic test	72-hour fecal fat determination	Antibody assays; small bowel biopsy
Association with DH	No	Yes

(DH = dermatitis herpetiformis)

9. Another cause of malabsorption is bacterial overgrowth in the small intestine. The diagnosis of bacterial overgrowth is suggested by a hydrogen breath test using glucose, lactulose, or xylose. Important causes of bacterial overgrowth include the following conditions:
   • Enteric bowel fistulas, as occurs in Crohn's disease
   • Liver disease, notably cirrhosis
   • Resection of small bowel

10. Several conditions are associated with *vitamin B$_{12}$ deficiency*. A Schilling test is used to differentiate among the various causes of vitamin B$_{12}$ malabsorption. A brief review of the *causes of vitamin B$_{12}$ malabsorption* follows:
   • Pernicious anemia caused by atrophic gastritis and anti–intrinsic factor antibodies
   • Gastrectomy with removal of the cells that produce intrinsic factor
   • Chronic pancreatitis
   • Disease of the ileum (e.g., Crohn's disease)
   • Bacterial overgrowth of the small bowel

Please see E 209.

ID, HEENT, PUL

E 216   Which of the following conditions is considered to be an anaerobic infection?
   A. Antibiotic-associated colitis
   B. Gas gangrene
   C. Aspiration-related lung abscess
   D. Botulism
   E. Bacterial vaginosis

Answer: A, B, C, D, and E
A is correct because the anaerobic *Clostridium difficile* is the infectious cause of antibiotic-associated colitis. B and D are correct because anaerobic *Clostridium* species cause gas gangrene and botulism. C is correct because aspiration of anaerobic flora from the oral cavity and gingiva into the lungs can cause development of lung abscess. E is correct because bacterial vaginosis is a polymicrobial disease in which anaerobic organisms appear to be dominant.

■ **You should know:**

1. Anaerobic bacteria causing human infection include the following:
   • Gram positive
     (1) Peptostreptococcus species
     (2) *Clostridium (C. difficile, C. perfringens, C. botulinum)*
   • Gram negative (these are normal flora in the gums, oropharynx, and nasopharynx)
     (1) *Bacteroides* species
     (2) *Fusobacterium*
     (3) *Prevotella*
     (4) *Porphyromonas*

2. Anaerobic organisms are important causes of dental infections, including gingivitis, periapical abscess, and necrotizing ulcerative gingivitis (Vincent angina). Vincent angina is common in young adults and is characterized by painful inflammation of the gums with necrosis and membrane formation.

Essentials is designed to promote critical thinking and enrich your knowledge base.
Therefore, many questions will have more than one correct answer.

3. Aspiration bacterial pneumonia is most common in those who experience loss of consciousness associated with an impaired gag or cough reflex. Examples include grand mal seizure and impaired consciousness caused by alcohol or drugs. The impaired reflexes enable organisms normally found in the mouth and on the gums to be aspirated into the lungs. The anaerobic bacteria cause development of one or more lung abscesses. (Remember that other causes of lung abscess include tricuspid endocarditis in which infected valvular vegetations embolize into the lungs and pneumonia caused by *Klebsiella* or *Staphylococcus aureus*.)

4. Gas gangrene is caused by anaerobic clostridia typically associated with wound infection. Wounds are swollen with foul-smelling drainage and development of gas in the soft tissues. Toxins that are produced may precipitate hemolysis and hemodynamic shock.

5. Tetanus is caused by *Clostridium tetani* bacteria that are found in the soil. Human infection is often associated with a puncture wound or human bite. The neurotoxin released by the bacteria causes spasm of jaw muscles ("lockjaw") followed by spasms in the neck, back, and abdomen. The patient who has tetanus should be treated with tetanus immune globulin followed by tetanus toxoid.

6. Clinical manifestations of botulism are caused by a neurotoxin produced by the anaerobic *Clostridium botulinum*. The alert, responsive patient has the acute onset of bilateral cranial nerve palsies followed by weakness moving peripherally to the extremities. (In contrast, the patient who has Guillain-Barré syndrome usually has weakness starting peripherally in the toes or fingers and then moving proximally.)

7. There are antitoxins and botulinum immune globulin for treatment of botulism in infants and adults. Antibiotics are used in selected cases of botulism.

8. Human bites cause infection by both anaerobic and aerobic bacteria. A clenched fist injury is particularly likely to become infected. In addition to local wound care, antibiotics should be given to all patients with human bites.

9. Antibiotics that are used in the treatment of anaerobic infections include the following:
   - Metronidazole
     (1) Metronidazole is used in treatment of infections caused by anaerobic bacteria and protozoans (e.g., *Giardia*, *Trichomonas*, *Entamoeba*, and topically in treatment of rosacea).
   - Beta-lactam plus beta-lactamase inhibitors
   - Chloramphenicol

GI/N, HEME/ONC

E 217   A 48-year-old well-nourished man who generally drinks 1 to 2 ounces of alcohol per week suddenly goes on a 2-day binge of heavy alcohol intake after receiving emotionally disturbing news. Which of the following is a likely complication of the acute heavy binge drinking?

A. Acute pancreatitis
B. Paroxysmal atrial fibrillation
C. Fatty liver
D. Gastritis
E. Gout

Answer: A, B, C, D, and E

A is correct because acute pancreatitis can occur in hours to 2 days after acute binge drinking. B is correct because atrial fibrillation occurs in 60% of binge drinkers with or without underlying heart disease. C is correct because a fatty liver can occur within hours after a large alcohol binge. Fatty liver can occur after a *single* large binge. D is correct because alcohol can cause development of hemorrhagic gastritis and ulcers. E is correct because alcohol ingestion increases urate production and decreases renal clearance of uric acid, thus precipitating acute gout.

You should know:

1. Generally, patients who have any form of alcoholic liver disease have disproportionate elevation of serum aspartate aminotransferase (AST) compared to serum alanine aminotransferase (ALT).

2. Fatty liver is caused by a direct effect of alcohol on hepatocytes. The patient may be asymptomatic or have right upper quadrant abdominal pain. A fatty liver does not predict progression to cirrhosis. Other causes of fatty liver include starvation and drug toxicity, notably tetracycline, valproic acid, and the antiviral medicines zidovudine and dideoxyinosine.

3. The adverse effects of alcohol may be arbitrarily divided into two categories:
   • Binge drinking without *chronic* heavy alcohol intake (see above)
   • Chronic heavy alcohol abuse

4. *Chronic heavy alcohol abuse* may lead to development of the following conditions:
   • Alcohol cardiomyopathy (dilated cardiomyopathy with systolic heart failure, atrial and ventricular arrhythmias)
   • Chronic pancreatitis (with malabsorption syndrome and hyperglycemia)
   • Mallory-Weiss syndrome (most patients have a history of chronic alcohol abuse; acute retching leads to distal esophageal and proximal gastric tears with epigastric or back pain and acute bleeding)
   • Alcoholic hepatitis (manifest by fever, jaundice, and hepatomegaly; liver biopsy shows presence of Mallory bodies)
   • Cirrhosis
   • Liver cancer
   • Alcoholic ketoacidosis (manifest by high anion gap metabolic acidosis; plasma glucose may be low, normal, or slightly elevated)
   • Alcohol hypoglycemia (related to poor nutrition and depleted glycogen stores)
   • Peripheral sensorimotor neuropathy (manifest by paresthesias, muscle cramps, and weakness; examination shows decreased sense of touch and vibration)
   • Wernicke encephalopathy (thiamine deficiency manifest by encephalopathy, oculomotor nerve palsy and nystagmus, and ataxic wide-based, slow gait)
   • Korsakoff psychosis (manifest primarily by amnesia)
   • Folate deficiency megaloblastic anemia (alcohol abuse is the most common cause of folate deficiency in the United States)

5. The clinician should be aware that acute binge drinking is common in preteens and adolescents. In contrast to adults, ethanol-related hypoglycemia in children occurs despite adequate nourishment.

Essentials is designed to promote critical thinking and enrich your knowledge base. Therefore, many questions will have more than one correct answer.

CV

E 218   A 15-year-old boy has had two episodes, each occurring while running, of anterior chest pressure radiating into the neck. With rest the discomfort spontaneously ends in 3 to 4 minutes. Angina pectoris is diagnosed. Which of the following conditions may be associated with angina pectoris in a child or adolescent?

A. Hypertrophic obstructive cardiomyopathy
B. Anomalous origin of a coronary artery
C. Preexcitation syndrome
D. Long QT interval syndrome
E. Coarctation of the aorta

Answer: A and B
A is correct because 30% of patients with hypertrophic obstructive cardiomyopathy (HOCM) have angina pectoris. The angina pectoris is related to increased oxygen demand of the hypertrophic myocardium. The other two classic manifestations of HOCM are dyspnea (caused by diastolic heart failure) and syncope. B is correct because patients born with anomalous origin of a coronary artery may develop angina pectoris during later childhood or teenage years.

You should know:

1. Anomalous origin of a coronary artery, often a coronary artery arising from a *pulmonary artery*, causes myocardial ischemia at birth resulting in myocardial infarction or heart failure. However, if collateral circulation is adequate, the clinical manifestations of angina pectoris or dilated cardiomyopathy may start at approximately age 10 years or even in early adulthood.

2. *The physical examination in a patient who has HOCM while asymptomatic is very variable*:
   • From a normal cardiac examination to
   • Apical lift with S4 gallop to
   • Apical lift, S4 gallop, ejection murmur at the apex and lower left sternal border, and bisferiens carotid arterial pulse

3. If HOCM is suspected and the cardiac examination is normal or shows only an apical S4 gallop with apical lift, maneuvers are indicated. These include:
   • Abrupt standing
   • Valsalva strain
     (1) Both of which would likely elicit an ejection murmur

4. Syncope in HOCM typically occurs during or immediately after exercise.

5. The following are mechanisms causing syncope in HOCM:
   • Ventricular arrhythmia
   • Left ventricular outflow obstruction caused by a bulging ventricular septum that impedes flow of blood from the left ventricle into the aorta
   • Decreased cardiac output related to inadequate left ventricular filling during diastole
   • Inappropriate peripheral vasodilation during exercise. Some patients with HOCM will have *an abnormal decrease in blood pressure* during exercise. The

decrease in blood pressure is related to inappropriate *dilation of arterioles in nonexercising muscles.*

6. Congenital long QT interval syndrome and preexcitation syndrome are congenital, nonstructural heart disorders that may cause syncope or sudden cardiac death. They do not cause angina pectoris.

7. Kawasaki disease is a vasculitis of childhood. The classic manifestations are fever, nonexudative conjunctivitis, erythema and cracking of the lips, erythema of the oral mucosa, diffuse erythema of the palms and soles, and occasionally cervical lymphadenopathy. Cardiac complications include coronary artery aneurysm formation, myocardial infarction, and heart failure. Administration of intravenous immune globulin (IVIG) reduces the incidence of aneurysm formation. The IVIG is given together with aspirin.

8. A brief review of IVIG:
   • IVIG is immunoglobulins; primarily IgG, derived from pooled human plasma.
   • IVIG is used in the treatment of the following conditions:
     (1) Primary antibody deficiency states (e.g., primary agammaglobulinemia)
     (2) Secondary antibody deficiency states (e.g., HIV, parvovirus B19)
     (3) Neurologic diseases (e.g., myasthenia gravis, Guillain-Barré syndrome, Lambert-Eaton syndrome, multifocal motor neuropathy)
     (4) Hematologic disease (e.g., idiopathic thrombocytopenic purpura)

REPRO, GU

E 219 In which of the following conditions is there an elevated serum human chorionic gonadotropin (hCG) level?
   A. Pregnancy
   B. Hydatidiform mole
   C. Nonseminoma germ cell testicular tumor
   D. Panhypopituitarism
   E. Polycystic ovary syndrome

Answer: A, B, and C
A is correct because in pregnancy, both intrauterine and ectopic, there is an increased serum level of hCG. B is correct because a hydatidiform mole, a tumor of trophoblastic tissue in the placenta, produces hCG. C is correct because 95% of nonseminoma germ cell tumors of the testis produce hCG and alpha-fetoprotein.

■ **You should know:**

1. Human chorionic gonadotropin (hCG) is secreted by the trophoblast and can be detected in maternal blood and urine approximately 8 to 10 days after fertilization. The primary function of hCG is to maintain the corpus luteum until the placenta is developed to assume production of progesterone. (The trophoblasts are the precursor cells of the placenta. These cells differentiate into the other cell types found in the placenta.)

2. In a viable pregnancy the hCG concentration doubles every 1 to 2 days during the initial 30 days of pregnancy.

3. All pregnancy tests rely upon production of hCG by the placenta.

4. Serum hCG is elevated in the following conditions:
   • The placenta produces the hCG
      (1) Pregnancy
      (2) Hydatidiform mole
      (3) Choriocarcinoma
   • The tumor produces the hCG
      (1) Germ cell (nonseminoma) tumor of testis
      (2) Rarely, nontrophoblastic tumors produce hCG:
         (a) Cervix
         (b) Ovary
         (c) Gastrointestinal tract
         (d) Lung
         (e) Breast

5. The cardinal manifestations of ectopic pregnancy include abdominal pain, amenorrhea, and vaginal bleeding. The diagnosis is based upon transvaginal ultrasound and serial serum hCG levels.

6. In the patient who has polycystic ovary syndrome the serum testosterone and luteinizing hormone (LH) concentrations are elevated.

ID, HEENT

E 220   A 6-year-old girl has the sudden onset of fever (39°C), painful swallowing, and severe sore throat. Upon inspection the patient is drooling, sitting in a tripod position with her jaw protruding and neck extended. Her speech is muffled. Which of the following is the most likely diagnosis?

A. Foreign body aspiration
B. Croup
C. Diphtheria
D. Epiglottitis
E. Pertussis

Answer: D
D is correct because epiglottitis is characterized by the sudden onset of high fever, sore throat and painful swallowing, muffled speech ("hot potato"), and drooling.

■ You should know:

1. Primary immunization against *Haemophilus influenzae* infection is the *H. influenzae* type b conjugate vaccine (Hib). Although vaccination schedules vary based upon vaccine preparation, two or three doses are administered starting after age 6 weeks. Commonly, a three-dose schedule would be administered at ages 2, 4, and 6 months. A booster dose should be given at age 12 to 15 months.

2. Routine immunization against pertussis is the diphtheria, tetanus toxoids, and pertussis vaccine (DTaP). It should be administered at ages 2, 4, 6, and 15 to 18 months and 4 to 6 years of age.

3. Epiglottitis is an infectious disease and *medical emergency* most commonly caused by *Haemophilus influenzae* type b (Hib), even in immunized children. Other, less frequent, infecting organisms include *Streptococcus* and *Staphylococcus aureus* (methicillin sensitive and resistant).

4. Epiglottitis is diagnosed by the following:
   • Visualization of the epiglottis (by an experienced clinician with emergency airway procedures immediately available)
      (1) At the bedside, avoid intraoral examination of the pharynx with a tongue blade when the patient is in moderate or severe distress
   • Lateral soft tissue radiograph of the neck showing an enlarged epiglottis ("thumb" sign)
   • Culture of the epiglottis

5. Before the specific causative organism has been identified, empiric antibiotic therapy in epiglottitis should include coverage for *Staphylococcus*. Initial therapy may include ceftriaxone or cefotaxime plus clindamycin or vancomycin.

6. Other important elements in the treatment of epiglottitis include the following:
   • Hospitalization with *very close monitoring of airway* (intubation may be necessary)
   • Supplemental humidified oxygen

7. *Croup* is an infectious laryngotracheitis caused by viruses. The most common infecting organism is parainfluenza virus type 1, followed by respiratory syncytial virus and adenovirus. It is most prevalent during the fall and early winter months.

8. The usual clinical presentation of croup is fever, coryza, followed by hoarseness, barking cough, and stridor. Examination usually shows nasal congestion but no evidence of or minimal pharyngitis. Upper airway obstruction with stridor may be the key physical signs.

9. Soft tissue posterior-anterior radiography of the neck shows the "steeple sign"—namely, tapering of the upper trachea. Confirmation of the diagnosis of croup is generally not necessary. If necessary, viral culture or tests for viral antigens may be performed.

10. *Pertussis* (whooping cough) is caused by the bacterium *Bordetella pertussis*. It may occur in vaccinated children. In fact, despite vaccination, it is increasing in frequency in both children and young adults. The classic presentation includes paroxysmal coughing followed by a long, forced inspiratory effort producing a "whoop" sound.

Essentials is designed to promote critical thinking and enrich your knowledge base.
Therefore, many questions will have more than one correct answer.

11. Treatment of pertussis includes a macrolide antibiotic, inhaled beta agonist, and microbial prophylaxis for close contacts. In view of the increasing prevalence of pertussis in adults, the U.S. Advisory Committee on Immunization Practices recommends a single dose of vaccine containing tetanus toxoid, diphtheria toxoid, and acellular pertussis vaccine (Tdap) to adults aged 19 to 64 years and, in selected cases, to others.

12. The following table compares and contrasts epiglottitis, croup, and pertussis:

	Epiglottitis	Croup	Pertussis
Clinical features	*H. influenzae* type b Drooling, tripod posture, "hot potato" voice	Viruses Barking cough, stridor	*Bordetella pertussis* Paroxysmal cough, whooping
Radiography	"Thumb" sign on lateral radiograph of neck	"Steeple" sign on PA radiograph of neck	Chest radiograph may be normal or peribronchial cuffing
Treatment	Cefotaxime or ceftriaxone + vancomycin or clindamycin	Corticosteroids, nebulized epinephrine, humidified air	Macrolide, trial of inhaled beta agonist; avoid cough suppressant
Diagnosis	Laryngoscopy, C+S	Clinical diagnosis; infrequently, viral culture or tests for viral antigens	C+S, polymerase chain reaction (Centers for Disease Control and Prevention)

CV

E 221   Without prodromal symptoms, an 83-year-old man suddenly faints. The electrocardiographic (ECG) rhythm strip taken by rescue squad personnel is depicted below. Which of the following is the ECG abnormality that is demonstrated?

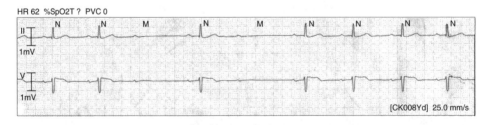

    A. Sinus arrest
    B. Complete (3rd-degree) atrioventricular block
    C. Sinus bradycardia with junctional escape beat
    D. 2nd-degree atrioventricular block
    E. Intermittent conduction through accessory pathways

Answer: D

D is correct because the basic rhythm is sinus bradycardia. The third and fifth P waves are not conducted to the ventricles. The P waves that are conducted have a fixed PR interval of 0.24 second.

■ **You should know:**

1. The common denominator in patients who faint (syncope) is *transient generalized cerebral ischemia.*

2. Syncope has many causes, including the following:
   - Arrhythmia (bradycardia or tachycardia)
   - Structural heart or lung disease that obstructs blood flow (pulmonary embolism, aortic valve stenosis, hypertrophic obstructive cardiomyopathy, atrial myxoma)
   - Orthostatic hypotension (autonomic insufficiency or hypovolemia)
   - Neutrally mediated syncope (vasovagal, carotid sinus hypersensitivity, situational)

3. Typically, syncope caused by an arrhythmia is not associated with prodromal symptoms except for the bradycardia associated with vasovagal fainting when the patient has nausea, sweating, and pallor.

4. Delayed atrioventricular (AV) conduction may be *anatomic* or *functional.* In the patient who has a diseased heart, AV block is commonly related to structural anatomic fibrosis in the atrioventricular node. This occurs in ischemic or valvular heart disease or in idiopathic myocardial fibrosis. The AV block is permanent in those whose AV block is caused by structural disease.

5. *Functional* slowing of AV conduction is caused by heightened parasympathetic (vagal) tone or by medication. This is a transient phenomenon. Medicines that slow AV conduction and can cause AV block include beta-adrenergic blockers, digoxin, the calcium channel blockers verapamil and diltiazem, and amiodarone.

Essentials is designed to promote critical thinking and enrich your knowledge base.
Therefore, many questions will have more than one correct answer.

CV

E 222   A 79-year-old woman has 1 hour of severe anterior chest pain associated with sweating and dyspnea. Electrocardiography (see tracing below) shows an acute ST segment elevation anterior wall myocardial infarction (STEMI). Which of the following is another electrocardiographic abnormality on the tracing?

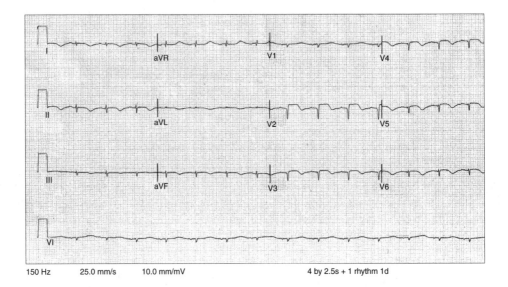

150 Hz   25.0 mm/s   10.0 mm/mV   4 by 2.5s + 1 rhythm 1d

   A. Left ventricular hypertrophy
   B. Prolonged QT interval
   C. Old inferior wall myocardial infarction
   D. Hyperkalemia
   E. Left atrial enlargement

Answer: B

This electrocardiogram (ECG) shows diffuse T-wave inversion with a prolonged QT interval. Hypocalcemia is an electrolyte abnormality that causes a prolonged QT interval. Although the ECG manifestations of hypokalemia or hypomagnesemia are depression of the ST segment, decreased amplitude of the T wave, and increased amplitude of the U wave, many include these in the etiology of prolonged QT interval.

■ **You should know:**

   1. Prolongation of the QT interval, whether congenital or acquired, can cause torsades de pointes (Tdp), a polymorphous ventricular tachycardia that may precipitate syncope or sudden cardiac death.

   2. *Congenital* long QT interval is a genetic inherited disorder of ion channel repolarization in a structurally normal heart that predisposes to torsades de pointes.

   3. The classic precipitating event in provoking Tdp is activation of the sympathetic nervous system, either by emotional upset or physical exertion.

   4. *Acquired* long QT interval occurs in those with a genetic predisposition who ingest many medications or who have hypokalemia, hypomagnesemia, or hypocalcemia.

Please see E 203.

CV

E 223   A 42-year-old woman awakens at 2 a.m. with anterior chest pressure radiating down the left arm. Electrocardiography performed during the pain is depicted below. Which of the following is the most likely diagnosis?

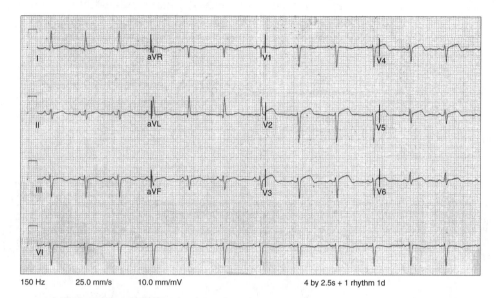

150 Hz   25.0 mm/s   10.0 mm/mV   4 by 2.5s + 1 rhythm 1d

   A. Subendocardial myocardial ischemia
   B. Nutcracker esophagus
   C. Variant angina
   D. Acute pericarditis
   E. Hyponatremia

Answer: C

C is correct because electrocardiography performed in a patient with variant angina *during the myocardial ischemia with angina pectoris* shows ST segment elevation.

▨ **You should know:**

1. The myocardial ischemia in variant angina is *transmyocardial ischemia; therefore, the ST segment is **elevated** during the anginal discomfort.*

2. In contrast, myocardial ischemia related to atherosclerotic narrowing of a coronary artery or myocardial hypertrophy is *subendocardial ischemia,* for the subendocardial layer of the myocardium is most susceptible to insufficient perfusion. Subendocardial ischemia is *manifest by ST segment **depression**.*

CV

E 224   An 82-year-old woman has a 1-week history of progressively worsening short-ness of breath without associated cough, hemoptysis, or anginal discomfort. Blood pressure is 102/66 mm Hg; pulse, 126/min; respirations, 27/min. Auscultation of the lungs is clear. Heart size is indeterminate. No murmur or gallop is heard. There is no peripheral edema. The patient's electrocardiogram is depicted below. Which of the following is the preferred initial medication to be administered?

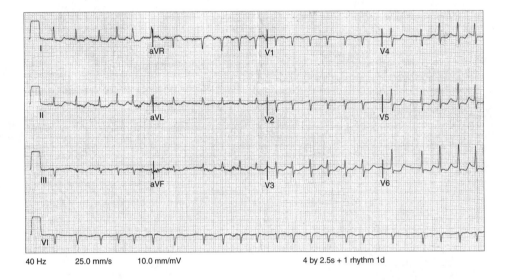

40 Hz   25.0 mm/s   10.0 mm/mV   4 by 2.5s + 1 rhythm 1d

    A. Furosemide
    B. Heparin
    C. Nifedipine
    D. Adenosine
    E. Isosorbide dinitrate

Answer: B
B is correct because anticoagulation for stroke prevention is a primary consideration in the patient who is in atrial fibrillation (AF). In this patient, the duration of AF is unknown; therefore, anticoagulation with heparin is indicated. In addition to heparin, the patient should receive a medication to slow the ventricular rate.

▨ **You should know:**

    1. Electrocardiography shows the patient to be in atrial fibrillation (AF) with a fast ventricular response (approximately 140/min).

    2. In AF there are no discrete P waves. Rather, fibrillatory waves at a frequency of 400 to 600/min are present in the atria, varying in amplitude and morphology.

    3. Conduction through the atrioventricular (AV) node is very irregular as many of the fibrillatory waves find the AV nodal tissue in a refractory state. Thus, the ventricular response is *irregularly irregular*.

4. The primary elements in management of atrial fibrillation include the following:
   - Ventricular rate control
   - Anticoagulation
   - Consideration of reversion to normal sinus rhythm

5. In the above patient, nifedipine, furosemide, and adenosine are not appropriate therapy:
   - Nifedipine does not slow atrioventricular conduction.
   - The vagal effect of adenosine lasts only seconds and therefore is of no clinical value.
   - There is no clinical evidence of heart failure. Administration of furosemide would decrease circulating blood volume and precipitate hypotension.
   - The patient is not having symptoms of myocardial ischemia. Administration of isosorbide dinitrate would lower arterial pressure and further increase heart rate.

6. Medicines that slow AV conduction and thus slow the ventricular response in the patient who has AF include the following:
   - Nondihydropyridine calcium channel blockers verapamil and diltiazem
   - Beta-adrenergic blockers
   - Digoxin

7. Once slowing of the ventricular response has been achieved, the decision whether to attempt conversion to normal sinus rhythm is made on an individual patient basis.

8. Heparinization is indicated in an effort to prevent systemic embolization and stroke. Oral warfarin therapy is initiated at the same time. When the INR is therapeutic, the heparin is discontinued.

9. The duration of warfarin anticoagulation is dependent upon multiple clinical factors, including valvular disease and the CHADS2 score for stroke risk that considers hypertension, history of stroke, transient ischemic attack or thromboembolism, heart failure, diabetes mellitus, and age equal to or greater than 75 years.

Please see question E 199.

DERM, ID

E 225   One week after completing therapy with a sulfonamide, a 22-year-old woman has fever, diffuse myalgia, oral pain with painful swallowing, and a diffuse, tender rash with target lesions. The rash involving the lips is shown in the photograph. Which of the following is the most likely diagnosis?

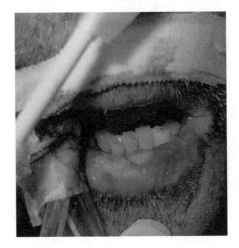

A. Stevens-Johnson syndrome
B. Pemphigus
C. Lichen planus
D. Churg-Strauss vasculitis
E. Herxheimer reaction

Answer: A
A is correct because Stevens-Johnson syndrome is an idiosyncratic reaction commonly related to medicines including sulfonamides. It causes target skin lesions and vesicles and bullae on the lips and mouth.

■ **You should know:**

1. Please see Essentials question E 190 for a full description of Stevens-Johnson syndrome and its comparison to erythema multiforme.

2. Churg-Strauss disease is a vasculitis in which inflammation of small arteries occurs. Early manifestations include rhinosinusitis, asthma, and eosinophilia. Later, involvement of the heart (heart failure), kidneys (glomerulonephritis), skin (nodular ulceration), and nervous system (peripheral neuropathy) may occur.

E 226   Three days after bruising his upper arm, a 28-year-old man has fever, pain, and a rash in the affected area. A photograph of the rash is shown. Which of the following is the most likely diagnosis?

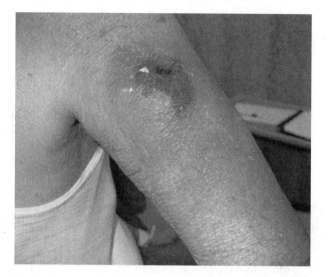

    A. Cellulitis
    B. Carbuncle
    C. Herpes zoster
    D. Erythema migrans
    E. Impetigo

Answer: A

A is correct because the clinical presentation of cellulitis commonly includes a break in the skin barrier (e.g., abrasion) followed by diffuse erythema without a clearly defined margin, edema, and increased skin temperature.

▨ **You should know:**

1. Cellulitis and erysipelas are skin infections that are most commonly caused by beta-hemolytic streptococci. However, cellulitis is frequently caused by *Staphylococcus aureus*, both methicillin sensitive and resistant, and less commonly by many other organisms.

2. *Common denominators* related to cellulitis and erysipelas include the following:
   - Beta-hemolytic streptococci are the most common infecting organism.
   - Predisposing factors are similar and include:
     (1) A break in the skin allowing entry of bacteria into the dermis. Skin disruption may be due to the following:
        (a) A penetrating wound including needle injection.
        (b) Skin infection (e.g., tinea pedis). Toe web intertrigo, an infection between the toes caused by fungi and many bacteria, is a very common predisposing cause of cellulitis. The intertrigo must be treated in order to prevent recurrent cellulitis.

    (c) Skin inflammation as may occur during radiation therapy.

    (d) Chronic edema as may occur in venous insufficiency.

- Treatment
  - (1) Initial therapy is intravenous antibiotics effective against beta-hemolytic streptococci and staphylococcus.

3. There are important *clinical differences* between cellulitis and erysipelas:
   - Onset of symptoms:
     - (1) Cellulitis has a more indolent course with development of local symptoms over a few days.
     - (2) Erysipelas has a more acute onset with fever and chills.
   - Depth of the infection:
     - (1) Cellulitis involves deeper dermis and subcutaneous fat. There is no sharp demarcation between infected and noninfected skin.
     - (2) Erysipelas involves the upper dermis and superficial lymphatics. There is a sharp demarcation between infected and noninfected skin, and the lesions are raised above the surrounding skin. Erysipelas commonly affects the face and ears.
   - Complication
     - (1) Cellulitis may develop bullae and become purulent (i.e., form pus).
     - (2) Erysipelas does not become purulent.

4. The differential diagnosis of cellulitis includes deep vein thrombosis (DVT) and necrotizing fasciitis. Similar to cellulitis, DVT may present with warmth, tenderness, erythema, and edema. Venous duplex ultrasonography is used to differentiate DVT from cellulitis.

Please see Essentials question E 210 for a discussion of necrotizing fasciitis and streptococcal shock syndrome.

E 227   One week after completing antibiotic therapy for streptococcal pharyngitis, a 7-year-old girl has diffuse, persistent abdominal pain and nausea followed by the onset of a rash on both lower legs. Urinalysis shows 1+ proteinuria and red blood cell casts. A photograph of the rash is shown. Which of the following is the most likely diagnosis?

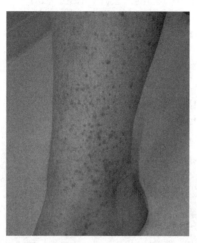

   A. Rocky Mountain spotted fever
   B. Idiopathic thrombocytopenic purpura
   C. Systemic lupus erythematosus
   D. Henoch-Schönlein purpura
   E. Acute granulocytic leukemia

Answer: D
D is correct because the Henoch-Schönlein purpura (HSP) is a vasculitis that commonly presents after streptococcal infection and is characterized by abdominal pain, arthritis or arthralgia, purpuric rash, and hematuria.

▓ You should know:

1. HSP is of unknown etiology but in half the cases is preceded by an upper respiratory infection, especially a streptococcal infection. There is no specific test for HSP. Serum IgA levels are elevated in approximately half of cases.

2. HSP is a vasculitis characterized by deposition of IgA in the walls of skin venules and in the mesangium of the kidney glomerulus.

3. The clinical presentation of HSP includes the following:
   • Arthritis or arthralgia: Most commonly affects the hips, knees, and ankles; the joints are generally not warm or erythematous on examination; there is no chronic joint damage.
   • Purpura: An *elevated* purpura that symmetrically involves the legs or buttocks. *An important clinical point: The platelet count and prothrombin time are normal in the patient with HSP.*
   • Abdominal pain: Gastrointestinal manifestations may vary from *mild*, with nausea and abdominal discomfort, to *severe*, with bowel necrosis, intussusception, and bowel perforation. Intussusception is the most common gastrointestinal complication of HSP.

Essentials is designed to promote critical thinking and enrich your knowledge base. Therefore, many questions will have more than one correct answer.

- Kidney disease: Manifestations vary from asymptomatic gross or microscopic hematuria to severe complications including nephrotic syndrome, renal insufficiency, and hypertension.
- Scrotal pain mimicking testicular torsion occurs in approximately 25% of boys with HSP.

4. Prognosis is generally excellent in children who have HSP. Most cases are treated with bed rest, hydration, and analgesics (e.g., nonaspirin nonsteroidal anti-inflammatory agent) for joint or abdominal pain. Nephrology consultation is indicated for significant renal involvement.

ID, DERM

E 228   A 7-year-old boy has a 2-day history of fever, sore mouth, and rash. Examination shows vesicles in the mouth. A photograph of the rash is shown. Which of the following is the most likely diagnosis?

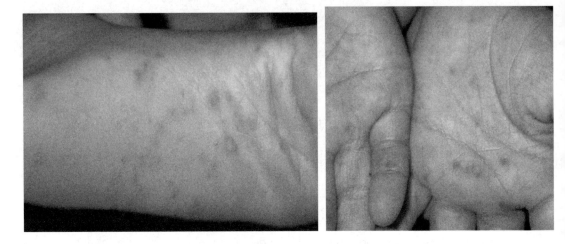

A. Rocky Mountain spotted fever
B. Meningococcal meningitis
C. Congenital syphilis
D. Hand-foot-and-mouth syndrome
E. Varicella

Answer: D

D is correct because hand-foot-and-mouth syndrome (HFM) causes a vesicular rash on the buccal mucosa, tongue, and gingiva and a maculopapular or tender vesicular rash on the palms, soles, and buttocks.

▪ **You should know:**

1. HFM is an infectious disease most commonly caused by group A coxsackievirus and less frequently by enterovirus 71.

2. It is usually a self-limited disease with resolution in 2 to 3 days. Rarely, myocarditis or aseptic meningitis may occur as a complication.

3. HFM is contagious and is spread by the following:
   - Fecal-oral route
   - Nasal discharge
   - Saliva

4. The virus may persist in the stool for weeks after resolution of symptoms; the patient is still contagious. Nonetheless, in an effort to prevent spread of the disease, the following measures are recommended:
   - Hand washing by patient
   - Removal from school or group setting while oral lesions or skin rash is present
   - A pregnant woman near term should be advised to avoid contact with the patient in an effort to prevent intrauterine death.

5. The following table is a review of diseases that cause *fever, rash, and meningitis*:

Disease	Rash
Meningococcemia	Petechiae on skin, conjunctivae, soft palate
Cryptococcosis	Variable; purpura, plaques, umbilicated papules; primarily in immunocompromised patients
Enterovirus/coxsackievirus	Vesicular or maculopapular; involves palms and soles
Lyme disease	Erythema migrans
Rocky Mountain spotted fever	Maculopapular, then petechiae; involves palms
Secondary syphilis	Maculopapular; involves palms and soles

Photos for questions E 178, E 179, E 182, E 183, E 184, E 225, E 226, E 227, and E 228 from: Barankin, B, and Freiman, A. *Derm Notes: Clinical Dermatology Pocket Guide.* Philadelphia: F.A. Davis Company, 2006.

Part Two

Performance: Gauging Your Test Success

The **PERFORMANCE** section provides you with clinical questions that relate to the medical topics in **ESSENTIALS**. In this carefully constructed manner, Performance is linked to Essentials and "You Should Know." As a result, you are learning much more about clinical medicine, not just learning isolated facts about a disease.

The questions are purposely not arranged by organ system. Rather, the questions are haphazard in their order in an effort to prepare the candidate for PANCE and PANRE questions. Thus, the test-book reader must quickly direct his or her critical thinking from Cardiology to Reproductive to Endocrinology, and so on.

Each question is labeled by organ system. This text is constructed in a way so that you may retrieve questions related to a specific organ system. In order to promote the learning process, some questions have multiple organ system labels. For example, a question on endocarditis prophylaxis will be labeled ID (Infectious Disease) and CV (Cardiovascular). A question on melasma will be labeled DERM (Dermatology) and REPRO (Reproductive).

Section One

Performance Test

CV

P 001 A 75-year-old man with chronic mitral regurgitation has dyspnea for 2 hours. Blood pressure is 90/70 mm Hg right arm sitting; respiratory rate, 28/min; and pulse, 130/min irregularly irregular. Cardiac examination shows a dilated left ventricle and apical holosystolic murmur. Bibasilar rales are heard. Electrocardiography indicates atrial fibrillation. Chest radiograph shows bilateral pulmonary congestion. In addition to metoprolol, which of the following is the preferred medicine to control the ventricular rate?

    A. Digoxin
    B. Verapamil
    C. Ibutilide
    D. Adenosine
    E. Captopril

NEURO, PSY/LE

P 002 A 56-year-old man has dementia associated with chronic alcohol abuse. In addition to efforts to prevent continuing alcohol intake, which of the following therapeutic measures should be taken?

    A. Oral administration of B-complex vitamins
    B. Intravenous infusion of octreotide
    C. Oral administration of levodopa
    D. Oral administration of diazepam
    E. Serial subcutaneous injections of vitamin B_{12}

CV

P 003   A 14-year-old boy has a 2-week history of exertional dyspnea without associated cough, wheezing, or sputum production. Blood pressure is 120/80 mm Hg right arm sitting; pulse, 72/min regular; and respirations, 17/min. A bisferiens carotid pulse is felt. An apical heave is felt. A diagnosis of hypertrophic cardiomyopathy is confirmed. In addition to administration of a diuretic, which of the following medications should be prescribed?

A. Oral digoxin
B. Oral verapamil
C. Oral captopril
D. Oral isosorbide dinitrate
E. Inhaled albuterol

NEURO

P 004   A 78-year-old man has a 2-month history of increasing memory loss and impaired judgment. He admits to recent urinary incontinence. Vital signs are normal. Examination shows an alert man with evidence of recent memory loss and impaired arithmetic calculations. Gait is wide based. Which of the following is the most likely diagnosis?

A. Alzheimer's disease
B. Chronic subdural hematoma
C. Normal pressure hydrocephalus
D. Encephalitis
E. Mad cow disease

HEME, GI/N

P 005   A 20-year-old African American soldier is started on primaquine for malarial prophylaxis. One week later he notes jaundice and dark brown urine. Laboratory values include hemoglobin, 10 g/dL; total bilirubin, 3.8 mg/dL; and unconjugated bilirubin, 3.1 mg/dL. Which of the following is the most likely diagnosis?

A. *Mycoplasma* infection
B. Sickle cell anemia
C. Thalassemia
D. Glucose-6-phosphate dehydrogenase deficiency
E. Acute granulocytic leukemia

ENDO

P 006   A 56-year-old woman has a 2-month history of worsening memory, constipation, weakness, and cold intolerance. Examination shows a lethargic woman who is oriented to time and place. She has dry skin and thinning of the outer third of the eyelids. Deep tendon reflex relaxation is slow. Which of the following is an expected serum laboratory value?

A. Fasting blood sugar 42 mg/dL
B. Sodium 118 mEq/L
C. Total cholesterol 146 mg/dL
D. Thyroid-stimulating hormone 22 microU/mL
E. Albumin 2.0 g/dL

CV

P 007 A 54-year-old man with chronic hypertension has a 2-week history of exertional breathlessness without associated cough, wheezing, or sputum production. There is no history of allergy. Blood pressure is 150/90 mm Hg sitting; pulse, 90/min regular; and respiratory rate, 20/min. Examination shows an apical lift and S4 gallop, but no murmur is present. Bibasilar crackles are heard. Which of the following is the most likely diagnosis?

A. Asthma
B. Psychogenic dyspnea
C. Diastolic heart failure
D. Cystic fibrosis
E. Dissection of the aorta

CV

P 008 A 57-year-old man has a 3-week history of increasing exertional dyspnea without cough, wheezing, or chest discomfort. At rest, vital signs and cardiopulmonary examination are normal. During treadmill exercise testing, the patient has dyspnea without anginal discomfort. At that time, the electrocardiogram shows horizontal ST segment depression. Which of the following is the most likely diagnosis?

A. Unstable angina pectoris
B. Variant angina pectoris
C. Anginal equivalent
D. Noncardiac dyspnea
E. Anxiety reaction

CV

P 009 A 14-year-old boy has anterior chest pressure radiating down the left arm and shortness of breath when he is playing basketball. The symptoms cease within 3 minutes of rest. Blood pressure is 130/90 mm Hg sitting; pulse, 70/min regular; and respirations, 18/min. Examination shows an apical heave, 2/6 left lower sternal border ejection murmur, and apical S4 gallop. There is no chest wall tenderness. Which of the following is the most likely diagnosis?

A. Anomalous origin of a coronary artery
B. Atherosclerotic heart disease
C. Mitral valve prolapse
D. Hypertrophic obstructive cardiomyopathy
E. Rheumatic mitral regurgitation

ENDO, MS

P 010 A 43-year-old man with a history of gout is to start therapy for dyslipidemia. Which of the following medications should not be prescribed?

A. Niacin
B. Cholestyramine
C. Simvastatin
D. Clofibrate
E. Ezetimibe

The Performance section is like a PANCE or PANRE. There is only *one* best answer.

CV

P 011   Five minutes after inhaling cocaine, an 18-year-old man has severe anterior chest pressure and sweating for which he is taken to the emergency department. The patient is alert, pink, and tremulous. Blood pressure is 230/120 mm Hg recumbent; pulse rate, 130/min regular; and respiratory rate, 28/min. Lung examination is normal. An apical S4 gallop is heard. Electrocardiography shows ST segment elevation in leads V1-V4. In addition to nitrates, which of the following medications should be given?

A. Propranolol
B. Verapamil
C. Hydralazine
D. Adenosine
E. Captopril

GI/N

P 012   A 57-year-old man with a long history of alcohol abuse has cirrhosis. He suddenly vomits a massive amount of red blood. Which of the following is the preferred initial therapeutic measure?

A. Insertion of Sengstaken-Blakemore tube
B. Intravenous administration of metoprolol
C. Intravenous administration of octreotide
D. Rectal administration of lactulose
E. Nasogastric administration of omeprazole

CV

P 013   A 78-year-old man has stable angina pectoris and chronic hypertension for which he takes lisinopril, verapamil, and nitroglycerin. The patient suddenly has a syncopal episode lasting 30 seconds. Blood pressure is 90/70 mm Hg; pulse, 46/min; and respiratory rate, 24/min. Electrocardiogram reveals Mobitz I atrioventricular block. Which of the following is the most likely cause of the syncope?

A. Adverse effect of verapamil
B. Vasovagal reaction
C. Orthostatic hypotension
D. Hypovolemia
E. Carotid artery stenosis

HEME, CV

P 014   A 66-year-old man has a 2-week history of increasing facial swelling. Vital signs are normal. The face is suffused and edematous. There is dilatation of arm and chest veins. Jugular venous pressure is elevated. There is no peripheral edema. Bilateral cervical, axillary, and inguinal nodes are felt. Which of the following is the most likely diagnosis?

A. Sarcoidosis
B. Non-Hodgkin's lymphoma
C. Right heart failure
D. Constrictive pericarditis
E. Angioneurotic edema

CV, GI/N

P 015 A 47-year-old woman has a 2-week history of increasing abdominal distention and peripheral edema. Four years earlier she had received chest radiotherapy for carcinoma of the breast. Blood pressure is 100/70 mm Hg sitting; pulse, 96/min regular; and respiratory rate, 18/min. Jugular venous pressure is elevated. Lungs are clear. No murmur or gallop is heard. Ascites and bilateral ankle edema are present. Which of the following is the most likely diagnosis?

A. Right heart failure
B. Pulmonary embolism
C. Mitral valve stenosis
D. Constrictive pericarditis
E. Superior vena cava syndrome

CV

P 016 A 68-year-old woman with chronic hypertension suddenly has severe, tearing pain in the anterior chest lasting 30 minutes. Supine blood pressure is 180/100 mm Hg left arm and 140/90 mm Hg right arm. Pulse is 100/min regular, and respiratory rate is 30/min. A new 2/6 right sternal border diastolic decrescendo murmur is heard. Which of the following is the preferred initial test?

A. Transesophageal echocardiogram
B. Aortogram
C. Chest radiograph
D. Cardiac enzyme profile
E. Ventilation-perfusion scan

GI/N

P 017 A 35-year-old man with long-standing Crohn's disease has 3 hours of right upper quadrant abdominal pain associated with nausea but without vomiting. Blood pressure is 120/82 mm Hg recumbent; pulse, 100/min regular; and respiratory rate, 18/min. Examination shows the patient to be nonicteric. The abdomen is flat and symmetrical. Moderate epigastric tenderness is present. No mass is felt, and bowel sounds are hypoactive. Serum laboratory values are amylase, 200 units/L; alanine aminotransferase, 106 units/L; and alkaline phosphatase, 130 units/L. Which of the following is the most likely diagnosis?

A. Acute cholecystitis
B. Acute pancreatitis
C. Peritonitis secondary to bowel perforation
D. Mesenteric ischemia
E. Acute intermittent porphyria

The Performance section is like a PANCE or PANRE. There is only *one* best answer.

P 018   A 45-year-old woman has a 1-month history of fatigue and a 2-week history of pruritus without rash. She takes no medication. Vital signs are normal. Examination shows generalized hyperpigmentation and hepatomegaly. Serum alkaline phosphatase is 300 units/L, gamma-glutamyl transpeptidase is 130 units/L, and total bilirubin is 1.2 mg/dL. Which of the following is the most likely diagnosis?

A. Metastatic carcinoma to bone
B. Primary biliary cirrhosis
C. Carcinoma of the pancreas
D. Chronic fatigue syndrome
E. Ischemic hepatic insufficiency

P 019   A 45-year-old man with type 1 diabetes mellitus now has proteinuria. Serum creatinine is 1.0 mg/dL, and blood urea nitrogen is 18 mg/dL. Blood pressure is 140/80 mm Hg sitting. Which of the following is recommended therapy?

A. Initiate thiazide therapy
B. Initiate angiotensin-converting enzyme inhibitor therapy
C. Observation for onset of azotemia
D. Initiate hydralazine therapy
E. Reduce insulin dosage

P 020   A 40-year-old woman has the acute onset of severe, anterior chest pain that is eased by sitting forward and increased during swallowing and changes in body position. For the past 3 weeks, the patient has had fatigue and generalized arthralgia. Examination shows the presence of a pericardial friction rub. White blood cell count is 2,200/microL. Which of the following is the most likely diagnosis?

A. Pericarditis due to coxsackievirus
B. Pericarditis due to *Staphylococcus* infection
C. Systemic lupus erythematosus
D. Constrictive pericarditis
E. Superior vena cava syndrome

P 021   A 65-year-old man has lightheadedness when arising from bed. In the sitting position, blood pressure is 130/70 mm Hg with pulse 70/min regular. Standing blood pressure is 100/50 mm Hg, and pulse is 71/min regular. Oral temperature is 98.6°F. Which of the following is the most likely etiology of the patient's symptoms?

A. Hypovolemia due to excessive diuresis
B. Addison's disease
C. Autonomic insufficiency
D. Pheochromocytoma
E. Gram-negative sepsis

MS

P 022   A 57-year-old woman is to begin alendronate as treatment for osteoporosis. Which of the following instructions should be given to the patient?

A. Take medication at bedtime
B. Do not eat for 60 minutes after taking medication
C. Take medication with an aluminum-containing antacid
D. Stand or sit upright for 30 minutes after taking medication
E. Check daily for signs of purpura

ENDO

P 023   Niacin therapy is initiated for dyslipidemia in a 56-year-old man with
type 1 diabetes mellitus. Which of the following instructions should be
given to the patient?

A. Insulin dosage may increase due to hyperglycemic effect of niacin
B. Proteinuria may occur as a side effect of medication
C. Do not ingest niacin within 2 hours of insulin administration
D. Take niacin with psyllium preparation
E. Angioedema is a common adverse effect of medication

NEURO

P 024   A 48-year-old woman has a 2-month history of progressively worsening
tremor of both hands. Examination shows a marked tremor when
holding a glass of water with a stationary outstretched arm. The tremor
worsens when bringing the glass to her lips. Neurologic examination
is otherwise normal. Which of the following is the preferred initial
therapy?

A. Levodopa
B. Prostigmine
C. Diazepam
D. Propranolol
E. Carbamazepine

CV

P 025   A 57-year-old man has a history of remote myocardial infarction. He has
an elevated serum C-reactive protein level that places him in the upper
quartile compared to normal values. The patient should be advised that
he is at increased risk for which of the following?

A. Carcinoma of the colon
B. Venous thrombosis
C. Rheumatoid arthritis
D. Recurrent myocardial infarction
E. Glaucoma

The Performance section is like a PANCE or PANRE. There is only *one* best answer.

GI/N, DERM

P 026   A 44-year-old woman has fatigue and generalized pruritus. A diagnosis of primary biliary cirrhosis is made. Presence in the serum of antibodies to which of the following is most likely?

A. Smooth muscle
B. Mitochondria
C. Acetylcholine receptors
D. Gastric parietal cells
E. Endotoxin

GI/N

P 027   A 56-year-old man has cirrhosis due to chronic alcohol abuse. An increase in which of the following serum levels raises suspicion of hepatocellular carcinoma?

A. Beta carotene
B. Alpha-fetoprotein
C. Alpha-tocopherol
D. Beta globin
E. CA 125

CV, HEME

P 028   A 36-year-old woman has acute pericarditis. A diagnosis of systemic lupus erythematosus is made. Which of the following laboratory values would be expected in this patient?

A. Platelet count 625,000/microL
B. Hemoglobin 17 g/dL
C. White blood cell count 2,100/microL
D. Fasting blood sugar 170 mg/dL
E. Serum ferritin 120 ng/mL

ENDO, CV

P 029   A 40-year-old woman has a 1-month history of paroxysmal sweating and palpitations. Examination shows a sitting blood pressure 180/120 mm Hg and pulse 100/min regular. In the standing position, blood pressure is 150/104 mm Hg with pulse of 114/min. Which of the following is the most likely etiology of the hypertension?

A. Essential hypertension
B. Hypercortisolism
C. Primary hyperaldosteronism
D. Pheochromocytoma
E. Coarctation of the aorta

ENDO, GI/N

P 030   A 60-year-old woman has a 2-month history of fatigue, nausea, anorexia, and a 6-pound weight loss. Which of the following is the preferred laboratory test to establish a diagnosis of Addison's disease?

A. Dexamethasone suppression test
B. Plasma renin activity
C. Schilling test
D. Cosyntropin stimulation test
E. 24-hour urinary sodium excretion value

NEURO, CV

P 031   A 79-year-old woman faints while sitting in a chair. Upon awakening, she has mild nausea. Examination in the emergency department shows the patient to be alert and pink. Blood pressure is 110/70 mm Hg right arm recumbent, pulse is 96/min regular, and respiratory rate is 17/min. Which of the following is the preferred initial diagnostic test?

A. Electroencephalogram
B. Ambulatory cardiac monitoring
C. CT imaging of the brain
D. Carotid ultrasound study
E. Serum creatine kinase and troponin levels

PUL, CV

P 032   A 54-year-old man with a 40 pack-year history of cigarette smoking has a chronic productive cough and dyspnea. In the past 2 weeks, he has swelling of both lower legs and abdominal distention. Examination shows elevated jugular venous pressure, an enlarged, smooth, tender liver, and 2+ bilateral lower leg edema. Which of the following is the most likely diagnosis?

A. Left heart failure
B. Constrictive pericarditis
C. Right heart failure
D. Superior vena cava syndrome
E. High cardiac output heart failure

PSY/LE, ENDO

P 033   Lithium therapy is initiated in a 27-year-old woman who has bipolar disorder. Which of the following is recommended in the management of the patient?

A. Obtain serum electrolyte values every 3 to 4 months
B. Obtain thyroid function values every 3 to 4 months
C. Advise patient to take oral potassium supplement
D. Obtain lipid profile values every 3 to 4 months
E. Advise patient to take medication on an empty stomach

The Performance section is like a PANCE or PANRE. There is only *one* best answer.

P 034   A 76-year-old woman has had three episodes of blurred vision in her right eye in the past week. Each episode lasts approximately 2 minutes and is described as "a curtain coming down over my eye." There are no associated symptoms. Vital signs are normal. When the patient is asymptomatic, the neurologic examination is normal. Which of the following is the most likely diagnosis?

    A. Multiple sclerosis
    B. Vertebrobasilar artery insufficiency
    C. Amaurosis fugax
    D. Petit mal seizures
    E. Transient 3rd-degree atrioventricular block

P 035   A 6-year-old boy has impulsivity, distractiveness, and inattentiveness that cause behavioral problems in school. He now has involuntary, repetitive momentary coughs and facial grimacing and is beginning to repeat sentences spoken by the teacher. Which of the following is the most likely diagnosis?

    A. Oppositional defiant behavior syndrome
    B. Tourette's syndrome
    C. Fetal alcohol syndrome
    D. Fragile X syndrome
    E. Hyperactive autism

P 036   A 2-year-old girl has a 3-week history of recurrent hives, flushing, and diarrhea approximately 30 minutes after eating. The mother is instructed to keep a diary of the child's food intake. Which of the following is least likely to precipitate the symptoms?

    A. Wheat
    B. Eggs
    C. Soy
    D. Milk
    E. Oats

P 037   Immediately after witnessing a serious automobile accident, a 17-year-old girl has a cold sweat and nausea followed by fainting. Pulse is 32/min regular, and blood pressure is 70/40 mm Hg recumbent. Which of the following is the pathophysiologic mechanism causing the faint?

    A. Orthostatic hypotension
    B. Heightened vagal tone
    C. Increased ventricular preload
    D. Systemic hypoxemia
    E. Increased prostaglandin secretion

PUL, CV

P 038 A 61-year-old woman with a 40 pack-year history of cigarette smoking has chronic dyspnea and productive cough. In the past 3 weeks, she has had worsening breathlessness, swelling of both lower legs, and abdominal distention. Examination shows central cyanosis, elevated jugular venous pressure, an enlarged, tender, smooth liver, and 2+ bilateral ankle edema. Which of the following is the primary pathophysiologic abnormality?

A. Decreased right ventricular preload
B. Increased cardiac output
C. Respiratory alkalosis
D. Pulmonary hypertension
E. Increased mean left atrial pressure

GI/N

P 039 A newborn infant fails to pass meconium followed by progressive abdominal distention and vomiting. Which of the following is the preferred test in the diagnosis of Hirschsprung's disease?

A. Abdominal ultrasonography
B. Inferior mesenteric arteriography
C. Spiral CT scan of the abdomen
D. Anorectal manometry
E. Small bowel contrast study via nasogastric tube

EENT, MS

P 040 A 34-year-old woman has been taking prednisone for 3 years as therapy for rheumatoid arthritis. She now notes the slow onset of painless, persistently blurred vision in both eyes. Which of the following is the most likely cause of the ocular symptoms?

A. Vertebrobasilar artery insufficiency
B. Open-angle glaucoma
C. Uveitis
D. Cataracts
E. Myasthenia gravis

PSY/LE, REPRO

P 041 Lithium therapy is initiated in a 21-year-old woman for the treatment of bipolar disorder. Which of the following instructions should be given to the patient?

A. Advise patient to ingest a high-carbohydrate, low-fat diet
B. Advise patient to avoid pregnancy while taking lithium
C. Advise patient to avoid nonsteroidal anti-inflammatory medicines
D. Advise patient of risk of nasal polyps
E. Advise patient to take daily oral potassium supplement

The Performance section is like a PANCE or PANRE. There is only *one* best answer.

P 042   A 67-year-old woman has a 1-month history of a 12-pound weight loss, anorexia, progressive weakness, and new skin lesions. Examination shows a wasted woman with bilateral axillary patches of thickened dark brown skin having prominent skin lines. Which of the following is the most likely diagnosis?

A. Adenocarcinoma of the stomach
B. Addison's disease
C. Diabetes insipidus
D. Adenocarcinoma of the ovary
E. Adenocarcinoma of the pancreas

P 043   A 6-year-old child has cholera with severe diarrhea. Which of the following laboratory abnormalities is the most likely to occur?

A. Hyperglycemia
B. Hypokalemia
C. Hypernatremia
D. Metabolic alkalosis
E. Hypertriglyceridemia

P 044   A 16-year-old girl has a 3-day history of sore throat, fever, and malaise. Examination shows tonsillar inflammation with white exudates and diffuse adenopathy. A diagnosis of infectious mononucleosis is made. Which of the following is the most likely complication?

A. Aseptic meningitis
B. Endocarditis
C. Nephrotic syndrome
D. Megaloblastic anemia
E. Uveitis

P 045   An 18-year-old woman is prescribed contact lens in place of eyeglasses. She should be advised that the most frequent complication is which of the following?

A. Optic neuritis
B. Adenovirus conjunctivitis
C. Corneal ulceration
D. Herpes simplex keratitis
E. Closed-angle glaucoma

MS, GI/N

P 046   A 40-year-old woman has a 2-year history of Raynaud's phenomenon. She now has heartburn and dysphagia to both solids and liquids. Vital signs are normal. Examination shows thickening of the skin of the fingers with loss of creases. Which of the following is the most likely diagnosis?

A. Sjögren's syndrome
B. Achalasia
C. Squamous cell carcinoma of the esophagus
D. Carcinoma of the lung with paraneoplastic syndrome
E. Scleroderma

ID, NEURO

P 047   An 18-year-old man living in Connecticut has the sudden onset of bilateral Bell's palsy. Two months earlier, he had a flulike illness with fever, chills, and myalgia. At that time, he had noted a slightly raised, red rash on his thigh. Which of the following tests is the preferred initial diagnostic test?

A. ELISA test
B. Biopsy of skin in area of rash, with culture
C. Assay of serum immunoglobulin A
D. Dark field microscopic examination of blood
E. Blood culture in anaerobic medium

HEME

P 048   A 55-year-old man with aggressive stage IV non-Hodgkin's lymphoma is to begin chemotherapy. Initiation of which of the following prophylactic interventions is indicated?

A. Oral acetazolamide
B. Oral ammonium chloride
C. Oral allopurinol
D. Intravenous hypotonic glucose
E. Intravenous lidocaine

PUL, GI/N

P 049   A 43-year-old African American woman has a 2-week history of malaise and dry cough. Examination shows bilateral enlargement of the parotid glands and enlargement of the submandibular and axillary lymph nodes. Chest radiograph shows bilateral hilar enlargement. Which of the following is an expected serum abnormality?

A. Elevated immunoglobulin A
B. Elevated angiotensin-converting enzyme
C. Reduced calcium
D. Elevated gastrin
E. Reduced norepinephrine

The Performance section is like a PANCE or PANRE. There is only *one* best answer.

EENT

P 050   An 18-year-old woman is to start wearing contact lens for correction of a refractive error. Which of the following is the proper advice to be given to the patient?

A. Hard lens are better tolerated than soft lens
B. Sterilization is best accomplished through antibiotic solutions
C. Avoid extended wear of the soft lens
D. At 3-month intervals, do not wear contact lens for 2 weeks
E. Disposable lens do not cause corneal ulceration

ENDO, EENT, NEURO

P 051   A 66-year-old man awakens and suddenly is aware of double vision when both eyes are open. Vital signs are normal. Examination shows an alert, cooperative man. There is ptosis of the left eyelid with lateral deviation of the eye. The pupil size of the affected eye is normal. Which of the following is the most likely underlying disorder?

A. Cerebral aneurysm
B. Diabetes mellitus
C. Wernicke's encephalopathy
D. Cataract
E. Hypothyroidism

CV

P 052   A 78-year-old man with chronic hypertension has acute onset of severe, tearing upper posterior chest pain lasting 40 minutes. Blood pressure is 170/100 mm Hg right arm recumbent and 130/80 mm Hg left arm recumbent. Pulse is 110/min regular, and respiratory rate is 30/min. Electrocardiography shows left ventricular hypertrophy. Which of the following is the most likely diagnosis?

A. Acute myocardial infarction
B. Acute occlusion of the innominate artery
C. Superior vena cava syndrome
D. Acute dissection of the thoracic aorta
E. Subclavian steal syndrome

NEURO, EENT

P 053   A 71-year-old woman has had three episodes of blurred vision in her left eye in the past week. Each episode lasts 1 to 2 minutes followed by spontaneous return of normal vision. There are no associated symptoms. Vital signs are normal. Neurologic examination is normal. Which of the following is the preferred initial intervention?

A. Initiate propranolol therapy
B. Obtain serum antiphospholipid antibody level
C. Perform duplex carotid artery ultrasound
D. Obtain erythrocyte sedimentation rate value
E. Trial of sumatriptan when episode recurs

MS

P 054   A 37-year-old woman has been taking prednisone for 4 years as therapy for rheumatoid arthritis. A bone density study now shows significant osteopenia. In addition to oral calcium supplementation, which of the following is recommended?

A. Initiate therapy with a thiazide diuretic
B. Initiate therapy with fluoride
C. Initiate therapy with a bisphosphonate
D. Obtain 24-hour urinary calcium level
E. Initiate high-protein diet

CV, GU

P 055   A 78-year-old man has chronic systolic heart failure for which he takes metoprolol, furosemide, digoxin, and lisinopril. His electrocardiogram now shows frequent ventricular ectopic beats due to digoxin toxicity. Which of the following is the most likely precipitating factor causing the toxicity?

A. Metabolic acidosis
B. Hypokalemia
C. Hypermagnesemia
D. Hyponatremia
E. Hyperosmolality

GU, CV

P 056   A 66-year-old man has a 3-hour history of increasing weakness. He takes lisinopril for hypertension and, for the past 2 days, has used artificial salt on his food. In the emergency department, serum potassium is 6.8 mEq/L, serum creatinine is 1.3 mg/dL, and blood urea nitrogen is 22 mg/dL. The electrocardiogram shows peaked T waves. Which of the following is the preferred initial therapy?

A. Emergent hemodialysis
B. Administration of intravenous calcium
C. Administration of intravenous glucose and insulin
D. Sodium polystyrene sulfonate enema
E. Administration of intravenous epinephrine

GI/N, DERM

P 057   A 52-year-old man has a 4-month history of progressive exertional breathlessness without associated cough or angina pectoris. He now has dysphagia to both solids and liquids. Blood pressure is 140/90 mm Hg sitting; pulse, 96/min regular; and respiratory rate, 28/min. Examination shows thickening of the skin of the face and hands. Telangiectasia is noted on the face. Chest radiograph shows diffuse pulmonary fibrosis. Which of the following is the most likely diagnosis?

A. Sarcoidosis
B. Chronic pulmonary embolic disease
C. Asbestosis
D. Scleroderma
E. Silo-filler's disease

The Performance section is like a PANCE or PANRE. There is only *one* best answer.

P 058   A 42-year-old man has exertional dyspnea and dry cough due to sarcoidosis. Chest radiograph shows diffuse interstitial fibrosis. Which of the following systemic arterial blood gas values would be expected?

A. pH 7.48, Pao_2 66 mm Hg, $Paco_2$ 28 mm Hg
B. pH 7.40, Pao_2 100 mm Hg, $Paco_2$ 40 mm Hg
C. pH 7.48, Pao_2 100 mm Hg, $Paco_2$ 48 mm Hg
D. pH 7.34, Pao_2 66 mm Hg, $Paco_2$ 28 mm Hg
E. pH 7.34, Pao_2 100 mm Hg, $Paco_2$ 28 mm Hg

P 059   A 66-year-old man has exertional dyspnea and dry cough due to idiopathic diffuse pulmonary fibrosis. Which of the following is an expected abnormality on pulmonary function testing?

A. Decreased forced expiratory volume 1 second/forced vital capacity ratio (FEV1/FVC)
B. Increased residual volume
C. Decreased carbon monoxide diffusing capacity
D. Decreased forced expiratory flow rate
E. Increased vital capacity

P 060   Presence of which of the following would be expected on examination of a peripheral blood smear in a patient who has pernicious anemia?

A. Microcytosis
B. Hypersegmented neutrophils
C. Target red blood cells
D. Blast cells
E. Increased number of platelets

P 061   After having had diffuse joint aching for 4 days, a 6-year-old girl now has diffuse abdominal pain and a rash on her legs. Vital signs are normal. Abdominal examination shows diffuse tenderness with normal bowel sounds. Palpable purpura is noted on both legs. Urinalysis shows 10 to 15 RBCs per high-power field and red blood cell casts. Which of the following is the most likely diagnosis?

A. Systemic lupus erythematosus
B. Serum sickness
C. Acute rheumatic fever
D. Endocarditis
E. Henoch-Schönlein purpura

NEURO, HEME

P 062 A 73-year-old woman has paresthesia and ataxia. Peripheral blood examination shows macrocytosis. The serum vitamin B_{12} level is borderline abnormal. Which of the following serum values should be obtained in order to confirm a diagnosis of pernicious anemia?

A. C-reactive protein
B. 5-Hydroxytryptamine
C. Methylmalonic acid
D. Anti-mitochondrial antibodies
E. Antiphospholipid antibody

CV

P 063 A 31-year-old woman with Marfan syndrome has the sudden onset of severe, ripping anterior chest pain followed by collapse. Blood pressure is 70/40 mm Hg both arms recumbent; pulse, 140/min regular; and respiratory rate, 38/min. The patient is cold and pale. Jugular venous pressure is elevated. Which of the following is the preferred initial diagnostic test?

A. Aortography
B. Positron emission tomography
C. Transesophageal echocardiography
D. Thoracentesis
E. Magnetic resonance venography

PUL, ID

P 064 A 66-year-old man has an acute exacerbation of chronic bronchitis for which tetracycline is prescribed. Which of the following is proper counseling to be given to the patient?

A. Take medication with milk
B. Do not take medication with antacids
C. Medication may cause ecchymosis
D. Medication may cause rectal bleeding
E. Avoid intake of tea while taking medication

CV

P 065 A 69-year-old woman has the sudden onset of tearing anterior chest pain lasting 1 hour. Blood pressure is 180/110 mm Hg both arms recumbent; pulse, 120/min regular; and respiratory rate, 24/min. Jugular venous pressure is normal. Cardiac examination shows an apical lift and new 2/6 left sternal border diastolic murmur. In addition to intravenous nitroprusside, which of the following medicines should be administered intravenously?

A. Hydralazine
B. Metoprolol
C. Diazoxide
D. Low molecular weight heparin
E. Tirofiban

The Performance section is like a PANCE or PANRE. There is only *one* best answer.

P 066   Presence of which of the following differentiates pernicious anemia from folic acid deficiency anemia?

    A. Hypersegmented neutrophils
    B. Abnormal position sense
    C. Megaloblastic bone marrow
    D. Hypertension
    E. Antiphospholipid antibodies

GI/N

P 067   Which of the following is proper counseling for a patient who has Crohn's disease with extensive involvement of the small bowel?

    A. Avoid acetaminophen intake
    B. Avoid cephalosporin intake
    C. Receive monthly vitamin B_{12} injections
    D. Receive annual pneumococcal vaccine
    E. Avoid the sun's direct rays as much as possible

GI/N, HEME

P 068   Which of the following is the mechanism by which gastrectomy causes megaloblastic anemia?

    A. Dumping syndrome
    B. Alkalinity in the small bowel
    C. Lack of intrinsic factor production
    D. Reduced parasympathomimetic intestinal tone
    E. Lack of gastrin production

GI/N, PUL, ENDO

P 069   A 52-year-old man has a 3-week history of pain in both hands and both ankles. There is no associated swelling or increased temperature. Hypertrophic osteoarthropathy is diagnosed. Which of the following is the most likely underlying condition?

    A. Hyperthyroidism
    B. Adenocarcinoma of the lung
    C. Angiodysplasia of the colon
    D. Acromegaly
    E. Hyperparathyroidism

CV

P 070   Which of the following is the pathophysiologic basis for the increased pulse pressure associated with aging?

    A. Decreased arterial compliance
    B. Increased stroke volume
    C. Decreased ventricular contractility
    D. Decreased preload
    E. Decreased cardiac output

CV

P 071 A 76-year-old asymptomatic man has had four blood pressure measurements over a 2-week period. The blood pressure range is 158–170/70–78 mm Hg. He takes no medication. Which of the following is the preferred management?

A. Initiate methyldopa therapy
B. No medicinal therapy
C. Initiate thiazide therapy
D. Initiate fish oil supplementation
E. Initiate beta-adrenergic blocker therapy

HEME, NEURO

P 072 A 77-year-old woman has a 2-month history of bilateral leg paresthesias. Blood examination shows anemia, macrocytosis, and hypersegmented neutrophils. Which of the following neurologic signs would be expected to be abnormal in this patient?

A. Pupillary response to light
B. Extraocular muscle movement
C. Romberg test
D. Stereognosis
E. Cranial nerve VII function

ENDO, CV

P 073 A 69-year-old woman has a 1-month history of generalized weakness and a 6-pound weight loss. She now presents in the emergency department with new-onset atrial fibrillation. Which of the following is the most likely diagnosis?

A. Adrenal insufficiency
B. Hypercortisolism
C. Hyperthyroidism
D. Hyperparathyroidism
E. Zollinger-Ellison syndrome

NEURO, ENDO, CV

P 074 A 67-year-old man with type 1 diabetes mellitus has symptomatic orthostatic hypotension. His medications include insulin, aspirin, and simvastatin. Which of the following is the most likely pathophysiologic mechanism causing the orthostatic hypotension?

A. Hypovolemia
B. Autonomic insufficiency
C. Decreased number of serotonin receptors
D. Decreased cardiac output
E. Metabolic acidosis

The Performance section is like a PANCE or PANRE. There is only *one* best answer.

NEURO, CV

P 075   A 54-year-old woman has lightheadedness and graying of vision upon arising from bed. Blood pressure is 114/72 mm Hg with pulse 78/min in the sitting position. Upon arising, blood pressure is 92/58 mm Hg with pulse 106/min. Which of the following is the most likely cause?

A. Autonomic insufficiency
B. Decreased left ventricular compliance
C. Decreased serum norepinephrine level
D. Hypovolemia
E. Hypo-osmolar serum

NEURO, ENDO, CV

P 076   A 49-year-old man faints when arising from bed. Blood pressure is 118/74 mm Hg with pulse 84/min in the sitting position. Upon arising, blood pressure is 78/48 mm Hg with pulse of 85/min. Which of the following is the most likely underlying diagnosis?

A. Chronic adrenal insufficiency
B. Excessive diuresis
C. Diabetes mellitus
D. Nonfunctioning pituitary adenoma
E. Bleeding gastric ulcer

CV

P 077   Which of the following is the pathophysiologic mechanism that causes an increased plasma Nt-BNP level in patients who have heart failure?

A. Decreased glomerular filtration rate
B. Decreased systemic vascular resistance
C. Ventricular wall stretching
D. Stimulation of baroreceptors
E. Decreased plasma renin activity

PUL, CV

P 078   A 65-year-old man who has a long history of cigarette smoking and a 7-year history of hypertension now has worsening dyspnea over 1 week. Which of the following is the best indicator to exclude heart failure?

A. Normal jugular venous pressure
B. Absence of gallop sound
C. Normal urine osmolality
D. Normal plasma Nt-BNP
E. Normal serum C-reactive protein

ENDO, PUL

P 079   Which of the following is the most likely source of ectopic adrenocorticotropic hormone (ACTH)?

A. Villous adenoma of the colon
B. Medullary carcinoma of the thyroid
C. Parathyroid adenoma
D. Gastrinoma
E. Small cell carcinoma of the lung

PUL, ID

P 080   A 32-year-old man with cystic fibrosis has an acute, extensive pneumonia.
Which of the following is the most likely infecting organism?

A. *Escherichia coli*
B. Fusiform bacilli
C. Respiratory syncytial virus
D. *Chlamydia trachomatis*
E. *Pseudomonas aeruginosa*

CV, HEME

P 081   Unfractionated heparin therapy is initiated in a 67-year-old woman for
treatment of deep venous thrombosis. Which of the following should be
performed after 5 days of anticoagulation?

A. Prothrombin time
B. Platelet count
C. White blood cell count
D. Serum sodium level
E. Arterial blood gas determination

PUL

P 082   Which of the following is a pulmonary complication of cystic fibrosis?

A. Diffuse interstitial fibrosis
B. Granulomatous infiltration
C. Eisenmenger's syndrome
D. Bronchiectasis
E. Bullae formation

PSY/LE, CV

P 083   Lithium therapy is initiated in a 36-year-old man for treatment of bipolar
disorder. He should be counseled that which of the following medicines
will increase lithium blood levels?

A. Aspirin
B. Acetaminophen
C. Meclizine
D. Verapamil
E. Hydrochlorothiazide

The Performance section is like a PANCE or PANRE. There is only *one* best answer.

P 084   Lithium therapy is to be initiated in a 32-year-old woman for treatment of bipolar disorder. Which of the following is proper counseling for the patient?

A. Reduce ingestion of potassium-containing foods
B. Avoid pregnancy
C. Check complete blood count every 4 months
D. Wear gloves when holding frozen foods
E. Check blood pressure every 2 months

P 085   Presence of which of the following differentiates the visual symptoms of unilateral carotid artery stenosis from migraine?

A. Unilateral character of visual symptoms
B. Symptoms last more than 2 hours
C. Presence of "stars" and "sparks" in visual fields
D. Association with photophobia
E. Association with nausea and vomiting

P 086   A 44-year-old woman has painless, persistent blurred vision in both eyes. Cataracts are diagnosed. Intake of which of the following medicines is most likely to be associated with premature cataract formation?

A. Prednisone
B. Lithium
C. Diazepam
D. Radioactive iodine
E. Estrogen/progesterone combination

P 087   A 56-year-old woman develops acanthosis nigricans in the axillary areas. Which of the following is the most likely associated condition?

A. Chronic adrenal insufficiency
B. Hyperthyroidism
C. Crohn's disease
D. *H. pylori*–related peptic ulcer
E. Gastric adenocarcinoma

P 088   Which of the following is a pathophysiologic abnormality associated with acanthosis nigricans?

A. Deficiency of bile salts
B. Tissue insulin resistance
C. Ectopic adrenocorticotropic hormone production
D. Defective glycogenolysis
E. Increased somatostatin secretion

DERM, ID

P 089 Which of the following is the typical skin rash associated with Lyme disease?

   A. Erythema multiforme
   B. Erythema migrans
   C. Erysipelas
   D. Dermatitis herpetiformis
   E. Erythema marginatum

HEME, GU

P 090 A 14-year-old girl has acute leukemia for which chemotherapy is to be initiated. Which of the following is the appropriate prophylactic medication to be given to the patient in order to prevent tumor lysis syndrome?

   A. Oral theophylline
   B. Inhaled albuterol
   C. Intravenous potassium
   D. Oral allopurinol
   E. Intramuscular glucagons

PUL

P 091 Presence of which of the following differentiates idiopathic pulmonary fibrosis from chronic bronchitis?

   A. Decreased systemic arterial Pa_{O_2}
   B. Respiratory acidosis
   C. Increased tidal volume
   D. Normal FEV_1/FVC ratio
   E. Normal carbon monoxide diffusing capacity

HEME, GU

P 092 A 22-year-old man with bulky non-Hodgkin's lymphoma is to start chemotherapy. Prevention of which of the following is the reason to give prophylactic allopurinol to the patient?

   A. Dilated cardiomyopathy
   B. Hyperuricemic nephropathy
   C. Seizures
   D. Increased anion gap metabolic acidosis
   E. Mesenteric ischemia

CV

P 093 A 77-year-old man is diagnosed with chronic systolic heart failure. He is in normal sinus rhythm. In addition to furosemide and lisinopril, which of the following medicines should be taken by the patient?

   A. Warfarin
   B. Verapamil
   C. Metoprolol
   D. Doxazosin
   E. Levodopa

The Performance section is like a PANCE or PANRE. There is only *one* best answer.

P 094 Which of the following is the primary pharmacologic effect of nitroglycerin?

A. Increase ventricular contractility
B. Decrease ventricular preload
C. Slow atrioventricular conduction
D. Increase afterload
E. Decrease slope 4 of sinoatrial action potential

CV, GU

P 095 A 77-year-old hospitalized patient is found to have a prolonged QT interval on electrocardiography. Which of the following is the most likely cause of the QT prolongation?

A. Hypomagnesemia
B. Hyponatremia
C. Nitrate therapy
D. Angiotensin-converting enzyme inhibitor therapy
E. Hypercalcemia

NEURO

P 096 Presence of which of the following differentiates central cranial nerve VII palsy from peripheral cranial nerve VII palsy?

A. Ability to wrinkle forehead on affected side
B. Ability to close eye on affected side
C. Ataxia
D. Ability to taste on affected side
E. Nystagmus

CV, NEURO

P 097 A 12-year-old girl suddenly faints while playing soccer. Upon regaining consciousness, she is alert, pink, and asymptomatic. Blood pressure is 110/70 mm Hg; pulse, 80/min regular; and respirations, 14/min. Cardiac, lung, and neurologic examination is normal. Which of the following is the most likely cause of the syncope?

A. Vasovagal faint
B. 3rd-degree atrioventricular block
C. Long QT interval syndrome
D. Hypoglycemia
E. Hypertrophic obstructive cardiomyopathy

CV, PUL

P 098 A 47-year-old asthmatic woman suddenly has palpitations. Blood pressure is 110/70 mm Hg; pulse, 190/min regular; and respirations, 20/min. Lung examination is normal. No murmur or gallop is heard. Electrocardiography shows paroxysmal supraventricular tachycardia. Which of the following is the preferred initial therapy?

A. Adenosine
B. Metoprolol
C. Digoxin
D. Verapamil
E. Ibutilide

GU

P 099 A 34-year-old man has known polycystic kidney disease. Which of the following is the most likely complication?

A. Salt-losing nephropathy
B. Inappropriate ADH syndrome
C. Gout
D. Metabolic alkalosis
E. Hypertension

GU

P 100 A 14-year-old girl has a 3-day history of ankle and periorbital facial swelling in addition to dark urine. Which of the following urinary laboratory abnormalities is most suggestive of the diagnosis of acute glomerulonephritis?

A. White blood cell casts
B. Polyuria with fixed urine specific gravity
C. Oxalate crystals in urine
D. Red blood cell casts
E. Broad waxy casts in urine

ENDO, HEME

P 101 A 57-year-old woman has had treated hypothyroidism for 4 years. Which of the following conditions is most likely to arise in this patient?

A. Interstitial nephritis
B. Pernicious anemia
C. Inappropriate ADH syndrome
D. Polycythemia rubra vera
E. Acute lymphoblastic leukemia

P 102   A patient who has which of the following disorders will have gastric achlorhydria?

    A. *Helicobacter pylori* gastric ulcer
    B. Gastric lymphoma
    C. Pernicious anemia
    D. Achalasia of esophagus
    E. Gastroparesis

P 103   A patient who suffers from chronic alcohol abuse is most likely to show which of the following laboratory values?

    A. Macrocytosis
    B. Hypersegmented neutrophils
    C. Red blood cell casts in urine
    D. Elevated serum thyrotropin level
    E. Elevated plasma albumin level

P 104   Presence of which of the following differentiates primary from secondary adrenal insufficiency?

    A. Elevated plasma adrenocorticotropin level
    B. Hypokalemia
    C. Hypernatremia
    D. Weight loss
    E. Low plasma renin level

P 105   A 66-year-old man has a 2-month history of anorexia, 7-pound weight loss, nausea, and generalized weakness. He now has dizziness upon arising from bed. In the sitting position, blood pressure is 90/70 mm Hg with pulse rate 76/min. Upon standing, blood pressure is 70/52 mm Hg with pulse rate 98/min. Which of the following is the most likely diagnosis?

    A. Primary hyperaldosteronism
    B. Adrenal insufficiency
    C. Carcinoid syndrome
    D. Pheochromocytoma
    E. Celiac disease

P 106   A 34-year-old woman has the sudden onset of severe, constant anterior chest pain that is worsened by lying recumbent and eased by sitting and leaning forward. A malar rash is present. Which of the following laboratory values would be expected in this patient?

    A. Platelet count 450,000/microL
    B. Presence of serum anti–acetylcholine receptor antibodies
    C. White blood cell count 2,000/microL
    D. Presence of serum antiperoxidase antibodies
    E. White blood cell casts in urine

CV, DERM, HEME

P 107   A patient with systemic lupus erythematosus has a rash in the malar area and on the extremities. Which of the following is the appropriate counseling to be given to the patient?

A. Apply coal tar and salicylate gel topically on weekly basis
B. Avoid direct sunlight
C. Avoid sunscreen preparations
D. Take weekly cornstarch bath
E. Avoid hydrocortisone topical medications

MS, CV

P 108   A 27-year-old woman has a 2-week history of diffuse joint aching. She now has the sudden onset of severe, persistent anterior chest pain. A pericardial friction rub is heard. Which of the following is the preferred diagnostic test in this patient?

A. Serum C-reactive protein level
B. 24-hour urinary 5-hydroxytryptamine excretion
C. Presence of factor V Leiden mutation
D. 24-hour urinary calcium excretion
E. Serum antinuclear antibody titer

EENT

P 109   A 37-year-old man has a recurrence of seasonal hay fever symptoms. Which of the following is the preferred treatment?

A. Intranasal phenylephrine
B. Intranasal beclomethasone
C. Oral chlorpheniramine
D. Oral cromolyn
E. Intranasal ipratropium

CV

P 110   An 8-year-old boy has a bicuspid aortic valve. Which of the following associated conditions is the most likely to be present?

A. Patent ductus arteriosus
B. Coarctation of the aorta
C. Secundum atrial septal defect
D. Ebstein's anomaly
E. Polycystic kidney disease

CV, ID

P 111   A 6-year-old asymptomatic boy has a systolic ejection murmur and ejection click best heard near the apex. A bicuspid aortic valve is diagnosed. Which of the following is the most appropriate recommendation?

A. Avoid contact sports
B. Limit dietary calcium intake to 300 mg/day
C. Take daily penicillin G until age 12 years
D. No need for endocarditis prophylaxis
E. Have annual echocardiographic study

The Performance section is like a PANCE or PANRE. There is only *one* best answer.

CV

P 112   A 40-year-old woman has recurrent chest pain that awakens her in the early morning hours. Variant angina pectoris is diagnosed. Which of the following is the preferred therapy?

    A. Streptokinase
    B. Aspirin
    C. Metoprolol
    D. Simvastatin
    E. Verapamil

CV, ENDO

P 113   A 72-year-old man with hyperlipidemia has a 2-week history of exertional dyspnea without associated cough, chest discomfort, palpitations, or peripheral edema. Pulmonary function tests and chest radiography are normal. Which of the following is the preferred diagnostic test?

    A. Outpatient cardiac monitoring
    B. Thallium stress cardiac testing
    C. Bronchoscopy
    D. MRI scan of the chest
    E. Serum brain natriuretic peptide level

HEME, CV

P 114   A 66-year-old woman has a 2-week history of increasing facial swelling and edema of both arms. Superior vena cava syndrome is diagnosed. Which of the following is the most likely underlying condition?

    A. Non-Hodgkin's lymphoma
    B. Squamous cell carcinoma of the lung
    C. Thymoma
    D. Adenocarcinoma of the pharynx
    E. Medullary carcinoma of the thyroid

NEURO

P 115   Ability to perform which of the following is a test of cranial nerve V function?

    A. Close eyes tightly
    B. Raise shoulders against resistance
    C. Smile
    D. Move chin from side to side
    E. Move eyes to lateral gaze

MS, GI/N

P 116   A 71-year-old man has elevation of serum alkaline phosphatase but normal serum gamma-glutamyl transpeptidase (GGTP) and normal serum calcium. Which of the following is the most likely diagnosis?

    A. Pancreatic carcinoma
    B. Paget's disease of bone
    C. Chronic active hepatitis
    D. Hyperparathyroidism
    E. Metastatic tumor in the liver

CV

P 117   A 25-year-old asymptomatic man has a congenital bicuspid aortic valve. Which of the following is the most appropriate counseling for this patient?

A. Endocarditis prophylaxis is indicated
B. Significant aortic stenosis is likely to occur in adulthood
C. There is an 80% likelihood of his children having bicuspid aortic valve
D. Take daily oral penicillin G, 125 mg
E. Undergo genetic typing

CV, PUL

P 118   A patient with chronic obstructive lung disease now has atrial fibrillation. Which of the following is the preferred medicine to control the ventricular rate?

A. Esmolol
B. Metoprolol
C. Quinidine
D. Verapamil
E. Adenosine

CV

P 119   A patient who has diffuse atherosclerotic vascular disease and claudication of the legs now has atrial fibrillation. Which of the following is the preferred medicine to control the ventricular rate?

A. Diltiazem
B. Metoprolol
C. Nifedipine
D. Sotalol
E. Propafenone

MS

P 120   A 72-year-old man is incidentally found on radiography of the hip to have Paget's disease of bone. Which of the following is the expected laboratory value?

A. Hypercalcemia
B. Elevated urinary hydroxyproline
C. Elevated serum gamma-glutamyl transpeptidase
D. Normal serum alkaline phosphatase
E. Elevated serum aminotransferase

CV

P 121   A 73-year-old man has chronic nonvalvular atrial fibrillation for which he takes digoxin and warfarin. His ventricular rate is poorly controlled, with ventricular rates always greater than 100/min. Which of the following is the most likely complication?

A. Dilated cardiomyopathy
B. 3rd-degree atrioventricular block
C. Superior vena cava syndrome
D. Left atrial thrombus formation
E. Pulmonary infarction

The Performance section is like a PANCE or PANRE. There is only *one* best answer.

P 122   A 60-year-old man with cirrhosis and portal hypertension has an acute hemorrhage from ruptured esophageal varices. Which of the following is the preferred medicine to prevent recurrent bleeding?

A. Octreotide
B. Esomeprazole
C. Nadolol
D. Spironolactone
E. Nifedipine

P 123   A 56-year-old man has cirrhosis due to chronic alcohol abuse. Serial measurement of which of the following serum levels would be most predictive of development of hepatocellular carcinoma?

A. Gamma-glutamyl transpeptidase
B. C-reactive protein
C. CA 125
D. Alpha-fetoprotein
E. Alkaline phosphatase

P 124   A 44-year-old woman is diagnosed with variant angina. Which of the following is the expected finding on electrocardiography performed while the patient is having anginal discomfort?

A. ST segment depression
B. ST segment elevation
C. Isoelectric ST segments with T wave inversion
D. Widening of the QRS segments
E. Prolongation of the QT interval

P 125   A 32-year-old woman with diabetes mellitus is to begin angiotensin-converting enzyme inhibitor therapy for hypertension. Which of the following is the proper advice for this patient?

A. Do not become pregnant while on therapy
B. Do not take oral contraceptives while on therapy
C. Therapy increases the likelihood of twinning
D. Ensure daily intake of calcium greater than 1,000 mg/day
E. Use salt substitute for flavoring of food

P 126   A 34-year-old man has a rash on his elbows. Presence of which of the following is most suggestive of the diagnosis of psoriasis?

A. Symmetrical arthritis
B. Pitting of nails
C. Maculopapular eruption
D. Clubbing of fingers and toes
E. Raynaud's phenomenon

PSY/LE

P 127   A 24-year-old woman has had three episodes of sudden, intense fear associated with trembling, palpitations, and dyspnea. These have each lasted 10 to 15 minutes. Each occurred a few days before normal menses. Which of the following is the most likely diagnosis?

    A. Dissociative disorder
    B. Panic disorder
    C. Hypoglycemia
    D. Pheochromocytoma
    E. Carcinoid syndrome

CV

P 128   Which of the following is the proper advice to give a patient who is starting clonidine therapy for hypertension?

    A. Take medication with milk or antacid
    B. Do not take aspirin while on therapy
    C. Red meat ingestion lessens efficacy of medication
    D. Medication raises blood sugar
    E. Withdraw medication over 1 week if it is to be discontinued

MS

P 129   Presence of which of the following differentiates psoriatic arthritis from rheumatoid arthritis on radiographic imaging?

    A. Joint swelling
    B. Demineralization
    C. Joint space narrowing
    D. "Sharpened pencil" appearance of fingers
    E. Cartilaginous calcification

CV

P 130   A 72-year-old asymptomatic man with a history of remote myocardial infarction has new-onset hypertension. Left ventricular ejection fraction is 52%. Which of the following is the preferred initial class of medication for hypertensive therapy?

    A. Angiotensin-converting enzyme inhibitor
    B. Alpha-1-adrenergic blocker
    C. Loop diuretic
    D. Nondihydropine calcium channel blocker
    E. Alpha-2a-adrenergic agonist

ENDO, CV

P 131   A 78-year-old woman with type 1 diabetes mellitus develops hypertension. Which of the following is the preferred initial medication in hypertensive therapy?

    A. Verapamil
    B. Doxazosin
    C. Captopril
    D. Losartan
    E. Clonidine

The Performance section is like a PANCE or PANRE. There is only *one* best answer.

DERM

P 132   A 37-year-old woman has ringworm on her trunk. Which of the following is not a recommended therapy?

A. Betamethasone with clotrimazole (Lotrisone)
B. Miconazole (Lotrimin)
C. Econazole (Spectazole)
D. Butenafine (Mentax)
E. Terbinafine (Lamisil)

CV

P 133   A 42-year-old healthy woman has new-onset hypertension. Which of the following is the preferred initial medication in hypertensive therapy?

A. Hydrochlorothiazide
B. Clonidine
C. Doxazosin
D. Verapamil
E. Metoprolol

MS

P 134   A 61-year-old woman with osteoporosis has new-onset hypertension. Which of the following is the preferred initial medication for hypertensive therapy?

A. Captopril
B. Hydralazine
C. Diltiazem
D. Hydrochlorothiazide
E. Propranolol

CV

P 135   A 59-year-old asymptomatic man has new-onset hypertension. His hemoglobin is 14 g/dL; blood urea nitrogen, 12 mg/dL; serum creatinine, 0.9 mg/dL; and serum uric acid, 11 mg/dL. Which of the following classes of medication is contraindicated in this patient?

A. Angiotensin-converting enzyme inhibitor
B. Alpha-1-adrenergic blocker
C. Angiotensin-receptor blocker
D. Thiazide
E. Calcium channel blocker

ENDO

P 136   A 16-year-old boy has type 1 diabetes mellitus. Elevated plasma levels of which of the following would be expected?

A. Insulin
B. Glucagon
C. Epinephrine
D. 5-Hydroxytryptamine
E. Cholecystokinin

DERM

P 137   A 28-year-old woman has two round lesions on her left arm. Examination shows rings of erythema with an advancing scaling border and central clearing. Which of the following is the most appropriate initial diagnostic test?

A. Punch biopsy
B. Serologic test for syphilis
C. Antinuclear antibody titer
D. Potassium hydroxide preparation of scales
E. Culture and sensitivity of lesion scrapings

REPRO, GU

P 138   A 37-year-old man has a 2-month history of erectile dysfunction. Which of the following classes of medicine is the most likely cause of his sexual dysfunction?

A. Selective serotonin receptor inhibitors
B. Angiotensin-converting enzyme inhibitors
C. Dihydropyridine calcium channel blockers
D. H2 receptor blockers
E. Carbonic anhydrase inhibitors

CV, GU

P 139   A 66-year-old man has had erectile dysfunction for 2 years. He now has stable angina pectoris for which he is taking aspirin, metoprolol, and isosorbide dinitrate. He should be advised to avoid which of the following?

A. H2 receptor blockers
B. Proton pump inhibitors
C. Herpes zoster immunization
D. Selenium hair compounds
E. Phosphodiesterase-5 inhibitors

DERM

P 140   A 24-year-old man is diagnosed as having scabies. Which of the following is the proper advice for the patient?

A. Washed clothing should be dried on hangers
B. Place clothes worn before diagnosis in a plastic bag for 10 days
C. Spray recently worn clothes with peroxide
D. Destroy clothing worn for 10 days before diagnosis
E. Wear only white cotton clothing in contact with rash for 1 week

The Performance section is like a PANCE or PANRE. There is only *one* best answer.

ID

P 141   A 16-year-old boy has confirmed infectious mononucleosis. However, he does not get symptomatic relief of his sore throat using saline gargles and ibuprofen. A superimposed infection with which of the following organisms is most likely?

A. Cytomegalovirus
B. HHV-6
C. *Staphylococcus*
D. *Candida*
E. *Streptococcus*

DERM

P 142   A 40-year-old woman has a painful mouth. Examination shows violaceous papules with white streaks. Which of the following is the most likely diagnosis?

A. Psoriasis
B. Rosacea
C. Lichen planus
D. Erythema multiforme
E. Candidiasis

DERM

P 143   A 33-year-old man has an exacerbation of facial rosacea. Which of the following is the recommended topical therapy?

A. Triamcinolone cream
B. Nystatin cream
C. Metronidazole gel
D. Miconazole cream
E. Clotrimazole cream

ID

P 144   An 18-year-old man has just recovered from infectious mononucleosis. Which of the following is proper counseling to be given to the patient?

A. Avoid aspirin intake for 3 months
B. May now participate in contact sports
C. Take daily supplement of glucosamine and chondroitin sulfate
D. Take daily supplement of creatine
E. Saliva may remain contagious for 6 months

DERM

P 145   A 50-year-old man has rosacea. He should be counseled that which of the following will worsen the rash?

A. Milk ingestion
B. Alcohol ingestion
C. Angiotensin-converting enzyme inhibitor therapy
D. Alpha-adrenergic blocker therapy
E. St. John's wort ingestion

PUL, CV

P 146   A 56-year-old man with a 60 pack-year history of cigarette smoking has a 2-week history of worsening cough and dyspnea followed by the onset of abdominal distention and ankle swelling. Examination shows central cyanosis, elevated jugular venous pressure, scattered rhonchi, ascites, and peripheral edema. Which of the following is the most likely diagnosis?

   A. Primary pulmonary hypertension
   B. Cor pulmonale
   C. Legionnaires' disease
   D. Atrial septal defect
   E. Eisenmenger's syndrome

CV, NEURO

P 147   A 77-year-old woman with hypertension and angina pectoris has a syncopal episode. Blood pressure is 84/60 mm Hg; pulse, 48/min irregular; and respiratory rate, 19/min. Electrocardiography shows Mobitz I atrioventricular block. Which of the following is the most likely etiology of the syncopal episode?

   A. Aspirin
   B. Hydrochlorothiazide
   C. Verapamil
   D. Captopril
   E. Isosorbide dinitrate

PUL, CV

P 148   A 49-year-old, massively obese man has progressively worsening somnolence. Examination shows central cyanosis, elevated jugular venous pressure, and peripheral edema. Which of the following would be the expected systemic arterial blood gas values?

   A. Pao_2 90 mm Hg, $Paco_2$ 40 mm Hg
   B. Pao_2 60 mm Hg, $Paco_2$ 60 mm Hg
   C. Pao_2 98 mm Hg, $Paco_2$ 60 mm Hg
   D. Pao_2 90 mm Hg, $Paco_2$ 27 mm Hg
   E. Pao_2 65 mm Hg, $Paco_2$ 30 mm Hg

ID, CV

P 149   For which of the following cardiac conditions is endocarditis prophylaxis not recommended?

   A. Bioprosthetic heart valve
   B. Tetralogy of Fallot
   C. Mitral regurgitation in transplanted heart
   D. Prior history of endocarditis
   E. Mitral valve prolapse

The Performance section is like a PANCE or PANRE. There is only *one* best answer.

P 150   Sertraline (Zoloft) therapy is initiated in a 34-year-old woman for treatment of depression. She should be advised to avoid intake of which of the following?

A. Omega-3 fish oil
B. Aluminum-containing antacids
C. Spinach
D. St. John's wort
E. Ginseng

P 151   A 40-year-old man is transported to the emergency department. He is confused, constantly moves on the examining table, and exhibits spasmodic contractions of the facial and neck muscles. An adverse effect to which of the following is most likely?

A. Diazepam
B. Chlorpheniramine
C. Haloperidol
D. Ibuprofen
E. Nifedipine

P 152   In a patient with newly diagnosed hypertension, a thiazide is preferred therapy over a nonselective beta-adrenergic blocker in a patient who has which of the following?

A. Cholelithiasis
B. Diverticulosis
C. Hyperthyroidism
D. Chronic obstructive lung disease
E. Chronic lymphocytic leukemia

P 153   A 72-year-old woman with known diverticulosis has acute left lower quadrant abdominal pain, fever, and vomiting. Blood pressure is 78/60 mm Hg; pulse, 134/min; and respirations, 28/min. Examination shows a rigid abdomen without bowel sounds. Radiography shows free air under the left hemidiaphragm. Arterial blood gas determination indicates metabolic acidosis. Which of the following is the preferred initial treatment?

A. Infusion of dextrose 5% in water
B. Administration of intravenous norepinephrine
C. Insertion of intra-arterial balloon pump
D. Infusion of 0.9% saline
E. Administration of intravenous isoproterenol

P 154   A 42-year-old woman takes sertraline (Zoloft) for treatment of depression. For the past 2 days she has taken a sympathomimetic medication for treatment of an acute upper respiratory infection. She is now transported to the emergency department because of the acute onset of agitation, delirium, and diarrhea. Blood pressure is 200/120 mm Hg; pulse, 136/min; and respirations, 22/min. Examination shows delirium, dilation of the pupils, flushed skin, and bilateral extensor Babinski signs. Which of the following is the most likely diagnosis?

A. Delirium tremens
B. Serotonin syndrome
C. Disorganized schizophrenia
D. Pheochromocytoma
E. Acute intermittent porphyria

P 155   Which of the following is the primary pathophysiologic abnormality in type 1 diabetes mellitus?

A. Defect in compensatory insulin secretion
B. Defect in small bowel absorption of carbohydrate
C. Defect in urinary excretion of ketones
D. Exaggerated hepatic gluconeogenesis
E. Autoimmune destruction of pancreatic B cells

P 156   Indomethacin therapy is initiated in a 59-year-old man for treatment of hip osteoarthritis. He takes hydrochlorothiazide for hypertension. Which of the following is the most appropriate advice to give the patient?

A. Check serum sodium in 10 to 14 days
B. Check blood pressure in 10 to 14 days
C. Avoid ingestion of milk products while taking indomethacin
D. Avoid salt substitute
E. Take oral magnesium supplements

P 157   A 79-year-old man has systolic hypertension for which he takes hydrochlorothiazide. A recent blood urea nitrogen is 34 mg/dL, and serum creatinine is 1.6 mg/dL. He should be advised to avoid which of the following?

A. Omega-3 fish oil
B. Ginseng
C. Chlorpheniramine
D. Cimetidine
E. Indomethacin

The Performance section is like a PANCE or PANRE. There is only *one* best answer.

P 158   Methotrexate therapy is to be initiated in a 47-year-old woman for treatment of rheumatoid arthritis. The patient should be advised to do which
of the following?

    A. Have liver function tests performed every 4 to 8 weeks
    B. Have thyroid function tests performed every 4 months
    C. Have annual bone marrow examination performed
    D. Eat a high-purine diet
    E. Avoid intake of magnesium-containing antacids

P 159   An 81-year-old woman has dyslipidemia for which she takes simvastatin.
She is now advised to take acetaminophen for treatment of painful
osteoarthritis of her knees and fingers. Which of the following is proper
counseling for the patient?

    A. Do not take acetaminophen in a dosage greater than 2.0 g/day
    B. Acetaminophen must be taken with food
    C. Acetaminophen and simvastatin must be ingested at least 4 hours apart
    D. Stop acetaminophen if warfarin therapy is advised in the future
    E. Reduce simvastatin dosage to half of previously prescribed dosage

P 160   Endocarditis prophylaxis is recommended in a patient who has which of
the following?

    A. Mechanical heart valve in aortic position
    B. Bicuspid aortic valve
    C. Mitral valve prolapse with regurgitation
    D. Rheumatic mitral valve stenosis
    E. Hypertrophic obstructive cardiomyopathy

P 161   A 62-year-old man has had recurrent attacks of acute gout. Which of the
following is the primary factor that determines whether probenecid or
allopurinol should be prescribed for the patient?

    A. Level of 24-hour urinary excretion of uric acid
    B. Level of serum uric acid
    C. Urinary pH after overnight fast
    D. Urinary osmolality after overnight fast
    E. Level of 24-hour urinary protein excretion

P 162   A 59-year-old man who takes verapamil for hypertension has just
recovered from an attack of acute gout. Which of the following is
proper counseling for the patient?

    A. Discontinue the verapamil therapy
    B. Limit water intake to 24 ounces per day
    C. May continue to eat unlimited red meat and shellfish
    D. Strictly limit intake of milk products
    E. Avoid ingestion of alcohol

MS

P 163 During a physical examination, a healthy, asymptomatic 57-year-old man is found to have a serum uric acid of 9.0 mg/dL. He has never had an attack of gout. Which of the following is the most appropriate management?

A. Initiate allopurinol therapy
B. Initiate probenecid therapy
C. Limit intake of milk products
D. Reduce ingestion of red meat and shellfish
E. May drink beer; avoid hard spirits

CV

P 164 A thiazide diuretic is preferable to a beta-adrenergic blocker in a patient with newly diagnosed hypertension who has which of the following?

A. Angina pectoris
B. Leg claudication
C. Atrial fibrillation
D. Hyperuricemia
E. Acquired hemolytic anemia

REPRO, ENDO

P 165 Presence of which of the following differentiates polycystic ovary syndrome from metabolic syndrome?

A. Insulin resistance
B. Elevated serum estrogen
C. Reduced serum testosterone
D. Elevated serum luteinizing hormone
E. Low serum LDL cholesterol

ENDO

P 166 A 56-year-old woman has type 2 diabetes mellitus. Which of the following physical signs best correlates with insulin resistance in this patient?

A. Body mass index
B. Subcutaneous obesity
C. Leptin level in serum
D. Waist-to-hip fat ratio
E. Ankle-brachial index

ENDO

P 167 A 34-year-old man has type 1 diabetes mellitus. Presence of which of the following would be an expected hematologic finding?

A. HLA-DR3 gene
B. Anti-Smith antibody
C. Anti–neutrophilic cytoplasm antibody
D. Elevated serum IgA level
E. Elevated erythrocyte sedimentation rate

The Performance section is like a PANCE or PANRE. There is only *one* best answer.

P 168   On routine screening, an asymptomatic, vigorous man who takes no medication has a hemoglobin of 12 g/dL; blood urea nitrogen, 36 mg/dL; and
serum creatinine, 0.9 mg/dL. Which of the following is the most
appropriate test to be performed?

A. Creatinine clearance
B. Serum myoglobin level
C. 24-hour urinary sodium excretion
D. Stool for occult blood
E. 24-hour dietary protein intake measurement

P 169   A 24-year-old man has acute pancreatitis. He drinks no alcoholic beverages. Elevation in blood level of which of the following is most likely to
be found in the patient?

A. Ferritin
B. Alpha-fetoprotein
C. Triglycerides
D. HDL cholesterol
E. Antiphospholipid antibodies

P 170   A normal serum amylase level is most likely to be noted in a patient who
has which of the following?

A. Mumps
B. Ruptured ectopic pregnancy
C. Renal failure
D. Diverticulosis
E. Pancreatic adenocarcinoma

P 171   A 4-year-old girl has had a common cold for 5 days. She now has fever,
nonproductive cough, and chest soreness. Examination shows a noncyanotic, nontoxic patient with scattered rhonchi in both lung fields. Chest
radiography shows an infiltrate consistent with pneumonia. Which of the
following is the preferred therapy?

A. Doxycycline
B. Azithromycin
C. No antibiotic therapy
D. Penicillin G
E. Cephalexin

GI/N

P 172   An 18-year-old woman has protracted, severe diarrhea from enteritis. Which of the following is the best indicator of hypovolemia?

A. Serum sodium level
B. Urine specific gravity
C. Jugular venous pressure
D. Orthostatic hypotension
E. Resting heart rate

PSY/LE

P 173   A 20-year-old man is diagnosed as having panic disorder manifest by terror and chest pressure. Which of the following is the preferred urgent treatment of an episode?

A. Sublingual nitroglycerin
B. Oral temazepam (Restoril)
C. Oral hydroxyzine (Vistaril)
D. Oral phenobarbital
E. Sublingual lorazepam (Ativan)

GI/N, CV

P 174   A 56-year-old man with a history of alcohol abuse now has acute, severe pancreatitis. Blood pressure is 76/50 mm Hg; pulse, 140/min; and respirations, 30/min. Which of the following is the preferred initial intravenous therapy of the hemodynamic state?

A. Dopamine
B. Normal saline
C. Dextrose 5% in half-normal saline
D. Half-normal saline
E. Dextrose 2½% in half-normal saline

PUL, CV

P 175   One week after trauma to the left calf, a 56-year-old man has dyspnea without pleuritic chest pain or hemoptysis. Which of the following would make the diagnosis of pulmonary embolism very unlikely?

A. Normal oxygen saturation on pulse oximetry
B. Normal respiratory rate
C. Plasma fibrinogen level of 200 mg/mL
D. Normal systemic arterial P_{CO_2} (Pa_{CO_2})
E. Serum D-dimer level of 400 ng/mL

The Performance section is like a PANCE or PANRE. There is only *one* best answer.

ENDO, CV

P 176   Angiotensin-converting enzyme inhibitor (ACEI) therapy is initiated in a
34-year-old woman with type 1 diabetes mellitus for new-onset hypertension. Plasma blood urea nitrogen and serum creatinine levels are
normal. Which of the following is appropriate counseling for the patient?

A. Angioedema typically occurs after 4 months of therapy
B. Take the medication with milk
C. Avoid nonselective nonsteroidal anti-inflammatory medicines
D. ACEI therapy increases risk of developing atrial fibrillation
E. Avoid pregnancy

CV

P 177   A 34-year-old obese man has a 3-day history of left calf soreness. Examination shows no overlying erythema or palpable venous cord in the calf.
Which of the following would signify that a duplex ultrasound study may
be omitted from the diagnostic plan?

A. Negative Homans' sign
B. Lack of calf edema
C. Serum D-dimer level of 400 ng/mL
D. Equal skin temperature in both calves
E. Erythrocyte sedimentation rate of 20 mm/hr

CV

P 178   A 78-year-old man has an acute ST segment elevation anterior wall
myocardial infarction (STEMI). Blood pressure is 130/70 mm Hg; pulse,
90/min; and respirations, 21/min. There is no clinical evidence of heart
failure. In addition to nitroglycerin, aspirin, and alteplase, which of the
following medicines should be given to the patient?

A. Dabigatran (Pradaxa)
B. Tirofiban (Aggrastat)
C. Intravenous nitroprusside
D. Captopril
E. Digoxin

ID, PUL

P 179   A 39-year-old man in excellent health has a 2-day history of fever to 102°F,
productive cough, and chest soreness. Blood pressure is 120/70 mm Hg;
pulse, 112/min; and respirations, 26/min. Examination shows dullness to
percussion and bronchial breath sounds at the right lung base. Which of the
following is the preferred therapy?

A. Admit for intravenous penicillin therapy
B. Outpatient treatment with penicillin G
C. Outpatient treatment with clarithromycin
D. Admit for intravenous macrolide therapy
E. Obtain sputum and blood cultures; await results before starting
antibiotic

ID, PUL

P 180   A 28-year-old man with cystic fibrosis has a 3-day history of fever and productive cough. Chest radiography shows right lower lobe pneumonia with a small cavity containing fluid. Which of the following is the most likely infecting organism?

A. *Klebsiella pneumoniae*
B. Respiratory syncytial virus
C. *Chlamydia pneumoniae*
D. *Streptococcus pneumoniae*
E. *Pseudomonas aeruginosa*

PUL, CV

P 181   A 42-year-old woman who has allergic asthma now has new-onset hypertension. Angiotensin-converting enzyme inhibitor (ACEI) therapy is being considered. Which of the following is the most appropriate clinical statement about ACEI therapy in this patient?

A. Increased likelihood of ACEI causing cough
B. Increased likelihood of exacerbating airflow obstruction
C. Diminished antihypertensive effect due to underlying asthma
D. Tolerated as well as in nonasthmatic
E. Increased likelihood of causing hyperkalemia

ID, PUL

P 182   A localized outbreak of Legionnaires' disease has been identified. Which of the following is the most likely source?

A. Contaminated food in a restaurant
B. Sick cows on a local farm
C. Cough aerosols from sick colleagues
D. Hotel showers
E. Malfunction in community sanitation system

PUL, ID

P 183   A 72-year-old woman with chronic obstructive lung disease has a 4-day history of fever and productive cough. One week earlier, she had returned from a vacation resort where she had used the hot tubs on a daily basis. Examination shows the patient to be acutely ill with decreased breath sounds at the left lung base. Chest radiography demonstrates pneumonia with lung abscess. Which of the following is the most likely diagnosis?

A. Pneumococcal pneumonia
B. Anthrax pneumonia
C. Chlamydial pneumonia
D. Legionnaires' disease
E. Psittacosis

The Performance section is like a PANCE or PANRE. There is only *one* best answer.

CV, GI/N

P 184   A 64-year-old obese man has hypertension and remote history of myocardial infarction. Which of the following foods would not be considered part of a prudent diet?

A. Partially hydrogenated coffee creamer
B. Peanuts
C. Salmon
D. Olive oil
E. Salt substitute

PUL, ID

P 185   A 41-year-old woman has a 2-day history of fever, cough productive of green sputum, and left pleuritic chest pain. Examination shows dullness to percussion, decreased tactile fremitus, and decreased breath sounds over the lower one third of the left posterior chest. Which of the following is the most likely diagnosis?

A. Atelectasis of the left lower lobe
B. Left hemothorax
C. Bronchogenic carcinoma
D. Bronchiectasis
E. Pneumonia with effusion

CV

P 186   An 83-year-old man with a long history of hypertension has severe, prolonged chest pain. Acute myocardial infarction is diagnosed. Blood pressure is 220/126 mm Hg; pulse, 102/min; and respirations, 20/min. Examination shows clear lung fields and apical S4 gallop without murmur. Which of the following is contraindicated at this time?

A. t-PA
B. Metoprolol
C. Clopidogrel
D. Nitroglycerin
E. Captopril

PUL, ENDO

P 187   A 62-year-old woman has small cell carcinoma complicated by syndrome of inappropriate antidiuretic hormone (SIADH). Which of the following is the most likely laboratory abnormality to be noted?

A. Elevated serum osmolality
B. Pleural fluid glucose level of 120 mg/dL
C. Systemic arterial pH of 7.47
D. Hyperphosphatemia
E. Hyponatremia

MS, CV

P 188   A 74-year-old man has severe osteoarthritis of the hips. In addition, he has chronic heartburn. The patient should be counseled that there may be an increased risk of which of the following when celecoxib (Celebrex) therapy is initiated?

A. Seizures
B. Myocardial infarction
C. Hemolytic anemia
D. Adult respiratory distress syndrome
E. Paroxysmal atrial fibrillation

ENDO, GI/N

P 189   Despite studious efforts, a 63-year-old man with type 1 diabetes mellitus has repeated episodes of nausea, bloating, and wide swings in his plasma glucose levels. Which of the following is the most likely cause?

A. Gastroparesis
B. Malabsorption syndrome
C. Insulin resistance syndrome
D. Villous atrophy of small bowel
E. Hepatocellular carcinoma

PUL, GI/N

P 190   A 61-year-old man who has which of the following diseases is most likely to have a transudative pleural effusion?

A. Pneumococcal pneumonia
B. Adenocarcinoma of the lung
C. Pancreatitis
D. Nephrotic syndrome
E. Sarcoidosis

CV

P 191   A 76-year-old man has prolonged, severe anterior chest pressure. Extensive anterior myocardial infarction is diagnosed. The patient has a history of cerebral hemorrhage 4 years earlier. Blood pressure is 130/70 mm Hg; pulse, 100/min; and respirations, 20/min. There is no clinical evidence of heart failure. Which of the following is contraindicated?

A. Oral aspirin
B. Intravenous metoprolol
C. Intravenous nitroglycerin
D. Oral captopril
E. Intravenous alteplase

The Performance section is like a PANCE or PANRE. There is only *one* best answer.

GI/N, ENDO

P 192   A 55-year-old woman who has type 1 diabetes mellitus is suspected now to have gastroparesis. Which of the following is the preferred diagnostic test?

A. Upper gastrointestinal endoscopy
B. Nuclear scintigraphy after radioactive-labeled meal
C. 24-hour esophageal pH monitoring
D. Upper gastrointestinal series with Gastrografin
E. CT imaging of the abdomen after overnight fast

GU, ID

P 193   A 15-year-old boy has urethritis due to *Neisseria gonorrhoeae*. Which of the following is not recommended in the management of the patient?

A. Cefoxitin
B. Doxycycline
C. Ofloxacin
D. Spectinomycin
E. Azithromycin

DERM

P 194   A 56-year-old healthy man has a 1-day history of constant burning pain extending in a line from his back around to his right anterior chest. The pain does not increase with inspiration or bending. Examination of the skin, chest, lung, and heart is normal. The patient should be advised of which of the following?

A. Pleurodynia is most likely diagnosis
B. Bed rest for 48 hours is advised
C. Zoster rash may appear in 24 to 48 hours
D. Ventilation-perfusion scan is indicated
E. Serial cardiac enzyme determination is advised

GI/N

P 195   Which of the following determinations is most specific for defining portal hypertension as the cause of ascites in a patient?

A. Ascites fluid total protein level
B. Ascites fluid triglyceride level
C. Ascites fluid lactic dehydrogenase level
D. Serum to ascites albumin gradient
E. Ascites fluid glucose level

GI/N

P 196   A 62-year-old man with known cirrhosis complicated by portal hypertension and ascites has a 2-day history of fever and abdominal pain. Rectal temperature is 101°F; blood pressure, 90/72 mm Hg; pulse, 110/min; and respirations, 26/min. Examination shows ascites with diffuse abdominal tenderness. White blood cell count is 14,000/microL, and systemic arterial blood gas reveals a pH of 7.21. Which of the following is the most likely diagnosis?

   A. Carcinoma of pancreas
   B. Cholecystitis
   C. Mesenteric infarction
   D. Spontaneous bacterial peritonitis
   E. Angiodysplasia of the colon

ID, GI/N

P 197   Two days after returning from a mountain hiking trip, a 26-year-old man has profuse watery diarrhea, abdominal cramps, and nausea. No fever is present. Which of the following is the most likely infectious organism?

   A. Enterotoxigenic *Escherichia coli*
   B. *Campylobacter jejuni*
   C. Rotavirus
   D. *Giardia lamblia*
   E. Adenovirus

ID, GI/N

P 198   In a healthy patient, presence of which of the following differentiates enteritis due to *Campylobacter jejuni* from *Giardia lamblia*?

   A. Axillary temperature of 103.6°F
   B. Incubation period of 3 weeks
   C. Association with uveitis
   D. Fecal presence of leukocytes
   E. Fecal presence of eosinophils

GI/N, ID

P 199   A 3-year-old girl who has been swimming in a community pool has the sudden onset of watery diarrhea and infrequent vomiting. Which of the following is the most likely infecting organism?

   A. Rotavirus
   B. Norovirus
   C. Cytomegalovirus
   D. Enterotoxigenic *Escherichia coli*
   E. *Cryptosporidium*

The Performance section is like a PANCE or PANRE. There is only *one* best answer.

ID, GI/N

P 200   A 61-year-old man with which of the following underlying conditions should take antimicrobial prophylaxis to prevent traveler's diarrhea?

   A. History of remote myocardial infarction
   B. Irritable bowel syndrome
   C. Diabetes insipidus
   D. Paroxysmal atrial fibrillation
   E. Idiopathic pulmonary fibrosis

CV, ID

P 201   A 71-year-old woman has an indwelling intravenous catheter in her right forearm. She has a 1-day history of aching pain, redness in that arm, and chills. Oral temperature is 101°F. Examination shows induration, erythema, and a tender venous cord in the right forearm. White blood cell count is 13,200/microL. In addition to catheter removal, which of the following is the preferred therapy?

   A. Unfractionated heparin
   B. Application of cold compresses to affected area
   C. Low molecular weight heparin
   D. Nafcillin
   E. Splinting of right forearm and wrist

CV

P 202   A 36-year-old man has a 3-week history of worsening dyspnea without cough or wheezing. Three years earlier, he was shot in the right thigh. Blood pressure is 164/56 mm Hg; pulse, 121/min; and respirations, 30/min. Examination shows bounding pulses, bibasilar rales, and apical S3 gallop. A thrill is felt over the scar in the right thigh. Which of the following is the most likely diagnosis?

   A. Hyperthyroidism
   B. Beriberi
   C. Paget's disease of bone
   D. Iron deficiency anemia
   E. Arteriovenous fistula

ID, ENDO, REPRO

P 203   Live, attenuated influenza vaccine is recommended for which of the following persons?

   A. Healthy 22-year-old nurse
   B. Patient with diabetes mellitus
   C. Pregnant woman
   D. Heart failure patient
   E. Nephrotic syndrome patient

ENDO, HEME

P 204   Propylthiouracil therapy is initiated for a 40-year-old woman who has
        Graves' disease. Onset of which of the following is considered to be
        associated with agranulocytosis?

A. Insomnia
B. Palpitations
C. Headache
D. Puffiness of fingers
E. Sore throat

CV, ENDO

P 205   A 28-year-old woman has a 2-week history of dyspnea and bilateral ankle
        edema. Blood pressure is 166/58 mm Hg; pulse, 126/min; and respirations,
        26/min. Examination shows warm skin, lid lag, bounding pulses, bibasilar
        rales, and fine tremor. Which of the following is the most likely diagnosis?

A. Myasthenia gravis
B. Essential tremor
C. Mercury poisoning
D. Hyperthyroidism
E. Arteriovenous fistula

GI/N

P 206   Which of the following classes of medication may produce acute bloody
        diarrhea due to an inflammatory colitis?

A. Nonaspirin, nonselective, nonsteroidal anti-inflammatory
B. Angiotensin-converting enzyme inhibitor
C. Calcium channel blocker
D. Thyroid hormone
E. Thiazide

GU

P 207   A 34-year-old man has metabolic acidosis of indeterminate cause. The
        anion gap equals which of the following?

A. $Na - (Cl + HCO_3 + albumin)$
B. $(Na + K + Mg) - (Cl + HCO_3)$
C. P_{CO_2} in mm Hg $- HCO_3$ in mEq/L
D. $Na - (Cl + HCO_3)$
E. $(Na + K) - (Cl + HCO_3 + lactate)$

ID

P 208   Trivalent inactivated influenza vaccine is not recommended for which of
        the following patients?

A. 47-year-old healthy woman
B. Chronic obstructive lung disease patient
C. Heart failure patient
D. Hemoglobinopathy patient
E. Patient taking long-term warfarin therapy

The Performance section is like a PANCE or PANRE. There is only *one* best answer.

NEURO

P 209   A 34-year-old woman has the sudden onset of an intensely severe headache followed quickly by nausea and vomiting. Vital signs are normal. Examination shows nuchal rigidity. CT imaging of the brain is normal. Which of the following is the most appropriate next diagnostic test for suspected subarachnoid hemorrhage?

A. Cerebral angiography
B. Magnetic resonance angiography
C. MRI scan of the brain
D. Lumbar puncture
E. Electroencephalogram

NEURO

P 210   Twenty-four hours after a lumbar puncture, a 34-year-old woman has a persistent frontal headache. This is unresponsive to bed rest and oral analgesics. Administration of which of the following is the next preferred treatment?

A. Intramuscular adrenocorticotropic hormone
B. Oral caffeine
C. Intramuscular methylprednisolone
D. Epidural blood patch
E. Intramuscular morphine sulfate

REPRO, NEURO

P 211   A 28-year-old woman, in her 35th week of pregnancy, has recurrent pain and tingling in the first and second fingers of both hands. Symptoms are worse at night. Tinel's sign is positive. Which of the following is recommended management?

A. Indomethacin for 2 weeks
B. Corticosteroid injection into the carpal tunnel
C. Surgical decompression of the carpal tunnel
D. Electrophysiologic study of the median nerves
E. Assurance to patient that symptoms disappear after delivery

GI/N

P 212   A 24-year-old woman has diarrhea with gross rectal bleeding. She is diagnosed as having ulcerative colitis limited to the proctosigmoid area. Which of the following is the preferred therapy?

A. Oral sulfasalazine
B. 2-week course of tapering glucocorticoids
C. 1-week course of oral infliximab
D. Hydrocortisone foam enemas
E. Oral clindamycin

P 213   A 49-year-old woman has newly diagnosed Graves' disease. Presence of which of the following in the blood is most specific to confirm this diagnosis?

A. Antithyroglobulin antibodies
B. Th1 CD4+ lymphocytes
C. Anti–thyroid-stimulating hormone receptor antibodies
D. Anti–thyroid peroxidase antibodies
E. HLA-antigen complex

P 214   A 76-year-old woman is in septic shock due to gram-negative bacteremia. An increase in which of the following is the pathophysiologic basis for the metabolic acidosis that is present?

A. Loss of bicarbonate in stool
B. Production of lactic acid
C. Loss of bicarbonate in urine
D. Production of ketone bodies
E. Production of ammonia

P 215   A 34-year-old man has a 1-week history of recurrent bloody diarrhea and fecal urgency. He has taken no medication for 6 months and has not traveled outside the United States for 3 years. Which of the following is the preferred initial diagnostic test?

A. Flexible sigmoidoscopy
B. Barium enema
C. CT imaging of the colon
D. Mesenteric angiography
E. Stool assay for *Clostridium difficile* toxin

P 216   Over a period of 1 month, a 62-year-old woman has developed bilateral carpal tunnel syndrome. Which of the following is the preferred diagnostic test?

A. Serum C-reactive protein
B. Erythrocyte sedimentation rate
C. Serum antinuclear antibody titer
D. Serum thyroid-stimulating hormone level
E. Serum anti–Sm antibody titer

The Performance section is like a PANCE or PANRE. There is only *one* best answer.

P 217   A 42-year-old man with gastroesophageal reflux should be advised to avoid which of the following?

    A. Blueberries
    B. Rice pudding
    C. Bread pudding
    D. Raspberry sherbet
    E. Chocolate ice cream

P 218   A patient has end-stage renal disease due to diabetic nephropathy. Which of the following acid-base conditions would most likely be present?

    A. Increased anion gap metabolic acidosis
    B. Metabolic alkalosis
    C. Respiratory acidosis
    D. Normal systemic arterial pH
    E. Normal anion gap metabolic acidosis

P 219   A 72-year-old woman with known coronary artery disease has newly diagnosed hyperthyroidism due to a toxic adenoma of the thyroid. Which of the following is recommended therapy prior to administration of radioactive iodine?

    A. Iodine
    B. Thyroglobulin
    C. Prednisone
    D. Methimazole
    E. Doxazosin

P 220   A 62-year-old obese woman has a 3-week history of recurrent heartburn occurring, on average, twice each week. The symptoms are present only at night, awakening the patient approximately 3 hours after retiring. Which of the following is the preferred initial therapy?

    A. Calcium carbonate at bedtime
    B. Aluminum hydroxide/magnesium carbonate/alginate at bedtime
    C. Omeprazole before breakfast and dinner
    D. Ranitidine at bedtime
    E. Omeprazole and cimetidine before breakfast

P 221   Which of the following is considered to be the most sensitive test for the diagnosis of hyperthyroidism due to a toxic adenoma of the thyroid?

    A. Serum T_3 level
    B. Serum thyroid-stimulating hormone level
    C. T_3 resin uptake
    D. Free T_4 index
    E. Thyroid hormone binding ratio

GI/N

P 222   A 44-year-old woman has a long history of ulcerative colitis that involves the entire colon. Which of the following is the most likely potential long-term complication?

A. Aseptic necrosis of the femur
B. Colon cancer
C. Angiodysplasia of the colon
D. Gangrene of the colon
E. Cholelithiasis

EENT, GI/N

P 223   A 56-year-old obese man who has never smoked now has a 4-week history of hoarseness. He has no heartburn or dysphagia. He takes no medication. Which of the following is the most likely cause?

A. Zenker's diverticulum
B. Squamous cell carcinoma of esophagus
C. Postnasal drip
D. Epiglottitis
E. Gastroesophageal reflux

REPRO, CV

P 224   Presence of which of the following differentiates preeclampsia from gestational hypertension?

A. Fasting plasma glucose greater than 140 mg/dL
B. Proteinuria
C. Patient was normotensive prior to pregnancy
D. Onset of hypertension at 12th to 16th week of gestation
E. Recognized association with migraine headaches

REPRO

P 225   Presence of which of the following differentiates eclampsia from preeclampsia?

A. Hypertension
B. Proteinuria
C. Thrombocytopenia
D. Blurred vision
E. Seizures

REPRO

P 226   A 33-year-old woman is diagnosed as having antiphospholipid antibody syndrome. Which of the following is the most likely complication to occur in the patient if she were pregnant?

A. Subarachnoid hemorrhage
B. Nephrotic syndrome
C. Placenta previa
D. Gestational diabetes
E. Recurrent fetal loss

The Performance section is like a PANCE or PANRE. There is only *one* best answer.

P 227   Which of the following is the primary pathophysiologic mechanism thought to be responsible for the development of preeclampsia?

A. Vasodilation of the placental arteries
B. Excess secretion of catecholamines
C. Endothelial dysfunction
D. Downregulation of adrenergic receptors
E. Increased secretion of brain natriuretic peptide

P 228   Eight weeks after her last normal menstrual period, a 26-year-old woman has abdominal pain and vaginal bleeding. Which of the following diagnostic tests is preferred in order to differentiate between ectopic pregnancy and threatened abortion?

A. Serum hCG concentration
B. MRI scan of the pelvis
C. Serum progesterone level
D. Transvaginal ultrasonography
E. Fetal karyotype determination

P 229   Which of the following is considered to be the highest risk factor for ectopic pregnancy?

A. Maternal age older than 35 years
B. Current cigarette smoking
C. History of bipolar coagulation sterilization
D. In vitro fertilization
E. Regular vaginal douching

P 230   A 27-year-old woman has the following hepatitis B serologic markers:
HBs-Ag negative
Anti-HBc negative
Anti-HBs positive
Which of the following is the clinical status of the patient?

A. Acute hepatitis B infection
B. Chronic hepatitis B infection
C. Susceptible to hepatitis B infection
D. Immune due to hepatitis B vaccination
E. Immune due to natural infection

GI/N, PSY/LE

P 231   A 49-year-old man has jaundice determined to be due to intrahepatic cholestasis. Which of the following medicines is most likely to be the causative agent?

A. Risperidone (Risperdal)
B. Paroxetine (Paxil)
C. Chlorpromazine (Thorazine)
D. Sertraline (Zoloft)
E. Nortriptyline (Pamelor)

HEME, GI/N

P 232   A 19-year-old woman has jaundice of the sclera and palms. Total serum bilirubin is 3.2 mg/dL, conjugated bilirubin is 0.4 mg/dL, and unconjugated fraction is 2.8 mg/dL. Serum alanine aminotransferase is 40 units/L, and serum alkaline phosphatase is 45 units/L. Which of the following is the most likely diagnosis?

A. Hepatic sarcoidosis
B. Choledocholithiasis
C. Infectious mononucleosis
D. Systemic lupus erythematosus
E. Hemolytic anemia

GI/N, ID

P 233   A 57-year-old man has acute right upper quadrant abdominal pain radiating to his right shoulder, nausea, fever, and chills. Blood pressure is 104/70 mm Hg; pulse, 130/min; and rectal temperature, 103°F. Examination shows scleral icterus and right upper quadrant abdominal tenderness without rebound. White blood cell count is 31,000/microL with left shift. Which of the following is the most likely diagnosis?

A. Acute cholecystitis
B. Primary sclerosing cholangitis
C. Primary biliary cirrhosis
D. Viral hepatitis
E. Ascending cholangitis

GI/N

P 234   A 47-year-old woman has a 3-week history of worsening fatigue and pruritus. Examination shows scleral icterus. Presence of which of the following serum antibodies is most specific for the diagnosis of primary biliary cirrhosis?

A. Antinuclear
B. Anti-Sm
C. Anti–smooth muscle
D. Antimitochondrial
E. Antiactin

GI/N

P 235   A 63-year-old man has jaundice. Which of the following laboratory values is most suggestive of the diagnosis of alcoholic hepatitis?

A. Elevated serum globulins
B. Ratio of serum AST/ALT is greater than 2:1
C. Hypoalbuminemia
D. Elevated serum cholesterol
E. Presence of serum antimitochondrial antibodies

GU

P 236   A 23-year-old woman has recurrent episodes of severe lower abdominal cramping that starts with the onset of menstrual bleeding. Primary dysmenorrhea is diagnosed. In addition to heat application to the abdomen, oral administration of which of the following is the preferred therapy?

A. Oxycodone
B. Ibuprofen
C. Magnesium
D. Nifedipine
E. Vitamin B_6

GU, PSY/LE

P 237   A 33-year-old woman has premenstrual dysphoric disorder manifest primarily by depression and hopelessness. Which of the following classes of medicine is the preferred therapy?

A. Benzodiazepine
B. Carbonic anhydrase inhibitor
C. GnRH agonist
D. Androgen
E. Selective serotonin reuptake inhibitor

GU, ENDO, CV

P 238   A 76-year-old woman with a history of type 2 diabetes mellitus is hospitalized for treatment of lobar pneumonia. Twenty-four hours later, she has polyuria and polydipsia. Plasma glucose is 622 mg/dL, and serum osmolality is 315 mOsmol/kg. Which of the following is the least likely laboratory abnormality to be present?

A. Anion gap 18 mEq/L
B. Systemic arterial pH 7.37
C. Serum sodium 129 mEq/L
D. Serum potassium 3.9 mEq/L
E. Serum bicarbonate 24 mEq/L

GU, ENDO

P 239   An obese 61-year-old man has type 2 diabetes mellitus. His serum creatinine concentration is 1.6 mEq/dL. Initiation of metformin therapy in this patient increases the risk for which of the following?

   A. Sodium-losing nephropathy
   B. Acute pericarditis
   C. Altered awareness of hypoglycemia
   D. "Dawn" phenomenon
   E. Lactic acidosis

ENDO, GI/N

P 240   A 57-year-old woman with which of the following should not receive metformin therapy for type 2 diabetes mellitus?

   A. Heavy alcohol intake
   B. Greater than 20% overweight
   C. Hypertension
   D. Left ventricular ejection fraction less than 40%
   E. Sensitivity to iodide contrast media

GU, ENDO

P 241   A 67-year-old man who is receiving metformin therapy for type 2 diabetes mellitus is to undergo peripheral arteriography utilizing a radiocontrast agent. Which of the following is proper counseling for the patient?

   A. NPO for 12 hours prior to imaging study
   B. Do not take metformin on morning of study
   C. Take furosemide 40 mg orally at 6 a.m. on day of study
   D. Take potassium chloride 20 mEq at 6 a.m. on day of study
   E. Switch to a sulfonylurea agent 1 week prior to study

EENT, PUL

P 242   A healthy 33-year-old man has a 3-day history of nasal congestion, rhinorrhea, sore throat, and cough productive of mucoid sputum. The patient has not had fever. Vital signs are normal. Examination shows nasal congestion and scattered bilateral wheezes. Which of the following medicines should not be prescribed?

   A. Ipratropium
   B. Ibuprofen
   C. Aspirin
   D. Azithromycin
   E. Phenylephrine

The Performance section is like a PANCE or PANRE. There is only *one* best answer.

CV

P 243   A 78-year-old man has an acute myocardial infarction complicated by recurrent runs of ventricular tachycardia. In the intensive care unit, he becomes stuporous and confused. Vital signs are normal. Cardiac monitoring shows normal sinus rhythm. Which of the following medicines is the most likely cause of the mental change?

A. Streptokinase
B. Lidocaine
C. Aspirin
D. Metoprolol
E. Nitroglycerin

GU

P 244   A 57-year-old man with a history of chronic renal insufficiency has a serum potassium concentration of 6.5 mEq/L. Which of the following is the preferred initial therapy?

A. Subcutaneous administration of regular insulin
B. Retention enema of sodium polystyrene (Kayexalate)
C. Hemodialysis
D. Intravenous administration of verapamil
E. Administration of nebulized albuterol

CV, GI/N

P 245   A 51-year-old woman receives furosemide for treatment of portal hypertension with ascites. Which of the following on electrocardiography is most suggestive of hypokalemia?

A. Peaked T waves
B. Shortened QT interval
C. Mobitz I atrioventricular block
D. Flattening of T waves with prominent U waves
E. Absence of P waves with widening of QRS complex

NEURO

P 246   A 34-year-old woman has a 3-week history of intermittent weakness of her legs and diplopia. Presence of which of the following serum antibodies is most suggestive of myasthenia gravis?

A. Anti-acetylcholine receptor
B. Anti–parietal cell
C. Anti-Sm
D. Anti–double-stranded DNA
E. Anti–smooth muscle

ENDO

P 247   Presence of which of the following differentiates Graves' disease from hyperthyroidism due to a toxic thyroid nodule?

A. Atrial fibrillation
B. Decreased serum thyroid-stimulating hormone level
C. Lid lag
D. Increased cardiac output
E. Anti–thyroid-stimulating hormone receptor antibodies

GU

P 248   A 42-year-old man has nephrotic syndrome due to focal glomerulosclerosis. In addition to sodium restriction and diuretic therapy, which of the following should be received by the patient?

A. Oral calcium channel blocker
B. Oral alpha-adrenergic blocker
C. Intermittent intravenous infusion of albumin
D. Oral COX-2 nonsteroidal anti-inflammatory agent
E. Oral angiotensin-converting enzyme inhibitor

CV, GU

P 249   A 47-year-old woman has nephrotic syndrome. Which of the following is the most likely complication to occur?

A. Subdural hematoma
B. Deep vein thrombosis
C. Chronic pyelonephritis
D. Spontaneous bacterial peritonitis
E. Avascular necrosis of the femur

HEME

P 250   A 20-year-old man has a 3-week history of dry cough and 1-week history of night sweats. Vital signs are normal. Examination shows enlarged right cervical, left inguinal, and left supraclavicular lymph nodes. No murmur or gallop is heard. Which of the following is the most likely diagnosis?

A. Endocarditis
B. Adverse reaction to retinoid therapy
C. Hodgkin's disease
D. Primary tuberculosis
E. Sarcoidosis

NEURO

P 251   Presence of which of the following differentiates essential tremor from Parkinson's disease?

A. Asymmetrical pupil size
B. Drooling
C. Tremor of the lips
D. Normal gait
E. Orthostatic hypotension

The Performance section is like a PANCE or PANRE. There is only *one* best answer.

NEURO

P 252   Presence of which of the following differentiates amyotrophic lateral
        sclerosis from Parkinson's disease?

A. Tremor
B. Orthostatic hypotension
C. Loss of sweating
D. Absence of deep tendon reflexes
E. Fasciculations

CV, EENT, NEURO

P 253   A 79-year-old woman has had three episodes, each lasting 5 to 10 minutes,
        of blurred vision in both eyes; dizziness; and unstable gait. Blood pressure
        in the right arm sitting is 150/80 mm Hg and in the left arm sitting is
        118/74 mm Hg. Neurologic examination performed when the patient
        is asymptomatic is normal. Which of the following is the most likely
        diagnosis?

A. Takayasu's arteritis
B. Coarctation of aorta
C. Giant cell arteritis
D. Subclavian steal syndrome
E. Thrombosis of left common carotid artery

NEURO, CV

P 254   An 82-year-old man has a 3-week history of recurrent bilateral
        blurred vision, circumoral paresthesias, and dizziness. Subclavian steal
        syndrome is diagnosed. Which of the following is the preferred treat-
        ment?

A. Regional sympathetic nerve block
B. Administration of oral nifedipine
C. Administration of oral prednisone
D. Ventricular-atrial shunting procedure
E. Percutaneous luminal angioplasty

GU, ENDO

P 255   A 63-year-old woman with type 2 diabetes mellitus has nephrotic
        syndrome. In addition to sodium restriction and a diuretic, which of
        the following classes of medicine is appropriate therapy?

A. Glucocorticoid
B. Alpha-adrenergic blocker
C. Alkylating agent
D. Angiotensin-converting enzyme inhibitor
E. Interferon-alpha

REPRO

P 256 A 26-year-old woman wishes to become pregnant but is concerned because of a family history of sudden infant death syndrome (SIDS). Which of the following is the most important counseling for the patient with specific reference to SIDS?

A. Avoid gaining more than 16 pounds during pregnancy
B. Do not smoke during pregnancy
C. Have fasting blood sugar determination every 7 to 8 weeks during pregnancy
D. Fetal genetic typing should be performed during pregnancy
E. Patient should be checked for acetyl-CoA dehydrogenase deficiency

NEURO, CV

P 257 Which of the following adverse effects is common to levodopa-carbidopa, dopamine agonists, and catechol O-methyltransferase inhibitors used in therapy of Parkinson's disease?

A. Autoimmune hemolytic anemia
B. Colitis
C. Thrombocytosis
D. Atrioventricular block
E. Orthostatic hypotension

REPRO, GU

P 258 A 33-year-old woman should preferably take a progestin-only contraceptive if she has which of the following conditions?

A. History of deep vein thrombosis
B. Postpartum more than 21 days and not breastfeeding
C. Obesity
D. Epilepsy
E. HIV infection

ENDO, REPRO

P 259 A 36-year-old pregnant woman has gestational diabetes mellitus. A cardiovascular fitness program has resulted in normalization of her glucose tolerance. Which of the following is the primary physiologic mechanism by which exercise improves glucose control?

A. Increases tissue sensitivity to insulin
B. Decreases hepatic gluconeogenesis
C. Decreases glycogenolysis
D. Reduces cellular oxidative stress
E. Increases acetyl CoA protein

The Performance section is like a PANCE or PANRE. There is only *one* best answer.

P 260   A 34-year-old woman who takes a single dose of glyburide daily for treatment of type 2 diabetes mellitus wishes to become pregnant. Which of the following is the most appropriate counseling for the patient when she becomes pregnant?

  A. Glyburide should be taken twice daily
  B. Morning insulin therapy should be added to the glyburide
  C. A trial period of nonhypoglycemic treatment should be attempted
  D. Glyburide should be replaced by metformin therapy
  E. Glyburide therapy must be replaced by insulin

P 261   Presence of which of the following differentiates intravascular hemolysis from extravascular hemolysis?

  A. Hemosiderinuria
  B. Elevation of serum indirect bilirubin
  C. Absent serum haptoglobin
  D. Hypersegmented neutrophils on peripheral smear examination
  E. Nucleated red blood cells on peripheral smear examination

P 262   A 36-year-old woman who takes no medicines has persistent fatigue and weakness. Vital signs are normal. Hemoglobin is 11.4 g/dL, and white blood cell count is 4,700/microL. Serum electrolytes are normal. Which of the following serum values is most likely to be diagnostic in the patient?

  A. Lactic dehydrogenase 210 units/L
  B. Thyroid-stimulating hormone level 4 mU/mL
  C. Cholesterol 330 mg/dL
  D. Ferritin 8 ng/mL
  E. C-reactive protein 4 mg/L

P 263   Which of the following is the pathophysiologic mechanism that results in iron deficiency in the patient who has celiac disease?

  A. Gastrointestinal bleeding due to hypocoagulable state
  B. Extravascular hemolysis
  C. Decreased marrow hematopoiesis
  D. Release of phosphate from myeloid cells
  E. Decreased gastrointestinal absorption of iron

P 264   In the 21st week of gestation, a 33-year-old primigravida has persistent blood pressure levels of 160/102 mm Hg associated with proteinuria. Which of the following agents is contraindicated?

  A. Hydralazine
  B. Methyldopa
  C. Nifedipine
  D. Labetalol
  E. Captopril

MS

P 265   A 33-year-old woman has a 2-month history of disturbing drawing and pulling sensations in both lower legs. The discomfort occurs only at rest and is immediately relieved by movement. Which of the following is the most likely etiology?

A. Iron deficiency
B. Muscle glycogen deficiency
C. Heightened creatine kinase activity
D. Estrogen deficiency
E. Hypercortisolism

GU

P 266   A 22-year-old man has a testicular mass. A germ cell testicular tumor is most likely when there is an elevated serum concentration of which of the following?

A. Testosterone
B. Luteinizing hormone
C. Prolactin
D. Alpha-fetoprotein
E. Adrenocorticotropic hormone

GI/N

P 267   A 56-year-old man has alcoholic cirrhosis. Elevation in the serum concentration of which of the following is most suggestive of the development of hepatocellular carcinoma?

A. Alanine aminotransferase
B. Anti–smooth muscle antibodies
C. Antiactin antibodies
D. Alpha-fetoprotein
E. Monoclonal M protein

GU

P 268   A 62-year-old man has red-colored urine for 2 days. Urine dipstick is positive for blood. Microscopic examination of the urine sediment shows no red blood cells. Which of the following is the most likely diagnosis?

A. Beeturia
B. Phenazopyridine ingestion
C. Porphyria
D. Intravascular hemolysis
E. Carcinoma of the kidney

The Performance section is like a PANCE or PANRE. There is only *one* best answer.

DERM

P 269   A 10-year-old girl has a 1-week history of low-grade fever, rhinorrhea, and headache followed by onset of a bilateral erythematous malar rash and circumoral pallor. No other rash is present. Which of the following is the most likely diagnosis?

    A. Systemic lupus erythematosus
    B. Rubella
    C. Erythema infectiosum
    D. Herpangina
    E. Hypersensitivity vasculitis

ID

P 270   An asymptomatic 29-year-old man with positive HIV serology should be considered to have AIDS when which of the following is met?

    A. CD4 lymphocyte count is greater than 400 cells/microL
    B. HIV viral load is less than 200 copies
    C. Serum IgM concentration is less than 50 mg/dL
    D. CD lymphocyte percentage is greater than 20%
    E. CD lymphocyte count is less than 200 cells/microL

ID

P 271   A 33-year-old woman with AIDS has a CD4 count of 48 cells/microL. Her tuberculin skin test shows 7 mm induration. She is varicella-zoster seronegative. Which of the following is not a recommended prophylactic therapy?

    A. Zoster vaccination
    B. Trimethoprim-sulfamethoxazole
    C. Isoniazid
    D. Influenza vaccine
    E. Pneumococcal vaccine

NEURO, ENDO

P 272   A 71-year-old woman with diabetes mellitus has numbness and tingling of both feet and lower legs. Which of the following neurologic signs is least likely to be noted upon examination?

    A. Impaired proprioception
    B. Absent ankle deep tendon reflexes
    C. Loss of light touch
    D. Loss of vibratory sensation
    E. Extensor Babinski response

NEURO, ENDO

P 273   A 47-year-old man has the sudden onset of footdrop due to common peroneal nerve palsy. Which of the following is the most likely underlying condition?

    A. Graves' disease
    B. Syndrome of inappropriate antidiuretic hormone
    C. Guillain-Barré syndrome
    D. Diabetes mellitus
    E. Myasthenia gravis

GI/N, NEURO, ENDO

P 274 A 60-year-old man who has type 1 diabetes mellitus has autonomic neuropathy involving the gastrointestinal tract. Which of the following is the most likely manifestation?

A. Water brash
B. Hematochezia
C. Malabsorption syndrome
D. Small bowel obstruction
E. Nocturnal diarrhea

CV, ENDO

P 275 Clinical testing in a 67-year-old man with diabetes mellitus demonstrates a lack in variation of heart rate during deep breathing and Valsalva maneuvers. The patient is at increased risk for which of the following?

A. Unstable angina pectoris
B. Diastolic heart failure
C. 3rd-degree atrioventricular block
D. Sudden cardiac death
E. Respiratory acidosis

CV, NEURO, ENDO

P 276 A 67-year-old diabetic man has lightheadedness when arising from bed. While sitting, blood pressure is 116/78 mm Hg with a pulse of 80/min. Standing blood pressure is 90/62 mm Hg with a pulse of 81/min. Which of the following is the most likely pathophysiologic mechanism causing the observed hemodynamic response?

A. Autonomic insufficiency
B. Hypovolemia
C. Parasympathetic nervous system dysfunction
D. Deficiency of gamma aminobutyric acid receptors
E. Extrapyramidal nervous system dysfunction

REPRO

P 277 Presence of which of the following differentiates the typical presentation of abruptio placentae from placenta previa?

A. Passage of blood clots
B. 1st-trimester bleeding
C. Serum antiphospholipid antibodies
D. Uterine contractions
E. Thrombocytosis

The Performance section is like a PANCE or PANRE. There is only *one* best answer.

REPRO

P 278   A 29-year-old woman has had three spontaneous pregnancy losses in a row. Each pregnancy ended in the 11th to 13th week of gestation. Which of the following is the most likely underlying maternal condition?

A. Reactive hypoglycemia
B. Presence of anti–thyroid peroxidase antibodies
C. Presence of anti–parietal cell antibodies
D. Membranous ventricular septal defect
E. Presence of antiphospholipid antibodies

ID, HEME

P 279   A 14-year-old boy with sickle cell anemia has had repeated infarctions of his spleen. Which of the following is appropriate therapy?

A. Daily oral penicillin
B. Monthly intramuscular streptomycin
C. Annual herpes zoster vaccination
D. Annual parenteral pegfilgrastim (Neulasta)
E. Monthly parenteral erythropoietin

NEURO, GI/N

P 280   A 52-year-old man with advanced chronic liver disease has hepatic encephalopathy manifest by confusion. Neurologic examination shows bilateral asterixis. Which of the following is preferred initial therapy?

A. Administration of oral spironolactone
B. Administration of Kayexalate enema
C. Administration of oral clindamycin
D. Ingestion of diet containing 125 g protein daily
E. Administration of lactulose enema

GU, GI/N

P 281   A 56-year-old woman has severe chronic liver disease due to alcohol abuse. Which of the following conditions is most likely to precipitate hepatic encephalopathy?

A. Ingestion of low-protein diet
B. Inhalation of 40% oxygen
C. Intake of zinc-containing antacids
D. Hypokalemia
E. Development of ascites

GU

P 282   Upon completing a marathon run, a 29-year-old man has nausea and vomiting and is in a confused state. Serum sodium is 119 mEq/L. Which of the following is the most likely cause of the hyponatremia?

A. Inadequate renal reabsorption of sodium
B. Low sodium concentration in sweat
C. Ingestion of excess water during race
D. Ingestion of a nonsteroidal anti-inflammatory before the race
E. Ingestion of a high-protein diet before the race

NEURO

P 283   Presence of which of the following differentiates a seizure from a transient ischemic attack?

A. Numbness
B. Diplopia
C. Weakness
D. Headache
E. Visual hallucinations

ENDO, NEURO

P 284   A 46-year-old man has a subarachnoid hemorrhage due to rupture of a cerebral aneurysm. Ten hours later, his urinary volume increases to 425 mL/hr. Serum sodium is 156 mEq/L. Which of the following is the most likely complication of the hemorrhage?

A. Diabetes insipidus
B. Hyperglycemic, nonketotic state
C. Hyperhidrosis
D. Syndrome of inappropriate antidiuretic hormone secretion
E. Acute adrenal insufficiency

ENDO, NEURO

P 285   A 16-year-old boy has generalized seizures for which he is transported to the emergency department. Lorazepam, phenytoin, and phenobarbital do not end the seizure activity. Which of the following is the most likely diagnosis?

A. Epilepsy
B. Arteriovenous malformation in the brain
C. Multiple sclerosis
D. Hypoglycemia
E. Hypercalcemia

GI/N

P 286   Which of the following is considered to be the pathophysiologic mechanism causing symptoms in dumping syndrome?

A. Postprandial hypoglycemia
B. Shift of fluid from circulation into bowel
C. Heightened vagal tone
D. Excess secretion of serotonin
E. Decreased adrenal secretion of catecholamines

ID, DERM, GU

P 287   A 32-year-old woman has asymptomatic lesions on her vulva. Examination shows condyloma acuminata. Infection due to which of the following is most likely?

A. Herpes simplex virus
B. Coxsackievirus
C. *Haemophilus ducreyi*
D. *Donovania granulomatis*
E. Human papillomavirus

The Performance section is like a PANCE or PANRE. There is only *one* best answer.

P 288   Presence of which of the following differentiates delirium tremens from alcoholic hallucinosis?

A. Somnolence
B. Auditory hallucinations
C. Hypotension
D. Disorientation
E. Alcohol abstinence before onset

P 289   A 57-year-old man with a long history of chronic alcohol abuse has the acute onset of delirium tremens. In addition to benzodiazepine therapy, which of the following should be administered?

A. Vitamin B_{12}
B. Folinic acid
C. Bromocriptine
D. Paraldehyde
E. Thiamine

P 290   A 3-week-old male infant has postprandial vomiting. Hypertrophic pyloric stenosis is diagnosed. Neonatal ingestion of which of the following is most likely associated with this diagnosis?

A. Nonaspirin, nonselective nonsteroidal anti-inflammatory
B. Medium-chain fatty acid formula
C. Increased dietary proportion of whey to casein
D. Cephalosporin
E. Macrolide

P 291   Which of the following classes of hypoglycemic medicines reduces gastrointestinal absorption of carbohydrate?

A. Insulin
B. Sulfonylureas
C. Thiazolidines
D. Alpha-glucosidase inhibitors
E. Meglitinides

P 292   Which of the following is the mechanism of action of thiazolidinediones in therapy of type 2 diabetes mellitus?

A. Suppress hepatic glucose production
B. Reduce gastrointestinal absorption of carbohydrate
C. Increase sensitivity to insulin
D. Increase pancreatic secretion of insulin
E. Inhibit autoimmune destruction of pancreas

PUL

P 293 A 27-year-old man with asthma has increased dyspnea and wheezing 1 hour after having been a passenger on a 4-hour commercial airline flight. Which of the following environmental factors in the aircraft cabin is the most likely cause of the respiratory symptoms?

A. Reduced cabin pressure
B. Reduced oxygen pressure
C. Low humidity
D. Transmission of airborne pathogens
E. Vibration of aircraft

EENT, DERM, ID

P 294 A 7-year-old boy has a 5-day history of fever and photophobia. Examination shows conjunctivitis, "strawberry" tongue, and cracked, red lips. A diagnosis of Kawasaki disease is made. Which of the following is the preferred initial therapy?

A. Intravenous methylprednisolone
B. Intravenous immune globulin plus aspirin
C. Intravenous cyclophosphamide
D. Oral aspirin alone
E. Intravenous rituximab (Rituxan)

CV

P 295 Which of the following is the major complication of untreated Kawasaki disease?

A. Autoimmune hemolytic anemia
B. Cholestatic hepatitis
C. Necrotizing pneumonia
D. Coronary artery aneurysm
E. Renal papillary necrosis

REPRO

P 296 A 36-year-old woman who has hyperlipidemia and who smokes cigarettes seeks counseling concerning oral contraceptive therapy (OCT). Her aunt and mother both died of ovarian cancer. Which of the following is appropriate counseling for the patient concerning OCT?

A. OCT decreases risk of coronary heart disease
B. OCT decreases risk of ovarian cancer
C. OCT is appropriate for the patient
D. OCT lowers serum triglycerides
E. OCT lowers blood pressure

The Performance section is like a PANCE or PANRE. There is only *one* best answer.

REPRO, GU

P 297   A 34-year-old woman has a 7-month history of oligomenorrhea. Examination shows an obese, hirsute woman. Which of the following serum laboratory values would be consistent with a diagnosis of polycystic ovary syndrome?

    A. Increased luteinizing hormone
    B. Decreased testosterone
    C. Decreased estrogen
    D. Decreased insulin
    E. Increased serotonin

ENDO

P 298   A 61-year-old woman has a 4-month history of enlarging hands and feet. A diagnosis of acromegaly is made. In addition to increased secretion of growth hormone, there is increased secretion of which of the following?

    A. Thyroid-stimulating hormone
    B. Corticotropin
    C. Follicle-stimulating hormone
    D. Vasopressin
    E. Prolactin

CV

P 299   A 40-year-old woman has a 3-month history of paroxysmal episodes of diffuse headache, sweating, palpitations, and anxiety. Each episode lasts approximately 30 minutes. Examination shows sitting blood pressure 200/120 mm Hg with pulse rate of 100/min. Standing blood pressure is 170/106 mm Hg with pulse rate of 114/min. Which of the following is the most appropriate laboratory test?

    A. 24-hour urine assay for cortisol
    B. 24-hour urine assay for catecholamines
    C. 24-hour urine assay for sodium and potassium
    D. Plasma renin activity
    E. 2-hour glucose tolerance test

GU, PSY/LE

P 300   A 56-year-old man takes sildenafil for therapy of erectile dysfunction. He now has new-onset hypertension. Addition of which of the following medicines is considered to have the greatest risk of causing profound hypotension?

    A. Hydrochlorothiazide
    B. Captopril
    C. Verapamil
    D. Doxazosin
    E. Propranolol

MS, GU

P 301   A 72-year-old man with type 2 diabetes mellitus and coronary heart disease has a blood urea nitrogen value of 38 mg/dL and a serum creatinine concentration of 1.9 mg/dL. Which of the following is the most appropriate advice for the patient?

A. Avoid nonaspirin, nonselective, nonsteroidal anti-inflammatory agents
B. Avoid thiazide diuretics
C. Limit daily fluid intake to 1,000 mL
D. Avoid aspirin
E. Isometric exercise is preferable to rhythmic exercise

GU, CV

P 302   A 59-year-old woman has hypertension for which she takes lisinopril therapy. The patient now has painful osteoarthritis for which ibuprofen is prescribed. Which of the following is the most appropriate intervention to be taken in 10 to 14 days?

A. Check blood urea nitrogen/serum creatinine ratio
B. Check serum potassium concentration
C. Obtain complete blood count
D. Check fasting blood sugar level
E. Check urine for proteinuria

NEURO, EENT

P 303   Presence of which of the following differentiates positional vertigo from presyncope related to orthostatic hypotension?

A. Symptoms occur when arising from bed
B. Unstable gait
C. Vertigo occurs when bending head back to look up
D. Vertigo is associated with pallor
E. Vertigo is associated with dimmed vision

HEME

P 304   An 18-year-old man has a severe frontal headache after exposure to a poorly ventilated fuel-burning stove. A diagnosis of carbon monoxide poisoning is made. Which of the following is the preferred therapy?

A. High-flow inhalation of oxygen via face mask
B. Administration of intravenous methylene blue
C. Administration of intravenous sodium bicarbonate
D. Positive end-expiratory pressure breathing treatment
E. Administration of oral *N*-acetyl cysteine

The Performance section is like a PANCE or PANRE. There is only *one* best answer.

P 305 A 33-year-old healthy, nonpregnant woman has a 3-day history of vaginal burning and dysuria. A vaginal discharge then is noted. Presence of which of the following is most suggestive of *Trichomonas vaginalis?*

A. Clue cells on wet mount preparation
B. Pyuria
C. Inguinal adenopathy
D. Gram-negative cocci in vaginal specimen
E. Strawberry cervix on physical examination

P 306 A 29-year-old healthy, nonpregnant woman has a vaginal discharge. A diagnosis of bacterial vaginosis is made based upon the presence of clue cells. Which of the following best describes clue cells?

A. Macrophages containing gram-positive cocci
B. Atypical monocytes
C. Polymorphonuclear cells with inclusion bodies
D. Vaginal epithelium cells with adherent bacteria
E. Macrophages containing azure bodies

P 307 A 29-year-old healthy, nonpregnant woman has gonococcal urethritis. Which of the following is the preferred therapy?

A. Ceftriaxone plus doxycycline
B. Nafcillin
C. Ciprofloxacin
D. Ceftriaxone alone
E. Ceftriaxone plus trimethoprim-sulfamethoxazole

P 308 A 35-year-old man has a 2-day history of fever, urinary frequency, and perineal pain. Examination shows a very tender, swollen prostate. Urinalysis shows 25 leukocytes/high-power field. Culture of the urine indicates infection by *Escherichia coli.* Which of the following is the preferred oral regimen of therapy?

A. Ciprofloxacin for 5 weeks
B. Ampicillin for 10 days
C. Levofloxacin for 10 days
D. Cephalexin for 10 days
E. Cefaclor for 5 weeks

ID, GU

P 309   A 41-year-old man has acute bacterial prostatitis manifest by fever, dysuria, and urinary frequency. Which of the following is the most likely infecting organism?

A. *Yersinia*
B. *Neisseria*
C. *Gardnerella*
D. *Bacteroides*
E. *Proteus*

HEME, CV

P 310   A 74-year-old woman has acute dyspnea and hemoptysis. In the past 2 months, she has lost 8 pounds and has a poor appetite. Blood pressure is 112/72 mm Hg, pulse is 112/min, and respiratory rate is 23/min. Examination shows a thin, noncyanotic patient. Lungs are clear to auscultation. Examination of the heart and abdomen is normal. Which of the following is the most likely underlying diagnosis?

A. Systemic lupus erythematosus
B. Factor V Leiden mutation
C. Mural thrombus of the left ventricle
D. Adenocarcinoma of the pancreas
E. Idiopathic thrombocytopenic purpura

PSY/LE

P 311   A 72-year-old man has newly diagnosed Alzheimer's disease. Which of the following classes of medicines is the preferred initial therapy?

A. 5-Phosphodiesterase
B. Alpha-adrenergic blocker
C. Monoamine oxidase inhibitor
D. Antioxidant
E. Cholinesterase inhibitor

PSY/LE

P 312   Donepezil therapy is initiated in a 76-year-old woman in treatment of Alzheimer's disease. Her caregiver should be counseled that which of the following is the most likely adverse effect?

A. Orthostatic lightheadedness
B. Constipation
C. Nausea
D. Purpura
E. Night sweats

P 313   A 42-year-old man with Crohn's disease has a newly diagnosed anemia. An increased serum level of which of the following is most suggestive of vitamin B_{12} deficiency as the cause of the anemia?

    A. Methylmalonic acid

    B. Ceruloplasmin

    C. Calcitonin

    D. Coproporphyrin

    E. Unconjugated bilirubin

P 314   Lithium therapy is initiated in a 34-year-old woman for bipolar disorder. The patient should be counseled to have monitoring of which of the following serum levels while receiving the medication?

    A. Ferritin

    B. Thyroid-stimulating hormone

    C. Lactate dehydrogenase

    D. Folinic acid

    E. Cortisol

P 315   Radioactive iodine (RAI) therapy is to be given to a 66-year-old woman in treatment of hyperthyroidism related to a toxic nodule. She should be counseled to have serial monitoring of which of the following diagnostic tests?

    A. Presence of antithyroid peroxidase antibodies

    B. Presence of antiacetylcholine antibodies

    C. Serum thyroid-stimulating hormone level

    D. Left ventricular ejection fraction

    E. Serum calcitonin level

P 316   Oral amiodarone therapy is initiated in a 67-year-old man in treatment of paroxysmal atrial fibrillation. The patient should be counseled to have serial monitoring of which of the following diagnostic tests?

    A. Platelet count

    B. Thyroid-stimulating hormone

    C. Alpha-fetoprotein

    D. Brain natriuretic peptide

    E. Adrenocorticotropic hormone (ACTH)

P 317   Methotrexate therapy is to be initiated in a 17-year-old boy for acute leukemia. Which of the following should be administered in an effort to reduce the risk of methotrexate-induced hepatotoxicity?

    A. Pyridoxine (vitamin B_6)

    B. Leucovorin

    C. Interferon alfa

    D. Interleukin-6

    E. Prednisone

GI/N, HEME/ONC

P 318   A 6-year-old boy has sickle cell disease. He is at greatest risk of developing which of the following?

A. Acute lymphoblastic leukemia
B. Dilated cardiomyopathy
C. Autoimmune hypothyroidism
D. Bilirubin gallstones
E. Pulmonary bullae

GI/N, ID

P 319   A 56-year-old woman with cirrhosis and ascites has a 2-day history of fever, abdominal pain, and confusion. Presence of which of the following on examination of the ascitic fluid is most suggestive of spontaneous bacterial peritonitis?

A. Neutrophil count greater than 250/microL
B. Glucose greater than 150 mg/dL
C. Pressure of ascitic fluid greater than systemic arterial pressure
D. Total bilirubin greater than 5 mg/dL
E. Total protein greater than 4 g/dL

GI/N, NEURO

P 320   A 63-year-old woman who has cirrhosis and ascites has a 2-day history of fever, abdominal pain, and confusion. Ascitic fluid cell count is 300 neutrophils/microL. Spontaneous bacterial peritonitis is suspected while results of fluid culture are awaited. Which of the following is the most likely infecting organism?

A. *Klebsiella pneumoniae*
B. *Pseudomonas aeruginosa*
C. *Escherichia coli*
D. *Staphylococcus epidermidis*
E. Enterobacteriaceae

CV

P 321   A 77-year-old man has chronic atrial fibrillation treated with warfarin and metoprolol. Ambulatory cardiac monitoring persistently shows the ventricular rate to be greater than 100/min. Which of the following is the most likely complication of the persistent tachycardia?

A. Endocardial fibroelastosis
B. Rupture of chordate tendineae
C. Dilated cardiomyopathy
D. Autonomic insufficiency
E. Endocarditis

The Performance section is like a PANCE or PANRE. There is only *one* best answer.

CV

P 322   Presence of which of the following differentiates nephrotic syndrome from superior vena cava syndrome?

    A. Elevated jugular venous pressure
    B. Facial edema
    C. Systemic hypertension
    D. Edema of the feet
    E. Increased plasma oncotic pressure

HEME/ONC, PUL

P 323   Presence of which of the following differentiates polycythemia rubra vera from secondary erythrocytosis in the patient who has chronic bronchitis?

    A. Low systemic arterial oxygen saturation (Pao_2)
    B. Low red blood cell mass
    C. Low serum erythropoietin level
    D. Elevated storage iron in the bone marrow
    E. Elevated pulmonary artery pressure

MS

P 324   Which of the following is the primary mechanism of action of bisphos-phonates in the treatment of osteoporosis?

    A. Inhibition of osteoclastic bone resorption
    B. Stimulation of osteoblasts in the bone
    C. Reduce urinary calcium excretion
    D. Enhance intestinal absorption of calcium
    E. Enhance production of type 1 collagen in the bone marrow

ENDO, CV

P 325   Oral amiodarone therapy is initiated in a 47-year-old woman in treatment of paroxysmal atrial fibrillation. Which of the following serum levels should be serially monitored in the patient?

    A. Follicle-stimulating hormone (FSH)
    B. Thyroid-stimulating hormone (TSH)
    C. Estradiol
    D. Angiotensin-converting enzyme (ACE)
    E. Growth hormone

NEURO

P 326   Presence of which of the following differentiates a migraine headache from a transient ischemic attack?

    A. Polyuria
    B. Decrease in systemic arterial oxygen pressure (Pao_2)
    C. Starts with positive neurologic symptoms
    D. Symptoms are unilateral
    E. Association with transient cranial nerve III palsy

PSY/LE

P 327   The mother of a 7-year-old boy who has attention deficit hyperactivity disorder (ADHD) asks about the long-term prognosis for her child. Which of the following is most likely to be present during adulthood?

A. Bipolar disorder
B. Antisocial personality disorder
C. Dysthymia
D. Major depression
E. Conversion disorder

GI/N

P 328   A newborn infant has meconium ileus. Which of the following is the preferred initial test for cystic fibrosis?

A. Sweat chloride concentration
B. Stool osmotic gap
C. Blood immunoreactive trypsin (IRT)
D. Serum calcium concentration
E. Deoxycholic acid concentration in stool

ENDO

P 329   Which of the following is the common denominator in patients who have acanthosis nigricans that is not associated with malignancy?

A. Elevated serum concentration of vascular endothelial growth factor
B. Growth hormone insensitivity syndrome
C. Elevated erythrocyte concentration of carbonic anhydrase
D. Insulin resistance
E. Thyroid hormone resistance

EENT

P 330   A 34-year-old woman has a corneal abrasion secondary to contact lens wear. Which of the following should be avoided in treatment?

A. Oral nonsteroidal anti-inflammatory drugs (NSAIDs)
B. Topical quinolone antibiotics
C. Cold compresses
D. Eye patching
E. Topical aminoglycoside antibiotic

HEME/ONC, CV

P 331   The glycoprotein IIb/IIIa inhibitor abciximab is administered to a patient undergoing percutaneous coronary intervention with stent placement. Which of the following is the most likely adverse effect to be noted 2 hours later?

A. Thrombocytopenia
B. Fluctuating hypertension
C. Hyperglycemia
D. Abdominal distention caused by gastroparesis
E. Hypokalemia

The Performance section is like a PANCE or PANRE. There is only *one* best answer.

P 332   A 63-year-old man with type 2 diabetes mellitus has slowly progressive burning and numbness in both ankles and feet. Which of the following is the most likely sign to be noted upon examination?

A. Extensor Babinski sign bilaterally
B. Ankle clonus bilaterally
C. Absence of knee deep tendon reflexes bilaterally
D. Impaired stereognosis bilaterally
E. Impaired serial 7 subtraction

ID

P 333   A 14-year-old girl has fever, malaise, and sore throat. Infectious mononucleosis is diagnosed. Which of the following coexisting conditions is most likely to be present?

A. Pneumococcal otitis media
B. Tinea corporis
C. Rosacea
D. Molluscum contagiosum
E. Streptoccoccal pharyngitis

ENDO

P 334   Presence of which of the following differentiates primary from secondary adrenal insufficiency?

A. Weight loss
B. Hyperpigmentation
C. Orthostatic hypotension
D. Reduced serum adrenocorticotropin hormone (ACTH) level
E. Hypercalcemia

ENDO

P 335   Prednisone therapy is initiated in a 57-year-old woman in treatment of chronic adrenal insufficiency. Despite increasing doses of the medication, hyperkalemia persists. Addition of which of the following is the most appropriate therapy?

A. Oral hydrocortisone
B. Oral fludrocortisone
C. Oral triamterene
D. Oral hydrochlorothiazide
E. Inhaled albuterol

CV, ENDO

P 336   Prednisone therapy is initiated in a 57-year-old woman in treatment of chronic adrenal insufficiency. Despite increasing doses of the medication, orthostatic hypotension persists. Which of the following is the pathophysiologic abnormality causing the hypotension?

A. Autonomic insufficiency
B. Depletion of myocardial adrenergic receptors
C. Depletion of mineralocorticoid
D. Carotid sinus hypersensitivity
E. Degeneration of the amygdala in the brain

CV

P 337   A 77-year-old woman is in acute pulmonary edema and receives nesiritide as part of her therapy. Which of the following is the class of this medication?

A. Alpha-adrenergic agonist
B. Beta-adrenergic blocker
C. Loop diuretic
D. Brain natriuretic peptide
E. Calcium channel blocker

ID

P 338   The mother of a 2-year-old boy inquires about influenza vaccine. Her son has cystic fibrosis and is allergic to eggs. Which of the following is appropriate counseling?

A. Neither inactivated nor live attenuated vaccine contains egg protein
B. Only live attenuated vaccine contains egg protein
C. Only inactivated vaccine contains egg protein
D. Both inactivated and live vaccines are contraindicated
E. Inactivated vaccine should be considered

NEURO, ID

P 339   Presence of which of the following in the analysis of cerebrospinal fluid differentiates bacterial from viral meningitis?

A. Glucose level
B. Protein level
C. White blood count
D. Pressure measurement
E. Type of white blood cell in fluid

NEURO, ID

P 340   Presence of which of the following differentiates meningococcal meningitis from pneumococcal meningitis?

A. Focal neurologic signs
B. Elevated neutrophil count in cerebrospinal fluid
C. Petechial rash
D. Low glucose level in cerebrospinal fluid
E. Occurrence in asplenic patients

The Performance section is like a PANCE or PANRE. There is only *one* best answer.

REPRO

P 341   A 23-year-old woman has newly diagnosed primary dysmenorrhea. Gynecologic examination is normal. Which of the following diagnostic tests should be routinely performed?

    A. Transvaginal ultrasound
    B. Hepatitis serology
    C. Rh testing
    D. Chlamydia testing
    E. Cervical culture for *N. gonorrhoeae*

ENDO

P 342   Oral hypoglycemic therapy is to be initiated in a 62-year-old obese man who has type 2 diabetes mellitus. Blood urea nitrogen and serum creatinine values are normal. Which of the following is more likely to occur if the patient is treated with a sulfonylurea rather than metformin?

    A. Lactic acidosis
    B. Hypoglycemia
    C. Acute renal insufficiency
    D. Weight loss
    E. Hypokalemia

REPRO

P 343   A 22-year-old woman with a newborn male infant seeks counseling concerning sudden infant death syndrome (SIDS). Which of the following is the most appropriate advice in order to reduce the risk of SIDS?

    A. Baby should sleep in the prone position
    B. Use a soft mattress
    C. Wrap baby in blankets to minimize heat loss
    D. Delay initial vaccinations for 6 months
    E. Baby should use a pacifier

ENDO, ID

P 344   Levofloxacin therapy is to be initiated in a 24-year-old woman who has type 1 diabetes mellitus. Which of the following is appropriate counseling for the patient concerning the potential effect of taking the antibiotic and insulin?

    A. Increases likelihood of having nausea
    B. Increases likelihood of having urticaria
    C. Increases risk of having hypoglycemic episodes
    D. Increases risk of developing jaundice
    E. Increases likelihood of having tinnitus

ID

P 345   A 7-day-old infant has chlamydial conjunctivitis. Which of the following classes of medicine is the preferred initial treatment?

A. Macrolide
B. Cephalosporin
C. Tetracycline
D. Carbapenem
E. Fluoroquinolone

GI/N

P 346   Macrolide therapy is initiated in a 6-day-old male infant for treatment of chlamydial conjunctivitis. Which of the following is the condition that is most likely to develop in the infant?

A. Henoch-Schönlein purpura
B. Polymyositis
C. Nephrotic syndrome
D. Infantile pyloric stenosis
E. Meningismus

GI/N

P 347   A 4-week-old male infant has infantile pyloric stenosis. Which of the following signs is most likely to be noted upon physical examination?

A. Ejection murmur in the pulmonic area
B. Elevated jugular venous pressure
C. Inguinal adenopathy
D. Splenomegaly
E. Jaundice

CV

P 348   A 67-year-old man has type 2 diabetes mellitus. Presence of which of the following is a risk factor for sudden cardiac death in this patient?

A. Atrial premature beats
B. Orthostatic hypotension
C. Fixed heart rate during deep breathing
D. 1st-degree atrioventricular block on electrocardiography
E. S4 gallop on cardiac auscultation

CV

P 349   A 76-year-old man with hypertension has the sudden onset of severe, tearing anterior chest pain. Presence of which of the following on physical examination is most suggestive of dissection of the ascending aorta?

A. Cranial nerve III (oculomotor) palsy
B. Hypotension
C. S4 gallop on cardiac auscultation
D. Unequal blood pressure in the arms
E. Radial-femoral artery pulse lag

The Performance section is like a PANCE or PANRE. There is only *one* best answer.

NEURO

P 350   A 44-year-old man has a severe cluster headache. In addition to sumatriptan therapy, which of the following is the preferred management?

A. Inhalation of 100% oxygen
B. Administration of intravenous isotonic saline
C. Oral oxycodone
D. Oral propranolol
E. Oral dapsone

ID, GU

P 351   A 34-year-old man has dysuria and a urethral discharge. Which of the following is the preferred diagnostic test to confirm chlamydial infection?

A. Culture of urethral specimen
B. Direct immunofluorescence
C. ELISA
D. Nucleic acid amplification
E. Complement fixation

GU/ID

P 352   A 33-year-old man is hospitalized for treatment of acute bacterial prostatitis. On the second hospital day, he develops urinary retention. Which of the following is the preferred management of the urinary retention?

A. Suprapubic drainage of the urinary bladder
B. Insertion of a urethral catheter
C. Administration of oral prostigmine
D. Administration of oral phenazopyridine (Pyridium)
E. Manual abdominal compression of the urinary bladder

DERM

P 353   Presence of which of the following differentiates Stevens-Johnson syndrome from erythema multiforme?

A. Buccal mucosal lesions
B. Skin necrosis
C. Splinter hemorrhages
D. Lymphadenopathy
E. Target lesions

HEME/ONC

P 354   Dabigatran therapy is to be initiated in a 57-year-old man in treatment of nonvalvular atrial fibrillation. Which of the following is proper counseling for the patient?

A. Avoid intake of acetaminophen
B. Avoid intake of lithium
C. Slowing of urination is an adverse effect
D. Avoid intake of macrolide antibiotics
E. Keep medicine capsules in original bottle

HEME/ONC

P 355   After 6 days of continuous unfractionated heparin therapy, a 65-year-old woman has thrombocytopenia. Which of the following is the pathophysiologic mechanism causing the low platelet count?

A. Decreased bone marrow production
B. Generalized endothelial destruction
C. Antiplatelet antibodies
D. Splenic sequestration of platelets
E. Consumptive coagulopathy

CV

P 356   An 81-year-old man with diabetes mellitus and chronic hypertension has new-onset atrial fibrillation. Blood pressure is 140/76 mm Hg, and pulse is 82/min. Cardiac examination is normal. There is no clinical evidence of heart failure. After parenteral heparin therapy, which of the following is the most appropriate long-term management?

A. Oral warfarin
B. Oral clopidogrel
C. Oral aspirin
D. No long-term anticoagulant therapy is indicated
E. Intravenous abciximab (ReoPro)

CV, HEME/ONC

P 357   A 55-year-old woman with chronic hypertension and type 2 diabetes mellitus has her first episode of atrial fibrillation lasting 1 hour. Blood pressure is 134/72 mm Hg, and pulse is 76/min. The heart size is normal. No murmur or gallop is heard. There is no clinical evidence of heart failure. Which of the following is the most appropriate management?

A. Initiate oral dabigatran
B. Initiate oral clopidogrel
C. Initiate oral aspirin
D. No anticoagulant therapy
E. Perform in vitro assay for aspirin resistance

ENDO

P 358   Thyroxine therapy is to be initiated in a 57-year-old woman in treatment of hypothyroidism. Which of the following is proper counseling for the patient concerning thyroxine?

A. Take on empty stomach 1 hour before breakfast
B. Avoid intake of macrolide antibiotic
C. May cause painful urticaria
D. Proton pump inhibitors increase absorption
E. Sit on side of bed before standing

ENDO, CV

P 359   A 66-year-old woman has the sudden onset of very fast heartbeat. Electrocardiography shows atrial fibrillation with a ventricular rate of 148/min. Presence of which of the following signs is most likely to be associated with the tachyarrhythmia?

A. Lid lag
B. Xanthomas on extensor surface of elbows
C. Acanthosis nigricans
D. Dry coarse skin
E. Splenomegaly

ID, CV

P 360   A 62-year-old woman is in septic shock caused by perforated diverticulitis. Which of the following is the preferred initial intravenous solution to be administered?

A. Normal saline
B. ½ normal saline
C. 5% dextrose in water
D. Ringer's lactate
E. Mannitol

ID

P 361   A 71-year-old man is hypotensive with blood pressure of 70/44 mm Hg and pulse of 136/min. Presence of which of the following on clinical evaluation differentiates gram-negative septic shock from cardiogenic shock?

A. Confusion
B. Oliguria
C. Meiosis
D. Hyperreflexia
E. Warm, dry skin

ENDO

P 362   Presence of which of the following differentiates paresthesias caused by hypoglycemia from paresthesias caused by hypocalcemia?

A. Sweating
B. Metabolic alkalosis
C. Polyuria
D. Long QT on electrocardiography
E. Horner's syndrome

ID

P 363   A 56-year-old woman has a 1-day history of fever, chills, and jaundice. Ascending cholangitis is diagnosed. Which of the following is the most likely complication?

A. Thrombotic thrombocytopenic purpura
B. Cardiogenic shock
C. Gram-negative bacteremia
D. Meningismus
E. IgA glomerulonephritis

CV

P 364 A 17-year-old boy has newly diagnosed hypertrophic obstructive cardiomyopathy. Which of the following is the most appropriate counseling related to his 12-year-old brother who is asymptomatic?

A. Tilt table testing
B. Annual echocardiography until age 18 years
C. Cardiac catheterization
D. Treadmill exercise testing
E. Avoid contact sports

DERM

P 365 A 22-year-old woman has a 2-day history of target lesions on her trunk. Erythema multiforme is diagnosed. Which of the following is the most likely underlying cause?

A. *Streptococcus pyogenes* infection
B. Immune-mediated reaction
C. Antiphospholipid antibodies
D. Herpes simplex virus infection
E. *Histoplasma capsulatum* infection

ID, DERM

P 366 A 62-year-old man has newly diagnosed Lyme disease. Which of the following is most likely to be found upon physical examination?

A. Erythema marginatum
B. Erythema migrans
C. Erythema nodosum
D. Erythema multiforme
E. Bullous pemphigoid

HEME/ONC, GI/N

P 367 Clopidogrel (Plavix) therapy is initiated in a 71-year-old man after percutaneous coronary intervention (PCI) related to a non–ST segment elevation myocardial infarction. Which of the following is proper counseling for the patient regarding the clopidogrel?

A. Avoid intake of artificial sweeteners
B. Must be taken while fasting for at least 1 hour
C. Avoid intake of aspirin
D. May cause angioneurotic edema
E. Avoid intake of omeprazole

The Performance section is like a PANCE or PANRE. There is only *one* best answer.

P 368   Two weeks after a grand mal seizure, a 26-year-old man has fever, weakness, and cough productive of putrid sputum. Chest radiography shows a lung abscess. Which of the following is the most likely infecting organism causing the abscess?

    A. *Streptococcus pyogenes*
    B. *Staphylococcus aureus*
    C. *Bacteroides* species
    D. *Klebsiella pneumoniae*
    E. *Corynebacterium urealyticum*

P 369   Parenteral glucagon is administered to a 21-year-old woman with type 1 diabetes mellitus who has a hypoglycemic reaction to her injected insulin. Which of the following is the primary physiologic action of the glucagon?

    A. Promotes glycogenolysis and gluconeogenesis
    B. Promotes intestinal absorption of carbohydrate
    C. Depresses hepatic production of urea
    D. Stimulates cholecystokinin secretion
    E. Depresses oxidation of LDL cholesterol

P 370   A 22-year-old man notes painless enlargement of his right testis. An elevated serum concentration of which of the following is suggestive of a nonseminoma germ cell tumor?

    A. Human chorionic gonadotropin
    B. Prolactin
    C. IgA
    D. Testosterone
    E. Methylmalonic acid

P 371   A 30-year-old man notes painless enlargement of his left testis. An elevated serum concentration of which of the following is suggestive of a nonseminoma germ cell tumor?

    A. Alpha-fetoprotein
    B. IgM
    C. Calcitonin
    D. Serotonin
    E. Prolactin

CV

P 372   An 8-year-old child has fever and erythema of the lips, buccal mucosa, and palms. Kawasaki disease is diagnosed. Administration of which of the following reduces the incidence of coronary artery aneurysm formation?

A. Indomethacin
B. Penicillin G
C. Rituximab (Rituxan)
D. Prednisone
E. Intravenous immune globulin

DERM, MS

P 373   A 7-year-old girl has a 3-day history of hip and knee pain followed by onset of a purpuric rash on both lower legs. Henoch-Schönlein purpura is diagnosed. Deposition of which of the following in the walls of skin venules is most likely to be noted?

A. IgM
B. Amyloid
C. Mallory bodies
D. IgA
E. IgE

HEME/ONC, DERM

P 374   An 8-year-old boy has newly diagnosed Henoch-Schönlein purpura. Which of the following laboratory values would be expected in the patient?

A. Abnormally low erythrocyte sedimentation rate
B. Elevated prothrombin time
C. Normal platelet count
D. Elevated serum IgE concentration
E. Eosinophilia in peripheral blood

ID, DERM

P 375   A 7-year-old boy has newly diagnosed hand-foot-and-mouth syndrome with lesions on the tongue and extremities. Which of the following is appropriate counseling for the parent?

A. Child is not contagious at this time
B. Wash skin lesions with chlorhexidine
C. Apply petrolatum gel to skin lesions
D. Keep child out of school until rash clears
E. Avoid further immunizations for 1 year

The Performance section is like a PANCE or PANRE. There is only *one* best answer.

ID, DERM

P 376   A 28-year-old pregnant woman near term is to visit her nephew who is a 7-year-old boy who has hand-foot-and-mouth syndrome. Which of the following is appropriate counseling to the woman?

A. Avoid contact with the ill child
B. Take oral doxycycline during visit and for 3 days following
C. Take trimethoprim-sulfamethoxazole during visit
D. No precautions need to be taken during visit
E. Wear a face mask when in the same room with child

CV

P 377   A 9-year-old girl has congenital long QT syndrome. She is most likely to faint caused by polymorphous ventricular tachycardia (torsades de pointes) during which of the following?

A. Arising from bed
B. Urination
C. Argument
D. Ingestion of a frozen dessert
E. Using electric hair dryer

ENDO, REPRO

P 378   Which of the following is the primary physiologic basis for the infant of a diabetic mother to have macrosomia?

A. Excessive maternal growth hormone secretion
B. Increased fetal red cell mass
C. Suppressed renin-angiotensin activity in the fetus
D. Fetal hyperinsulinemia
E. Increased fetal cyclooxygenase activity

CV, GU

P 379   A 76-year-old woman has a 3-week history of weakness and muscle cramps. She is in chronic systolic heart failure for which she takes lisinopril, metoprolol, and furosemide. Which of the following is the most likely cause of the weakness and muscle cramps?

A. Hypomagnesemia
B. Hyperchloremia
C. Hypernatremia
D. Respiratory acidosis
E. Hypophosphatemia

Answers to Performance Questions

The symbol represents links to related questions and key information in the Essentials section.

P 001   (A) Digoxin
          Answer: E 013

P 002   (A) Oral administration of B-complex vitamins
          Answer: E 002

P 003   (B) Oral verapamil
          Answer: E 001

P 004   (C) Normal pressure hydrocephalus
          Answer: E 003

P 005   (D) Glucose-6-phosphate dehydrogenase deficiency
          Answer: E 006

P 006   (D) Thyroid-stimulating hormone 22 microU/mL
          Answer: E 003

P 007   (C) Diastolic heart failure
          Answer: E 001

P 008   (C) Anginal equivalent
          Answers: E 001 and E 007

P 009   (D) Hypertrophic obstructive cardiomyopathy
          Answers: E 001 and E 007

P 010   (A) Niacin
          Answer: E 008

P 011   (B) Verapamil
          ↩   Answer: E 009

P 012   (C) Intravenous administration of octreotide
          ↩   Answer: E 012

P 013   (A) Adverse effect of verapamil
          ↩   Answer: E 013

P 014   (B) Non-Hodgkin's lymphoma
          ↩   Answer: E 014

P 015   (D) Constrictive pericarditis
          ↩   Answer: E 014

P 016   (A) Transesophageal echocardiogram
          ↩   Answer: E 015

P 017   (A) Acute cholecystitis
          ↩   Answer: E 010

P 018   (B) Primary biliary cirrhosis
          ↩   Answer: E 016

P 019   (B) Initiate angiotensin-converting enzyme inhibitor therapy
          ↩   Answer: E 017

P 020   (C) Systemic lupus erythematosus
          ↩   Answer: E 018

P 021   (C) Autonomic insufficiency
          ↩   Answer: E 019

P 022   (D) Stand or sit upright for 30 minutes after taking medication
          ↩   Answer: E 020

P 023   (A) Insulin dosage may increase due to hyperglycemic effect of niacin
          ↩   Answer: E 008

P 024   (D) Propranolol
          ↩   Answer: E 021

P 025   (D) Recurrent myocardial infarction
          ↩   Answer: E 022

P 026   (B) Mitochondria
             ↩   Answer: E 016

P 027   (B) Alpha-fetoprotein
             ↩   Answer: E 012

P 028   (C) White blood cell count 2,100/microL
             ↩   Answer: E 018

P 029   (D) Pheochromocytoma
             ↩   Answer: E 019

P 030   (D) Cosyntropin stimulation test
             ↩   Answer: E 019

P 031   (E) Serum creatine kinase and troponin levels
             ↩   Answer: E 024

P 032   (C) Right heart failure
             ↩   Answer: E 025

P 033   (B) Obtain thyroid function values every 3 to 4 months
             ↩   Answer: E 026

P 034   (C) Amaurosis fugax
             ↩   Answer: E 027

P 035   (B) Tourette's syndrome
             ↩   Answer: E 028

P 036   (E) Oats
             ↩   Answer: E 029

P 037   (B) Heightened vagal tone
             ↩   Answer: E 023

P 038   (D) Pulmonary hypertension
             ↩   Answer: E 025

P 039   (D) Anorectal manometry
             ↩   Answer: E 030

P 040   (D) Cataracts
             ↩   Answer: E 031

P 041   (B) Avoid pregnancy while taking lithium
         ⟲   Answer: E 026

P 042   (A) Adenocarcinoma of the stomach
         ⟲   Answer: E 032

P 043   (B) Hypokalemia
         ⟲   Answer: E 033

P 044   (A) Aseptic meningitis
         ⟲   Answer: E 035

P 045   (C) Corneal ulceration
         ⟲   Answer: E 036

P 046   (E) Scleroderma
         ⟲   Answer: E 044

P 047   (A) ELISA test
         ⟲   Answer: E 037

P 048   (C) Oral allopurinol
         ⟲   Answer: E 038

P 049   (B) Elevated angiotensin-converting enzyme
         ⟲   Answer: E 039

P 050   (C) Avoid extended wear of the soft lens
         ⟲   Answer: E 036

P 051   (B) Diabetes mellitus
         ⟲   Answer: E 040

P 052   (D) Acute dissection of the thoracic aorta
         ⟲   Answer: E 042

P 053   (C) Perform duplex carotid artery ultrasound
         ⟲   Answer: E 027

P 054   (C) Initiate therapy with a bisphosphonate
         ⟲   Answer: E 031

P 055   (B) Hypokalemia
         ⟲   Answer: E 033

P 056   (C) Administration of intravenous glucose and insulin
             ↩ Answer: E 034

P 057   (D) Scleroderma
             ↩ Answer: E 044

P 058   (A) pH 7.48, Pao_2 66 mm Hg, $Paco_2$ 28 mm Hg
             ↩ Answer: E 039

P 059   (C) Decreased carbon monoxide diffusing capacity
             ↩ Answer: E 039

P 060   (B) Hypersegmented neutrophils
             ↩ Answer: E 051

P 061   (E) Henoch-Schönlein purpura
             ↩ Answer: E 049

P 062   (C) Methylmalonic acid
             ↩ Answer: E 051

P 063   (C) Transesophageal echocardiography
             ↩ Answer: E 042

P 064   (B) Do not take medication with antacids
             ↩ Answer: E 043

P 065   (B) Metoprolol
             ↩ Answer: E 042

P 066   (B) Abnormal position sense
             ↩ Answer: E 051

P 067   (C) Receive monthly vitamin B_{12} injections
             ↩ Answer: E 051

P 068   (C) Lack of intrinsic factor production
             ↩ Answer: E 051

P 069   (B) Adenocarcinoma of the lung
             ↩ Answer: E 058

P 070   (A) Decreased arterial compliance
             ↩ Answer: E 059

P 071   (C) Initiate thiazide therapy
          ↩   Answer: E 059

P 072   (C) Romberg test
          ↩   Answer: E 060

P 073   (C) Hyperthyroidism
          ↩   Answer: E 059

P 074   (B) Autonomic insufficiency
          ↩   Answer: E 054

P 075   (D) Hypovolemia
          ↩   Answer: E 054

P 076   (C) Diabetes mellitus
          ↩   Answer: E 054

P 077   (C) Ventricular wall stretching
          ↩   Answer: E 069

P 078   (D) Normal plasma Nt-BNP
          ↩   Answer: E 069

P 079   (E) Small cell carcinoma of the lung
          ↩   Answer: E 057

P 080   (E) *Pseudomonas aeruginosa*
          ↩   Answer: E 056

P 081   (B) Platelet count
          ↩   Answer: E 055

P 082   (D) Bronchiectasis
          ↩   Answer: E 056

P 083   (E) Hydrochlorothiazide
          ↩   Answer: E 026

P 084   (B) Avoid pregnancy
          ↩   Answer: E 026

P 085   (A) Unilateral character of visual symptoms
          ↩   Answer: E 027

P 086   (A) Prednisone
⟳   Answer: E 031

P 087   (E) Gastric adenocarcinoma
⟳   Answer: E 032

P 088   (B) Tissue insulin resistance
⟳   Answer: E 032

P 089   (B) Erythema migrans
⟳   Answer: E 037

P 090   (D) Oral allopurinol
⟳   Answer: E 038

P 091   (D) Normal FEV_1/FVC ratio
⟳   Answer: E 039

P 092   (B) Hyperuricemic nephropathy
⟳   Answer: E 038

P 093   (C) Metoprolol
⟳   Answer: E 045

P 094   (B) Decrease ventricular preload
⟳   Answer: E 046

P 095   (A) Hypomagnesemia
⟳   Answer: E 047

P 096   (A) Ability to wrinkle forehead on affected side
⟳   Answer: E 037

P 097   (C) Long QT interval syndrome
⟳   Answer: E 064

P 098   (D) Verapamil
⟳   Answer: E 048

P 099   (E) Hypertension
⟳   Answer: E 049

P 100   (D) Red blood cell casts
⟳   Answer: E 049

P 101   (B) Pernicious anemia
            ⤶   Answer: E 050

P 102   (C) Pernicious anemia
            ⤶   Answer: E 188

P 103   (A) Macrocytosis
            ⤶   Answer: E 050

P 104   (A) Elevated plasma adrenocorticotropin level
            ⤶   Answer: E 065

P 105   (B) Adrenal insufficiency
            ⤶   Answer: E 065

P 106   (C) White blood cell count 2,000/microL
            ⤶   Answers: E 018, E 052

P 107   (B) Avoid direct sunlight
            ⤶   Answer: E 052

P 108   (E) Serum antinuclear antibody titer
            ⤶   Answer: E 052

P 109   (B) Intranasal beclomethasone
            ⤶   Answer: E 053

P 110   (B) Coarctation of the aorta
            ⤶   Answers: E 057, E 170

P 111   (D) No need for endocarditis prophylaxis
            ⤶   Answer: E 079

P 112   (E) Verapamil
            ⤶   Answer: E 007

P 113   (B) Thallium stress cardiac testing
            ⤶   Answer: E 001

P 114   (A) Non-Hodgkin's lymphoma
            ⤶   Answer: E 014

P 115   (D) Move chin from side to side
            ⤶   Answer: E 037

P 116   (B) Paget's disease of bone
⮌   Answer: E 066

P 117   (B) Significant aortic stenosis is likely to occur in adulthood
⮌   Answer: E 057

P 118   (D) Verapamil
⮌   Answer: E 013

P 119   (A) Diltiazem
⮌   Answer: E 013

P 120   (B) Elevated urinary hydroxyproline
⮌   Answer: E 066

P 121   (A) Dilated cardiomyopathy
⮌   Answer: E 013

P 122   (C) Nadolol
⮌   Answer: E 012

P 123   (D) Alpha-fetoprotein
⮌   Answer: E 012

P 124   (B) ST segment elevation
⮌   Answer: E 007

P 125   (A) Do not become pregnant while on therapy
⮌   Answer: E 070

P 126   (B) Pitting of nails
⮌   Answer: E 082

P 127   (B) Panic disorder
⮌   Answer: E 093

P 128   (E) Withdraw medication over 1 week if it is to be discontinued
⮌   Answer: E 070

P 129   (D) "Sharpened pencil" appearance of fingers
⮌   Answer: E 082

P 130   (A) Angiotensin-converting enzyme inhibitor
⮌   Answer: E 070

P 131   (C) Captopril
⮌   Answer: E 070

P 132   (A) Betamethasone with clotrimazole (Lotrisone)
⮌   Answer: E 081

P 133   (A) Hydrochlorothiazide
⮌   Answer: E 070

P 134   (D) Hydrochlorothiazide
⮌   Answer: E 070

P 135   (D) Thiazide
⮌   Answer: E 070

P 136   (B) Glucagon
⮌   Answer: E 085

P 137   (D) Potassium hydroxide preparation of scales
⮌   Answer: E 081

P 138   (A) Selective serotonin receptor inhibitors
⮌   Answer: E 071

P 139   (E) Phosphodiesterase-5 inhibitors
⮌   Answer: E 071

P 140   (B) Place clothes worn before diagnosis in a plastic bag for 10 days
⮌   Answer: E 072

P 141   (E) *Streptococcus*
⮌   Answer: E 080

P 142   (C) Lichen planus
⮌   Answer: E 072

P 143   (C) Metronidazole gel
⮌   Answer: E 072

P 144   (E) Saliva may remain contagious for 6 months
⮌   Answer: E 080

P 145   (B) Alcohol ingestion
⮌   Answer: E 072

P 146   (B) Cor pulmonale
              ⮌   Answer: E 073

P 147   (C) Verapamil
              ⮌   Answers: E 013 and E 087

P 148   (B) Pao_2 60 mm Hg, $Paco_2$ 60 mm Hg
              ⮌   Answer: E 073

P 149   (E) Mitral valve prolapse
              ⮌   Answer: E 079

P 150   (D) St. John's wort
              ⮌   Answer: E 074

P 151   (C) Haloperidol
              ⮌   Answer: E 074

P 152   (D) Chronic obstructive lung disease
              ⮌   Answer: E 087

P 153   (D) Infusion of 0.9% saline
              ⮌   Answer: E 091

P 154   (B) Serotonin syndrome
              ⮌   Answer: E 074

P 155   (E) Autoimmune destruction of pancreatic B cells
              ⮌   Answer: E 085

P 156   (B) Check blood pressure in 10 to 14 days
              ⮌   Answers: E 016, E 075

P 157   (E) Indomethacin
              ⮌   Answer: E 075

P 158   (A) Have liver function tests performed every 4 to 8 weeks
              ⮌   Answer: E 076

P 159   (A) Do not take acetaminophen in a dosage greater than 2.0 g/day
              ⮌   Answer: E 077

P 160   (A) Mechanical heart valve in aortic position
              ⮌   Answer: E 079

P 161   (A) Level of 24-hour urinary excretion of uric acid
           ⟲   Answer: E 078

P 162   (E) Avoid ingestion of alcohol
           ⟲   Answer: E 078

P 163   (D) Reduce ingestion of red meat and shellfish
           ⟲   Answer: E 078

P 164   (B) Leg claudication
           ⟲   Answer: E 087

P 165   (D) Elevated serum luteinizing hormone
           ⟲   Answer: E 086

P 166   (D) Waist-to-hip fat ratio
           ⟲   Answer: E 085

P 167   (A) HLA-DR3 gene
           ⟲   Answer: E 085

P 168   (D) Stool for occult blood
           ⟲   Answer: E 084

P 169   (C) Triglycerides
           ⟲   Answer: E 083

P 170   (D) Diverticulosis
           ⟲   Answer: E 083

P 171   (C) No antibiotic therapy
           ⟲   Answer: E 088

P 172   (D) Orthostatic hypotension
           ⟲   Answer: E 092

P 173   (E) Sublingual lorazepam (Ativan)
           ⟲   Answer: E 093

P 174   (B) Normal saline
           ⟲   Answer: E 091

P 175   (E) Serum D-dimer level of 400 ng/mL
           ⟲   Answer: E 105

P 176   (E) Avoid pregnancy
              ⤺   Answer: E 103

P 177   (C) Serum D-dimer level of 400 ng/mL
              ⤺   Answer: E 105

P 178   (D) Captopril
              ⤺   Answer: E 103

P 179   (C) Outpatient treatment with clarithromycin
              ⤺   Answer: E 102

P 180   (E) *Pseudomonas aeruginosa*
              ⤺   Answer: E 102

P 181   (D) Tolerated as well as in nonasthmatic
              ⤺   Answer: E 101

P 182   (D) Hotel showers
              ⤺   Answer: E 102

P 183   (D) Legionnaires' disease
              ⤺   Answer: E 102

P 184   (A) Partially hydrogenated coffee creamer
              ⤺   Answer: E 100

P 185   (E) Pneumonia with effusion
              ⤺   Answer: E 104

P 186   (A) t-PA
              ⤺   Answer: E 097

P 187   (E) Hyponatremia
              ⤺   Answer: E 104

P 188   (B) Myocardial infarction
              ⤺   Answer: E 096

P 189   (A) Gastroparesis
              ⤺   Answer: E 095

P 190   (D) Nephrotic syndrome
              ⤺   Answer: E 104

P 191   (E) Intravenous alteplase
         ↩   Answer: E 097

P 192   (B) Nuclear scintigraphy after radioactive-labeled meal
         ↩   Answer: E 095

P 193   (C) Ofloxacin
         ↩   Answer: E 099

P 194   (C) Zoster rash may appear in 24 to 48 hours
         ↩   Answer: E 098

P 195   (D) Serum to ascites albumin gradient
         ↩   Answer: E 094

P 196   (D) Spontaneous bacterial peritonitis
         ↩   Answer: E 094

P 197   (D) *Giardia lamblia*
         ↩   Answer: E 113

P 198   (A) Axillary temperature of 103.6°F
         ↩   Answer: E 113

P 199   (E) *Cryptosporidium*
         ↩   Answer: E 113

P 200   (B) Irritable bowel syndrome
         ↩   Answer: E 113

P 201   (D) Nafcillin
         ↩   Answer: E 106

P 202   (E) Arteriovenous fistula
         ↩   Answer: E 107

P 203   (A) Healthy 22-year-old nurse
         ↩   Answer: E 110

P 204   (E) Sore throat
         ↩   Answer: E 111

P 205   (D) Hyperthyroidism
         ↩   Answer: E 107

P 206　(A)　Nonaspirin, nonselective, nonsteroidal anti-inflammatory
　　　　　↩　　Answer: E 114

P 207　(D)　Na − (Cl + HCO$_3$)
　　　　　↩　　Answer: E 108

P 208　(A)　47-year-old healthy woman
　　　　　↩　　Answer: E 110

P 209　(D)　Lumbar puncture
　　　　　↩　　Answer: E 112

P 210　(D)　Epidural blood patch
　　　　　↩　　Answer: E 112

P 211　(E)　Assurance to patient that symptoms disappear after delivery
　　　　　↩　　Answer: E 109

P 212　(D)　Hydrocortisone foam enemas
　　　　　↩　　Answer: E 114

P 213　(C)　Anti–thyroid-stimulating hormone receptor antibodies
　　　　　↩　　Answer: E 111

P 214　(B)　Production of lactic acid
　　　　　↩　　Answer: E 108

P 215　(A)　Flexible sigmoidoscopy
　　　　　↩　　Answer: E 114

P 216　(D)　Serum thyroid-stimulating hormone level
　　　　　↩　　Answer: E 109

P 217　(E)　Chocolate ice cream
　　　　　↩　　Answer: E 115

P 218　(A)　Increased anion gap metabolic acidosis
　　　　　↩　　Answer: E 108

P 219　(D)　Methimazole
　　　　　↩　　Answer: E 111

P 220　(D)　Ranitidine at bedtime
　　　　　↩　　Answer: E 115

P 221   (B) Serum thyroid-stimulating hormone level
⮌   Answer: E 111

P 222   (B) Colon cancer
⮌   Answer: E 114

P 223   (E) Gastroesophageal reflux
⮌   Answer: E 115

P 224   (B) Proteinuria
⮌   Answer: E 118

P 225   (E) Seizures
⮌   Answer: E 118

P 226   (E) Recurrent fetal loss
⮌   Answer: E 118

P 227   (C) Endothelial dysfunction
⮌   Answer: E 118

P 228   (D) Transvaginal ultrasonography
⮌   Answer: E 119

P 229   (C) History of bipolar coagulation sterilization
⮌   Answer: E 119

P 230   (D) Immune due to hepatitis B vaccination
⮌   Answer: E 120

P 231   (C) Chlorpromazine (Thorazine)
⮌   Answer: E 122

P 232   (E) Hemolytic anemia
⮌   Answer: E 122

P 233   (E) Ascending cholangitis
⮌   Answer: E 122

P 234   (D) Antimitochondrial
⮌   Answer: E 122

P 235   (B) Ratio of serum AST/ALT is greater than 2:1
⮌   Answer: E 122

P 236 (B) Ibuprofen

⮌ Answer: E 123

P 237 (E) Selective serotonin reuptake inhibitor

⮌ Answer: E 124

P 238 (A) Anion gap of 18 mEq/L

⮌ Answer: E 127

P 239 (E) Lactic acidosis

⮌ Answer: E 128

P 240 (A) Heavy alcohol intake

⮌ Answer: E 128

P 241 (B) Do not take metformin on morning of study

⮌ Answer: E 128

P 242 (D) Azithromycin

⮌ Answer: E 129

P 243 (B) Lidocaine

⮌ Answer: E 130

P 244 (E) Administration of nebulized albuterol

⮌ Answer: E 130

P 245 (D) Flattening of T waves with prominent U waves

⮌ Answer: E 130

P 246 (A) Anti-acetylcholine receptor

⮌ Answer: E 131

P 247 (E) Anti–thyroid-stimulating hormone receptor antibodies

⮌ Answer: E 131

P 248 (E) Oral angiotensin-converting enzyme inhibitor

⮌ Answer: E 132

P 249 (B) Deep vein thrombosis

⮌ Answer: E 132

P 250 (C) Hodgkin's disease

⮌ Answer: E 133

P 251   (D) Normal gait
               ⟲   Answer: E 134

P 252   (E) Fasciculations
               ⟲   Answer: E 134

P 253   (D) Subclavian steal syndrome
               ⟲   Answer: E 136

P 254   (E) Percutaneous luminal angioplasty
               ⟲   Answer: E 136

P 255   (D) Angiotensin-converting enzyme inhibitor
               ⟲   Answer: E 132

P 256   (B) Do not smoke during pregnancy
               ⟲   Answer: E 138

P 257   (E) Orthostatic hypotension
               ⟲   Answer: E 134

P 258   (A) History of deep vein thrombosis
               ⟲   Answer: E 139

P 259   (A) Increases tissue sensitivity to insulin
               ⟲   Answer: E 141

P 260   (E) Glyburide therapy must be replaced by insulin
               ⟲   Answer: E 141

P 261   (A) Hemosiderinuria
               ⟲   Answer: E 143

P 262   (D) Ferritin 8 ng/mL
               ⟲   Answer: E 143

P 263   (E) Decreased gastrointestinal absorption of iron
               ⟲   Answer: E 143

P 264   (E) Captopril
               ⟲   Answer: E 142

P 265   (A) Iron deficiency
               ⟲   Answer: E 143

P 266   (D) Alpha-fetoprotein
        ↩   Answer: E 144

P 267   (D) Alpha-fetoprotein
        ↩   Answer: E 144

P 268   (D) Intravascular hemolysis
        ↩   Answer: E 145

P 269   (C) Erythema infectiosum
        ↩   Answer: E 146

P 270   (E) CD lymphocyte count is less than 200 cells/microL
        ↩   Answer: E 147

P 271   (A) Zoster vaccination
        ↩   Answer: E 148

P 272   (E) Extensor Babinski response
        ↩   Answer: E 149

P 273   (D) Diabetes mellitus
        ↩   Answer: E 149

P 274   (E) Nocturnal diarrhea
        ↩   Answer: E 150

P 275   (D) Sudden cardiac death
        ↩   Answer: E 150

P 276   (A) Autonomic insufficiency
        ↩   Answer: E 150

P 277   (D) Uterine contractions
        ↩   Answer: E 151

P 278   (E) Presence of antiphospholipid antibodies
        ↩   Answer: E 151

P 279   (A) Daily oral penicillin
        ↩   Answer: E 152

P 280   (E) Administration of lactulose enema
        ↩   Answer: E 153

P 281   (D) Hypokalemia
⟳   Answer: E 153

P 282   (C) Ingestion of excess water during race
⟳   Answer: E 155

P 283   (E) Visual hallucinations
⟳   Answer: E 156

P 284   (A) Diabetes insipidus
⟳   Answer: E 157

P 285   (D) Hypoglycemia
⟳   Answer: E 158

P 286   (B) Shift of fluid from circulation into bowel
⟳   Answer: E 158

P 287   (E) Human papillomavirus
⟳   Answer: E 159

P 288   (D) Disorientation
⟳   Answer: E 160

P 289   (E) Thiamine
⟳   Answer: E 160

P 290   (E) Macrolide
⟳   Answer: E 161

P 291   (D) Alpha-glucosidase inhibitors
⟳   Answer: E 162

P 292   (C) Increase sensitivity to insulin
⟳   Answer: E 162

P 293   (C) Low humidity
⟳   Answer: E 163

P 294   (B) Intravenous immune globulin plus aspirin
⟳   Answer: E 164

P 295   (D) Coronary artery aneurysm
⟳   Answer: E 164

P 296   (B) Decreases risk of ovarian cancer
              ↩   Answer: E 166

P 297   (A) Increased luteinizing hormone
              ↩   Answer: E 167

P 298   (E) Prolactin
              ↩   Answer: E 167

P 299   (B) 24-hour urine assay for catecholamines
              ↩   Answer: E 167

P 300   (D) Doxazosin
              ↩   Answer: E 168

P 301   (A) Avoid nonaspirin, nonselective, nonsteroidal anti-inflammatory
              agents
              ↩   Answer: E 168

P 302   (B) Check serum potassium concentration
              ↩   Answer: E 168

P 303   (C) Vertigo occurs when bending head back to look up
              ↩   Answer: E 171

P 304   (A) High-flow inhalation of oxygen via face mask
              ↩   Answer: E 172

P 305   (E) Strawberry cervix on physical examination
              ↩   Answer: E 175

P 306   (D) Vaginal epithelium cells with adherent bacteria
              ↩   Answer: E 175

P 307   (A) Ceftriaxone plus doxycycline
              ↩   Answers: E 099, E 175

P 308   (A) Ciprofloxacin for 5 weeks
              ↩   Answer: E 176

P 309   (E) *Proteus*
              ↩   Answer: E 176

P 310   (D) Adenocarcinoma of the pancreas
              ↩   Answer: E 116

P 311   (E) Cholinesterase inhibitor
          ⮌   Answer: E 002

P 312   (C) Nausea
          ⮌   Answer: E 002

P 313   (A) Methylmalonic acid
          ⮌   Answer: E 003

P 314   (B) Thyroid-stimulating hormone
          ⮌   Answer: E 003

P 315   (C) Serum thyroid-stimulating hormone level
          ⮌   Answer: E 062

P 316   (B) Thyroid-stimulating hormone
          ⮌   Answer: E 003

P 317   (B)Leucovorin
          ⮌   Answer: E 008

P 318   (D) Bilirubin gallstones
          ⮌   Answer: E 010

P 319   (A) Neutrophil count greater than 250/microL
          ⮌   Answer: E 012

P 320   (C) *Escherichia coli*
          ⮌   Answer: E 012

P 321   (C) Dilated cardiomyopathy
          ⮌   Answer: E 013

P 322   (D) Edema of the feet
          ⮌   Answer: E 014

P 323   (C) Low serum erythropoietin level
          ⮌   Answer: E 016

P 324   (A) Inhibition of osteoclastic bone resorption
          ⮌   Answer: E 020

P 325   (B) Thyroid-stimulating hormone (TSH)
          ⮌   Answer: E 026

P 326   (C) Starts with positive neurologic symptoms
        ⟳   Answer: E 027

P 327   (B) Antisocial personality disorder
        ⟳   Answer: E 028

P 328   (C) Blood immunoreactive trypsin (IRT)
        ⟳   Answer: E 030

P 329   (D) Insulin resistance
        ⟳   Answer: E 032

P 330   (D) Eye patching
        ⟳   Answer: E 036

P 331   (A) Thrombocytopenia
        ⟳   Answer: E 055

P 332   (C) Absence of knee deep tendon reflexes bilaterally
        ⟳   Answer: E 061

P 333   (E) Streptoccoccal pharyngitis
        ⟳   Answer: E 035

P 334   (B) Hyperpigmentation
        ⟳   Answer: E 065

P 335   (B) Oral fludrocortisone
        ⟳   Answer: E 067

P 336   (C) Depletion of mineralocorticoid
        ⟳   Answer: E 067

P 337   (D) Brain natriuretic peptide
        ⟳   Answer: E 069

P 338   (E) Inactivated vaccine should be considered
        ⟳   Answer: E 110

P 339   (E) Type of white blood cell in fluid
        ⟳   Answer: E 112

P 340   (C) Petechial rash
        ⟳   Answer: E 112

P 341   (D) Chlamydia testing
            ↩   Answer: E 123

P 342   (B) Hypoglycemia
            ↩   Answer: E 128

P 343   (E) Baby should use a pacifier
            ↩   Answer: E 138

P 344   (C) Increases risk of having hypoglycemic episodes
            ↩   Answer: E 140

P 345   (A) Macrolide
            ↩   Answer: E 161

P 346   (D) Infantile pyloric stenosis
            ↩   Answer: E 161

P 347   (E) Jaundice
            ↩   Answer: E 161

P 348   (C) Fixed heart rate during deep breathing
            ↩   Answer: E 150

P 349   (D) Unequal blood pressure in the arms
            ↩   Answer: E 170

P 350   (A) Inhalation of 100% oxygen
            ↩   Answer: E 174

P 351   (D) Nucleic acid amplification
            ↩   Answer: E 175

P 352   (A) Suprapubic drainage of the urinary bladder
            ↩   Answer: E 176

P 353   (B) Skin necrosis
            ↩   Answer: E 190

P 354   (E) Keep medicine capsules in original bottle
            ↩   Answer: E 192

P 355   (C) Antiplatelet antibodies
            ↩   Answer: E 193

P 356   (A) Oral warfarin
        ⟳   Answer: E 199

P 357   (A) Initiate oral dabigatran
        ⟳   Answer: E 199

P 358   (A) Take on empty stomach 1 hour before breakfast
        ⟳   Answer: E 198

P 359   (A) Lid lag
        ⟳   Answer: E 198

P 360   (A) Normal saline
        ⟳   Answer: E 206

P 361   (E) Warm dry skin
        ⟳   Answer: E 206

P 362   (A) Sweating
        ⟳   Answer: E 186

P 363   (C) Gram-negative bacteremia
        ⟳   Answer: E 206

P 364   (B) Annual echocardiography until age 18 years
        ⟳   Answer: E 189

P 365   (D) Herpes simplex virus infection
        ⟳   Answer: E 190

P 366   (B) Erythema migrans
        ⟳   Answer: E 190

P 367   (E) Avoid intake of omeprazole
        ⟳   Answer: E 213

P 368   (C) *Bacteroides* species
        ⟳   Answer: E 216

P 369   (A) Promotes glycogenolysis and gluconeogenesis
        ⟳   Answer: E 215

P 370   (A) Human chorionic gonadotropin
        ⟳   Answer: E 219

P 371   (A) Alpha-fetoprotein
        ↩   Answer: E 219

P 372   (E) Intravenous immune globulin
        ↩   Answer: E 218

P 373   (D) IgA
        ↩   Answer: E 227

P 374   (C) Normal platelet count
        ↩   Answer: E 227

P 375   (D) Keep child out of school until rash clears
        ↩   Answer: E 228

P 376   (A) Avoid contact with the ill child
        ↩   Answer: E 228

P 377   (C) Argument
        ↩   Answer: E 203

P 378   (D) Fetal hyperinsulinemia
        ↩   Answer: E 200

P 379   (A) Hypomagnesemia
        ↩   Answer: E 204

Appendix

How You Can Use the NCCPA Content Blueprint to Improve Your Test Performance

The section in the National Commission on Certification of Physician Assistants (NCCPA) website entitled "Exams: Content Blueprint/Task Areas" deserves critical review. Careful consideration of the blueprint will, I believe, result in improved test performance.

The defined NCCPA Task Areas are Applying Basic Concepts, History Taking and Performing Physical Examinations, Using Laboratory and Diagnostic Studies, Formulating Most Likely Diagnosis, Health Maintenance, Clinical Intervention, and Pharmaceutical Therapeutics.

Note: After each Essentials question there is "You Should Know," a succinct and rich resource that will help you prepare for the Performance questions. Again, remember that Performance questions are crafted in the same structure as PANCE and PANRE questions.

Davis's PA Exam Review **is logically designed to best prepare you for success on your certifying examination.** *Essentials* **promotes your critical thinking;** *You Should Know* **enhances your knowledge; and** *Performance* **enables you to assess your strengths and weaknesses.**

Applying Basic Concepts

Understanding principles of physiology and pathophysiology should enable the test candidate to correctly answer many PANCE and PANRE questions.

Remember these basic concepts:

Concept 1: Cardiac Function

A cardinal determinant of ventricular function is preload, which relates to the volume of blood in a ventricle at end-diastole. A dilated left ventricle signifies increased preload. Increased preload and the dilated ventricle, in turn, lead to systolic heart failure (SHF). SHF is characterized by a decreased left ventricular ejection fraction and low cardiac output. Typically, the physical examination shows the apical impulse to be displaced to the left and downward in the chest and an S3 gallop is present. The cardinal symptom of SHF is fatigue/weakness.

In contrast, diastolic heart failure (DHF) is due to a stiff left ventricle (decreased compliance). The stiff ventricle is often, but not always, related to ventricular hypertrophy from increased afterload, a second physiologic determinant of ventricular function. Increased afterload is caused by either systemic hypertension or aortic valve stenosis. In order to fill the stiff ventricle during diastole, left atrial pressure must increase to propel the blood into the ventricle. This increased atrial pressure is transmitted back to the lungs, and the patient's symptom is dyspnea. The physical signs of DHF are an apical lift in the presence of left ventricular hypertrophy and an S4 gallop when the patient is in normal sinus rhythm. It is important to recognize that the left ventricle may be stiff *without left ventricular hypertrophy and without increased afterload.* Myocardial ischemia or infiltrative disease may cause the left ventricle to be stiff resulting in the patient having dyspnea related to diastolic heart failure.

Note the key difference:

- SHF = fatigue = dilated left ventricle = increased preload
- DHF = dyspnea = stiff (noncompliant) left ventricle = increased afterload (often)

You are now able to answer many questions: What is the primary pathophysiologic abnormality in systolic heart failure or diastolic heart failure? Which of the following physical signs is most likely to be noted in the patient who has systolic or diastolic heart failure? What is the pathophysiologic basis for dyspnea in the patient who has diastolic heart failure? A decreased left ventricular ejection fraction is most likely to be noted in a patient with which of the following signs upon cardiac examination?

Concept 2: Cor Pulmonale

Cor pulmonale is heart disease secondary to lung disease. To answer questions correctly, you must know these points:

a. Pulmonary *parenchymal* disease (pulmonary fibrosis or chronic bronchitis) and pulmonary *vascular* disease are the primary causes of cor pulmonale.

b. The basic pathophysiologic mechanism in cor pulmonale is increased pulmonary vascular resistance causing pulmonary hypertension.

You can now answer important questions: Which of the following is the basic pathophysiologic mechanism in cor pulmonale? Which of the following diseases is most likely to cause cor pulmonale? Which of the following hemodynamic abnormalities is characteristic of cor pulmonale?

Concept 3: Syncope

The basic principle in understanding syncope is that all patients who faint share a common pathophysiology—namely, decreased cerebral perfusion. The decreased cerebral blood flow may, in turn, be due to many causes. Cardiovascular causes of syncope include arrhythmia (bradycardia or tachycardia) and obstruction to blood flow (aortic valve stenosis, hypertrophic obstructive cardiomyopathy, pulmonary embolism). Reflex syncope is characteristically due to heightened vagal tone. Orthostatic hypotension causing faint may be due to autonomic insufficiency (a defect in the sympathetic reflex arc) or to hypovolemia. Finally, there are psychogenic causes of fainting as may occur in the hysterical patient.

The history then becomes critically important in helping to differentiate among these multiple causes of decreased cerebral perfusion. Syncope while shaving suggests a hypersensitive carotid sinus (vagal response). Heightened vagal tone, as in the anxious patient who is undergoing venipuncture, causes the common faint. Heightened vagal tone—namely, increased parasympathetic activity—is characterized by hypotension and bradycardia. Fainting during an argument or during physical exertion in an older patient raises the possibility of arrhythmia due to myocardial ischemia. In contrast, fainting during argument or exertion in a child or young adult suggests either long QT interval (on electrocardiography) or hypertrophic obstructive cardiomyopathy. Fainting when urinating or defecating is situational syncope related to vagal tone. Finally, syncope when arising from bed indicates orthostatic hypotension. Orthostatic hypotension may be caused by either autonomic insufficiency or hypovolemia. In autonomic insufficiency, the pulse rate does not increase when the standing blood pressure has dropped. In contrast, in hypovolemia, the standing pulse rate is considerably faster than the rate while the patient is recumbent. Here is a typical clinical example: An 81-year-old woman faints when arising from bed. Recumbent blood pressure is 120/70 mm Hg with a pulse of 62/min. Standing blood pressure is 80/58 mm Hg with a pulse of 63/min. In this case, orthostatic hypotension is due to an impaired sympathetic nervous system (autonomic insufficiency) that is commonly noted in the patient who has diabetes mellitus. In contrast, if the fall in blood pressure in this same patient was associated with an increase in pulse rate, for example, from 62/min to 98/min, then the cause is hypovolemia as occurs in adrenal insufficiency or hypovolemia due to excessive diuresis.

You are now able to answer many questions: What is the pathophysiologic basis of all patients who faint? What are the typical physical signs during vagal fainting? Which of the following is the most likely cause of syncope in a 14-year-old athlete who faints during a basketball game and in whom physical examination shows an apical lift and double carotid arterial upstroke (bisferiens pulse)? Presence of which of the following differentiates syncope due to autonomic insufficiency from syncope due to hypovolemia? Which of the following activities is most likely to provoke syncope due to carotid sinus hypersensitivity?

Concept 4: Transient Neurologic Symptoms

Transient (in most cases, minutes) neurologic symptoms may be due to transient ischemic attack (TIA), migraine, or seizures. You must understand the difference between "positive" symptoms and "negative" symptoms. Positive symptoms may involve sensory or motor nerves and indicate that the nerve is irritated. Examples of positive symptoms include tingling, burning, jerking, and visual hallucinations. Negative symptoms indicate loss of nerve function. Examples of negative neurologic symptoms include numbness, weakness, or loss of vision.

Transient ischemic attacks always cause *negative* symptoms. In contrast, migraine and seizure activity frequently are associated with *positive* symptoms such as bright lights in the visual fields, jerking, or tingling. Another very important clinical point: In transient ischemic attacks, the symptoms occur at the same time, whereas in migraine or some seizures, the symptoms progress over time. For example, a patient with a TIA has loss of vision and weakness starting at the same time. In contrast, the patient with migraine typically has visual scintillations that slowly progress over the visual fields, or the patient has tingling that starts in one finger and then slowly progresses to involve the hand and arm.

You are now able to answer important questions: Which of the following differentiates a transient ischemic attack from migraine? Negative/positive neurologic symptoms are characteristic of which of the following conditions?

Concept 5: Hypoxemia

Hypoxemia is decreased oxygen content in the systemic circulation. Some important mechanisms that cause hypoxemia include hypoventilation, ventilation-perfusion mismatch, and diffusion impairment.

Hypoventilation always causes an increase in $PaCO_2$ in the systemic circulation. In room air, hypoventilation is associated with hypoxemia. Clinical examples of hypoventilation include respiratory depression from drug overdose and brain lesions involving the respiratory center.

Ventilation-perfusion mismatch relates to the balance between lung ventilation and perfusion. Clinical examples of hypoxemia due to this imbalance include obstructive pulmonary disease, pulmonary fibrosis, and chronic pulmonary emboli.

Diffusion impairment results in hypoxemia because there is inefficient transfer of oxygen from alveoli to capillaries. Pulmonary fibrosis is the classic disease characterized by diffusion impairment. Pulmonary fibrosis is considered restrictive lung disease, in contrast to chronic bronchitis and emphysema, which are obstructive lung diseases.

How, then, does one differentiate between obstructive and restrictive lung disease? Obstructive lung disease is characterized by increased airway resistance. Restrictive lung disease is characterized by decreased pulmonary compliance. Therefore, a basic lung function test that differentiates between restrictive and obstructive is forced expiratory volume in 1 second/forced vital capacity (FEV_1/FVC). In restrictive disease, the ratio is increased, and in obstructive lung disease, the ratio is decreased.

You are now able to answer important questions: Which of the following is the pathophysiologic abnormality in restrictive/obstructive lung disease? Which of the following diagnostic tests is preferred to differentiate between restrictive and obstructive lung disease? A patient who has respiratory depression secondary to heroin overdose will have which of the following systemic arterial blood gas values?

Concept 6: Genetic Transmission

You should know the inheritance patterns of important disorders. The following table will help you answer questions.

Disorder	Genetic Inheritance
Marfan syndrome	Autosomal dominant
Polycystic kidney	Autosomal dominant
Hypertrophic cardiomyopathy	Autosomal dominant; also sporadic cases
Glucose-6-phosphate dehydrogenase deficiency	X-linked disorder
Cystic fibrosis	Autosomal recessive

History Taking and Performing Physical Examinations

The History in Differential Diagnosis

You are now aware that the history obtained from the patient can differentiate between TIA and migraine. The activity during which syncope occurs (e.g., arising from bed or during exercise) is extremely important in determining the cause of loss of consciousness.

A thoughtful history can differentiate between angina pectoris and chest pain of noncardiac origin. Angina is a discomfort, not a sharp pain, that lasts continuously for at least 1 minute. Noncardiac pain is often jabbing and momentary, not continuous. Angina pectoris is not associated with chest wall tenderness and is not affected by body position, swallowing, or respiration. In contrast, pericardial pain may be influenced by body position, swallowing, and respiratory movement.

The history is important in differentiating among the many causes of peripheral edema. Edema affecting only one extremity suggests venous or lymphatic obstruction. Bilateral peripheral edema in the patient who suffers from chronic alcohol abuse suggests cirrhosis, portal hypertension, and hypoalbuminemia. Bilateral peripheral edema in the patient with long-standing valvular disease or atherosclerotic heart disease suggests right heart failure. A past history of chest irradiation in a patient presenting with peripheral edema and ascites suggests constrictive pericarditis. The focused physical examination now becomes important. A normal jugular venous pressure (JVP) in the edematous patient suggests liver disease or nephrotic syndrome. However, increased JVP in the edematous patient points toward a diagnosis of right heart failure or constrictive pericarditis.

Here is an important question that tests your physical examination skills: Presence of which of the following differentiates between folate deficiency anemia and vitamin B_{12} deficiency anemia? Answer: normal vibratory sensation and proprioception.

Risk Factors in Disease

The clinician is expected to know risk factors for common diseases. The following table will be helpful to you.

Disorder	Important Risk Factors
Atherosclerotic diseases	Sex, age, family history, dyslipidemia, hypertension, diabetes mellitus, smoking, sedentary lifestyle, elevated serum C-reactive protein
Aorta dissection	Hypertension, Marfan syndrome, cocaine use

Inspection as Part of the Physical Examination

An appropriate exam question would determine your ability to link a physical examination sign upon inspection to a clinical disorder. Here are examples:

Sign Upon Inspection	Significance
Clubbing	Primary or metastatic lung cancer
	Cyanotic congenital heart disease
	Bronchiectasis, pulmonary fibrosis, lung abscess
	Crohn's disease
	Clubbing is not a sign of COPD
Jaundice	Hemolysis or obstructive liver disease
Petechiae	Thrombocytopenia of any etiology
	Vasculitis
Spider angiomata, palmar erythema	Advanced chronic liver disease
Malar rash in an adult female	Systemic lupus erythematosus
Pitting of nails	Psoriasis
Elevated jugular venous pressure	Right heart failure
	Constrictive pericarditis
	Pericardial tamponade
	Superior vena cava syndrome
Periorbital edema	Hypothyroidism, nephritic syndrome, nephrotic syndrome, trichinellosis
Round face; abdominal striae	Cushing's disease
Splinter hemorrhages	Endocarditis, trichinellosis, psoriasis

Using Laboratory and Diagnostic Studies

Complete Blood Count

The basic white blood cell count in the blood can be helpful in determining the diagnosis. Acute pericarditis in the patient with systemic lupus erythematosus is associated with leukopenia (often 2,500 to 3,500/microL), whereas pericarditis due to bacterial infection (purulent pericarditis) typically is characterized by marked leukocytosis (20,000 to 30,000/microL).

In a question that clearly relates to a patient who has a hematologic disorder, carefully look for the red blood cell volume. Microcytosis suggests iron deficiency anemia or thalassemia. Macrocytosis, importantly, may occur with or without a megaloblastic bone marrow. Megaloblastic anemia with macrocytosis is due to either folate or vitamin B_{12} deficiency. Macrocytosis without megaloblasts is due to hypothyroidism, alcohol intake, or liver disease.

Serum Potassium

a. Hyperkalemia—immediately think of the following causes: renal failure (acute or chronic) and medicines (angiotensin-converting enzyme inhibitors [ACEI], spironolactone, and triamterene)

b. Hypokalemia—immediately think of the following causes: loop diuretic therapy, diarrhea, tube drainage, and vomiting

You can now answer many questions: Lisinopril therapy is initiated in a 65-year-old man in treatment of hypertension. Which of the following laboratory tests should be performed in 10 days? Which of the following electrolyte abnormalities is most likely to be noted in a 44-year-old man with recurrent severe vomiting?

Diseases Associated With Antibodies

Laboratory studies provide an important clue to distinguish pernicious anemia (PA) from other causes of vitamin B_{12} deficiency anemia. Only pernicious anemia is an autoimmune disorder. Therefore, only in pernicious anemia does the patient's serum have antibodies to intrinsic factor or to gastric parietal cells.

Similarly, there are several diseases that cause hyperthyroidism. Only Graves' disease is autoimmune and is associated with extrathyroidal signs (e.g., pretibial myxedema). Solitary toxic thyroid nodule, toxic multinodular goiter, and exogenous hyperthyroidism are not autoimmune and therefore are not associated with autoantibody formation.

You should expect that the PANCE and PANRE examinations will have many questions related to diseases and their associated antibodies. The following table should be helpful to you.

Disease	Clinical Character	Antibodies
Systemic lupus	Arthritis, pericarditis, malar rash	Antinuclear, anti-Sm, anti-ds DNA
Rheumatoid arthritis	Symmetric, small joints, deformity	Rheumatoid factor, anti-citrullinated peptide (ACPA)
Graves' disease	Hyperthyroid, extrathyroidal signs	Anti-TSH receptor
Hashimoto's disease	Hypothyroid	Anti–thyroid peroxidase, antithyroglobulin
Myasthenia gravis	Skeletal muscle involvement Intermittent symptoms	Anti–acetylcholine receptor
Primary biliary cirrhosis	Middle-aged female Pruritus, high alkaline phosphatase	Antimitochondrial
Autoimmune hepatitis	Aminotransferase abnormality is greater than alkaline phosphatase	Anti–smooth muscle

(Continued)

Disease	Clinical Character	Antibodies
Sjögren's syndrome	95% female	Antinuclear, rheumatoid factor
	Dry mouth and eyes	
Scleroderma (systemic sclerosis)	Skin thickening	Antinuclear, anti-Scl70
	Pulmonary fibrosis	
	Raynaud's phenomenon	
	Cardiorenal disease	
Type 1 diabetes	Insulin-dependent	Islet cell autoantibodies (ICAs)
Celiac disease	Gastrointestinal symptoms, osteoporosis, iron deficiency	IgA anti–tissue transglutaminase, IgA endomysial, antigliadin

Enzymes in Clinical Diagnosis

Serum enzyme levels are commonly measured in the diagnosis of disease. A brief description of their role in specific disorders will help you answer exam questions.

Enzyme	Characteristic	Used in Diagnosis
Glucose-6-phosphate dehydrogenase (in RBCs)	X-linked genetic deficiency	Infection and medications (e.g., primaquine) may trigger hemolysis
Angiotensin-converting enzyme	Found in lung, endothelium	Elevated in 50% of sarcoid
Alkaline phosphatase	Found in liver and bone	Intra- and extra-hepatic obstruction; bone disease
Gamma-glutamyl transpeptidase (GGTP)	In liver, not in bone	Cholestatic disease
Aminotransferases	In liver, skeletal muscle	Hepatocellular injury
Amylase	Pancreatic, salivary	Pancreatic, gastrointestinal, gynecologic, parotid disorders
Creatine kinase	Skeletal and cardiac muscle	CK-MM in myositis
	Brain	CK-MB in myocardial infarction

A classic question: Laboratory values in a 77-year-old man show elevation of serum alkaline phosphatase but a normal serum gamma-glutamyl transpeptidase (GGTP) level. Which of the following is the most likely diagnosis? The answer will be bone disease (e.g., metastatic tumor in bone or Paget's disease of bone). In contrast, the serum alkaline phosphatase and GGTP levels will both be increased in cholestatic liver disease in which there is obstruction to bile flow. Alkaline phosphatase is found in liver and bone. GGTP is found only in the liver.

Other Important Selected Blood Diagnostic Tests

D-dimer is a degradation product of fibrin and therefore is used in the diagnosis of pulmonary embolism. D-dimer is of greater clinical significance when it is *normal*. If D-dimer by ELISA is normal, pulmonary embolism can be excluded with 95% accuracy.

Systemic arterial blood gas determinations define the acid-base status of the patient. Remember, in the patient with metabolic acidosis, always calculate the *anion gap*. Increased anion gap metabolic acidosis is characteristic of diabetic ketoacidosis, lactic acidosis, renal insufficiency, and poisoning due to salicylates, methanol, and ethylene glycol.

Brain natriuretic peptide (BNP) is released by myocardial cells in response to increased ventricular pressures. Therefore, in the patient who has dyspnea, BNP is used to differentiate between heart failure (cardiac) and pulmonary disease as the cause of the symptom.

Serologic tests for *Helicobacter pylori* are less accurate than fecal antigen immunoassay and C13 urea breath test.

A very important serum marker is alpha-fetoprotein. Alpha-fetoprotein is a serum marker in the pregnant woman that may indicate a neural tube defect in the fetus. It is elevated in 95% of males who have testicular germ cell gonadal tumors. In patients with cirrhosis, an increasing serum level of alpha-fetoprotein raises concern for hepatocellular carcinoma.

You are now able to answer many questions on PANCE and PANRE. These questions may ask you to select the serum enzyme that is most appropriate to order in a suspected condition. Alternatively, the question stem may give you the enzyme value and then ask you the most likely diagnosis.

Imaging Studies

In cardiology, the echocardiogram plays a key role in diagnosis. In addition to demonstrating chamber volume, valvular function, and wall thickness, from the echocardiogram one can determine aortic root dimension, left ventricular ejection fraction, and evidence of aortic dissection or pericardial tamponade. Consequently, many PANCE and PANRE questions may address the role of echocardiography in the diagnosis of chronic and acute cardiac disorders.

When you know the previous facts, you are able to answer many questions that relate to the laboratory or imaging studies that are performed in clinical diagnosis.

Formulating Most Likely Diagnosis

Making the diagnosis forces the test candidate to integrate the elements of history, physical examination, and laboratory/imaging studies. The **Essentials** section and **You Should Know** feature of this book are designed to help you link these factors in formulating the most likely diagnosis.

One clinical example: A 54-year-old woman has a 3-month history of progressive nausea and an 8-pound weight loss. Sitting blood pressure is 104/68 mm Hg, and standing pressure is 82/53 mm Hg. Examination shows hyperpigmentation of the skin creases. Serum sodium concentration is 124 mEq/L. Which of the following is the most likely diagnosis? The symptoms, presence of orthostatic hypotension, the physical examination sign (hyperpigmentation), and laboratory abnormality (hyponatremia), when linked together, make chronic adrenal insufficiency the most likely diagnosis.

When reading a test question, try to think of the one disease that will represent the sum of symptoms, vital signs, physical examination signs, and diagnostic testing.

PANCE and PANRE examinations will determine whether you know the most likely infecting organism in the patient who has a specific disease or exposure. Here are examples:

Underlying Disease/Exposure	Likely Infecting Organism(s)
Sickle cell anemia	Encapsulated bacteria, esp. *Pneumococcus*
Cystic fibrosis	*Staphylococcus aureus*
	Pseudomonas
Intravenous drug abuser	*Staphylococcus aureus*
Lung abscess	Anaerobic bacteria (e.g., *Fusiform bacilli, Bacteroides*); *Staphylococcus aureus, Klebsiella pneumoniae*
Contaminated water in showers	*Legionella pneumophila*
Swimming pools	*Cryptosporidium*
Ascites/spontaneous bacterial peritonitis	*E. coli, Klebsiella;* gram-positive organisms associated with intravenous catheters

Pharmaceutical Therapeutics/Clinical Intervention

These two tasks are interweaved because they represent management of the patient. The test candidate must know the actions of a medication, its clinical indications and contraindications, and important drug interactions. Here are some important examples:

Medicine	Clinical Intervention
Labetalol	Has alpha- and beta-adrenergic blocking properties; used to treat hemodynamic effects of cocaine
Aspirin	Primary and secondary prevention of atherosclerotic events
Beta-adrenergic blockers	Prevention of recurrent myocardial infarction
	Used in therapy of *chronic* systolic heart failure (HF), but *not in acute* HF
Warfarin	Paroxysmal or chronic atrial fibrillation
	Mechanical heart valves

In selecting the preferred medication in a patient's therapy, you must be aware of two very important factors—namely, the patient's coexisting disease and the patient's present medication. Here are a few examples:

Avoid niacin in the patient with dyslipidemia who has gout because niacin elevates serum uric acid concentration.

Avoid a thiazide diuretic in the patient with hypertension who has hyperuricemia because thiazides elevate serum uric acid concentration and may precipitate a gout attack.

Avoid beta-adrenergic blockers in the patient who has obstructive lung disease or peripheral claudication because beta blockers may exacerbate the pulmonary or extremity symptoms.

In the patient who takes warfarin therapy, remember that aspirin, acetaminophen, cephalosporins, erythromycin, omeprazole, influenza virus, and macrolide antibiotics (a partial list) increase warfarin's effect. Oppositely, nafcillin, haloperidol, vitamin K, and oral contraceptives decrease the warfarin effect.

Health Maintenance

Immunizations

Immunizations are important in prevention of communicable disease. You must know the immunization schedule for infants and small children.

Vaccine	Recommended for Those Persons
Meningococcal	College students living in dormitories; military recruits
Pneumococcal	All adults older than 65 years
	Younger persons having immunocompromised state
	Metabolic, liver, and cardiopulmonary diseases
	Alcohol abuse
	Sickle cell patients
Influenza	All persons 6 months of age or older. (Refer to three [3] Recommended Immunization Schedules, U.S., 2012: For Ages 0 through 6 Years; 7 Years through 18 Years; and Adult Immunization Schedule. CDC schedules delineate proper form of vaccine to be administered.) A pregnant woman can receive the trivalent, inactivated vaccine (TIV).

Complications of Disease State

Here are typical questions that will determine your knowledge of a disease complication:

Question 1: A 64-year-old man has chronic, severe heartburn due to gastroesophageal reflux. He is at increased risk for which of the following? The answer is Barrett's esophagus.

Question 2: A 64-year-old man who has Barrett's esophagus would be expected to show which of the following histologic changes upon esophageal biopsy? The answer is columnar epithelium.

Question 3: A patient with Barrett's esophagus is at increased risk to develop which of the following? The answer is adenocarcinoma of the esophagus.

Here are two questions that determine whether you know the complications of pathophysiologic states.

Patients who have cardiac disorders characterized by increased ventricular preload are at risk to develop which of the following? The answer is systolic heart failure.

Patients who have cardiac disorders characterized by increased ventricular afterload are at risk to develop which of the following? The answer is diastolic heart failure.

Counseling

You should expect questions that will determine your knowledge in counseling. Here are some important examples of counseling that would make appropriate questions:

Patient	Counseling
Woman taking ACE inhibitor	Avoid pregnancy
Woman taking lithium	Avoid pregnancy
	Medication should be taken with meals
Any patient taking lithium	Serial thyroid and renal function studies; thiazide increases lithium blood level
Marfan syndrome	Avoid contact sports
Hypertensive patient	Lose weight if obese
	Restrict salt and alcohol intake
	Aerobic activity
	Low saturated-fat diet

Parents of infants and small children properly have health concerns over their children's development. "What should my child be able to do at 6 months ... at 12 months?" You must know normal language and motor development milestones in infants and small children.

"My daughter has a stomach ache after drinking milk. Is it an allergy?" You must know that eggs, milk, wheat, peanuts, and soy are common allergens in young children. However, in older children and adolescents, fish, shellfish, and nuts are common allergens.

Index